Conditions in Occupational Therapy

EFFECT ON OCCUPATIONAL PERFORMANCE

Conditions in Occupational Therapy

EFFECT ON OCCUPATIONAL PERFORMANCE

Editors

RUTH A. HANSEN, Ph.D., O.T.R., F.A.O.T.A.

Associate Professor and Director
Occupational Therapy Program
Eastern Michigan University
Ypsilanti, Michigan

BEN ATCHISON, M.Ed., O.T.R., F.A.O.T.A.

Assistant Professor
Occupational Therapy Program
Eastern Michigan University
Ypsilanti, Michigan

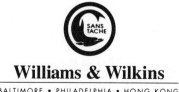

Williams & Wilkins

BALTIMORE • PHILADELPHIA • HONG KONG
LONDON • MUNICH • SYDNEY • TOKYO

A WAVERLY COMPANY

Editor: John P. Butler
Managing Editor: Linda Napora
Copy Editor: Anne K. Schwartz
Designer: Karen S. Klinedinst
Illustration Planner: Wayne Hubbel
Production Coordinator: Anne Stewart Seitz

Copyright (©) 1993
Williams & Wilkins
428 East Preston Street
Baltimore, Maryland 21202, USA

Accurate indications, adverse reactions, and dosage schedules for drugs are provided in this book, but it is possible that they may change. The reader is urged to review the package information data of the manufacturers of the medications mentioned.

Printed in the United States of America

Library of Congress Cataloging in Publication Data

Conditions in occupational therapy: effect on occupational performance / [edited by] Ruth A. Hansen, Ben Atchison.
    p. cm.
Includes index.
ISBN 0-683-03878-8
1. Occupational therapy. I. Hansen, Ruth Ann. II. Atchison, Ben.
[DNLM: 1. Occupational Therapy. 2. Rehabilitation, Vocational.
3. Work Capacity Evaluation. WB 555 C745]
RM735.C66 1993
615.8'515—dc20
DNLM/DLC
for Library of Congress
    92-15775
    CIP

94 95 96
2 3 4 5 6 7 8 9 10

Preface

This book is long overdue. Those of us who have been teaching occupational therapy have spent considerable time translating information from medical and pathophysiology texts for our conditions courses. Students, in turn, have struggled to interpret knowledge about diseases and impairments from the occupational therapy perspective.

This text has been organized into chapters that describe major conditions that cause difficulties in daily-living tasks for the individuals served by occupational therapists. The most frequently treated conditions were identified in the 1988 AOTA Membership Data Survey. Chapters 2 through 14 discuss these conditions. Each of these chapters includes basic information about the etiology, prognosis, and progression of the condition; a description of the routine diagnostic tests; and a discussion of medical management.

Each chapter synthesizes this information into an occupational performance perspective by answering the question, How might this condition inpinge upon each of the performance components—sensorimotor, psychosocial, and cognitive? To answer this question, each chapter systematically describes potential changes in each area and then, in turn, examines how these changes might affect the occupational performance areas of work, play/leisure, and activities of daily living. Most importantly, each chapter includes one or two case studies. These cases enable the reader to take the information in the first part of the chapter and apply it in an actual situation.

The method used in this book teaches the thinking process employed by occupational therapists to determine what occupational therapy services the individual patient/client needs. Each chapter provides a personal interpretation of the effects of the condition on occupational performance. This analysis is not absolute. Therapists may disagree about the importance of various disabilities and the secondary changes that might occur. We have provided the general descriptions regarding occupational dysfunction and the specific cases as material for discussion and deliberation.

We acknowledge the efforts of our contributors. We greatly appreciate their enthusiasm, cooperation, openness, and commitment. Also, we extend our gratitude to Jane Bird, our typist, and to Karen Khan, our student assistant and advisor. They provided moral and technical support and the attention to detail that is so essential in such an undertaking.

Ruth A. Hansen
Ben Atchison

Contributors

BEN ATCHISON, M.Ed., O.T.R., F.A.O.T.A.
Assistant Professor
Occupational Therapy Program
Eastern Michigan University
Ypsilanti, Michigan

CYNTHIA D. BATTS, O.T.R.
Director of Rehabilitation Services
Nederveld and Associates
Port Huron, Michigan

SUSAN NASSER BIERMAN, O.T.R.
Occupational Therapy Department
McLaren Rehabilitation Center
Flint, Michigan

GERRY E. CONTI, B.S., O.T.R.
Manager, Occupational Therapy
St. Joseph Mercy Hospital
Ann Arbor, Michigan

VIRGINIA ALLEN DICKIE, M.S., O.T.R.,
F.A.O.T.A.
Assistant Professor
Occupational Therapy Program
Eastern Michigan University
Ypsilanti, Michigan

CATHERINE HECK EDWARDS, O.T.R.
Senior Coordinator
Occupational Health Program
Ingham Medical Center
Lansing, Michigan

JOANNE PHILLIPS ESTES, M.S.,
O.T.R./L.
Consultant
Cincinnati, Ohio

JOYCE FRAKER, O.T.R
Washtenaw County Community Mental
  Health
Ypsilanti, Michigan

ELIZABETH FRANCIS-CONNOLLY,
M.S., O.T.R.
Instructor, Occupational Therapy Program
Eastern Michigan University
Ypsilanti, Michigan

RUTH A. HANSEN, Ph.D.,
O.T.R., F.A.O.T.A.
Associate Professor and Director
Occupational Therapy Program
Eastern Michigan University
Ypsilanti, Michigan

JACQUELINE McKILLOP, O.T.R.
Nittany Valley Rehabilitation Hospital
Pleasant Gap, Pennsylvania

ROXANNE McTURNER-GILL, M.S., O.T.R.
Manager, Occupational Therapy
Beyer Memorial Hospital
Ypsilanti, Michigan

LAURA VINCENT MILLER, M.S., O.T.R.
Director, Physical Medicine and
Rehabilitation
Detroit Receiving Hospital and
University Health Center
Detroit, Michigan

TRISHA MOZDZIERZ, O.T.R.
University of Michigan Medical Center
Ann Arbor, Michigan

YVONNE R. TESKE, Ph.D., O.T.R.,
F.A.O.T.A.
Professor Emeritus
Occupational Therapy Program
Eastern Michigan University
Ypsilanti, Michigan

MARY STEICHEN YAMAMOTO, M.S.,
O.T.R.
Consultant
Ann Arbor, Michigan

Contents

Thinking Like an O.T.

RUTH A. HANSEN AND BEN ATCHISON

It is more important to know what kind of person has the disease than what kind of disease the person has.

Sir William Osler

Address at Johns Hopkins University, February 1905

Susan is an occupational therapy student beginning her level II fieldwork experience. During the first week, she spent most of her time in orientation sessions and observing her supervising therapist treat patients. Now the time has come to have patients assigned to her and to take responsibility for initiating treatment. When she receives her first referral, she reads the diagnosis and begins to decide what to do next.

How does a student learn to correlate general information about a diagnosis with the needs of a particular person and identify the problems that require occupational therapy intervention? How does a staff therapist prioritize problems and decide which ones require immediate attention? How much problem identification can be done before the therapist actually sees the patient? How does a supervisor know when a student or therapist is doing a "good job" of screening referrals and anticipating the dysfunction that the patient might be experiencing? This book provides an explanation of this initial thinking/reasoning process from an occupational performance perspective.

What makes occupational therapy a unique health-care profession is the way that practitioners gather and use information to assist people in being self-sufficient in their daily activities. This data-gathering and analysis provides the therapist with the foundation for a treatment plan through a prioritized list of anticipated problems or dysfunctions for one individual. The purpose of this book is to give examples of how this process works. Each of the following 13 chapters uses the same systematic approach to examine selected conditions.

The general organization of each chapter is the same. First is a detailed description of the etiology, information about incidence and prevalence, signs and symptoms, progression or prognosis, and other information that is usually found in a medical or pathophysiology text. This book is unique because the authors have used these details to generate a description of the various aspects of occupational performance that might be affected. At the end of each chapter is a discussion of at least one case study. Cases provide specific details about how the condition might impinge upon the daily functioning of a particular person.

The occupational performance grid (Table 1.1) used in this book is adapted from the Uniform Terminology, second edition (1). Once you know the diagnosis and age of the person, you can use this grid to systematically examine the deficits that occur in the sensorimotor, psychosocial, and cognitive performance components,

as well as how these particular deficits can and do alter the person's ability to perform tasks in relevant areas of occupational performance (work, play-leisure, and activities of daily living). Appendix 1.1 at the end of this chapter includes complete definitions of all terms.

Occupational therapists have a unique and valuable view of an individual as an occupational being. All of us attach mean-

Table 1.1.
Occupational Performance Profile[a]

		Performance			
			Work Activities		
		Vocation	Education	Home Management	Care of Others
SENSORIMOTOR	**SENSORY INTEGRATION**				
	NEURO-MUSCULAR				
COGNITIVE	**MOTOR**				
	COGNITIVE				
	PSYCHO-LOGICAL				
PSYCHOSOCIAL	**SOCIAL**				
	SELF-MANAGEMENT				

(left margin, vertical: PERFORMANCE COMPONENTS)

EXTERNAL FACTORS WHICH INFLUENCE PERFORMANCE: CULTURE, ECONOMY, ENVIRONMENT

[a]Adapted from American Occupational Therapy Association. Uniform terminology for occupational therapy. 2nd ed. Am J Occup Ther 1989; 43.
Developed by the occupational therapy faculty at Eastern Michigan University.

ing to our lives and those of others through the activities and occupations that are part of our daily existence. Occupation, then, means more than just work. It is a much broader concept that refers to human involvement in activities that will result in productive and purposeful outcomes. It also includes leisure, rest, and self-care activities that some may not consider productive and purposeful.

For example, the occupations of a 3-month-old infant include activities that could be categorized under the general headings of play or activities of daily living. Activities such as play exploration and performance, feeding, socialization, and

Client initials: _____
Diagnosis: _____
Age: _____

Areas							
Play or Leisure Activities		Activities of Daily Living					
Exploration	Performance	Self-Care	Social-ization	Functional Communi-cation	Functional Mobility	Sexual Expression	

functional communication are critical at this age.

The complexity of occupation changes dramatically as the infant progresses toward preschool and school age. It is interesting to observe the rapid addition of new occupational roles and expectations as the child enters school. Many aspects of occupational development are emerging. For example, a 7-year-old engaging in classroom activities is involved in a type of work. Being on time, turning in assignments that are completed properly, good grooming, and getting along with others are all behaviors that will be important as the child approaches adulthood.

Adults are expected to assume, independently pursue, and maintain all relevant occupations. In general, adults spend the greater portion of their waking hours engaged in some type of work activity. This work may be a job or vocation that is done for pay, organized volunteer activities, or home management. The percentage of time spent in each area is largely determined by the role the individual assumes. In addition, adults spend a portion of their time exploring and performing leisure activities. Activities of daily living, particularly socialization, sexual expression, grooming, and eating are all important for adults.

BELIEF STATEMENTS

According to Reed and Sanderson in their book *Concepts of Occupational Therapy*, second edition, occupational therapy is based upon numerous assumptions (2). Of particular note are those about human beings: about occupational performance; about health, wellness, and illness; and most particularly, about occupational therapy itself. At the risk of oversimplifying their concepts, the following is a synthesis of their main ideas about the common professional values that occupational therapy practitioners share.

First, occupational therapists believe that each person possesses many complex and variable characteristics. A human being is biological, psychological, and social, and all of these attributes intertwine in various combinations to make us unique individuals. Because of the individual's needs and interaction with the environment, changes occur. If the person has good coping skills, adaptation occurs. Another concept is that each of us has responsibilities to ourselves and others, basic rights to fulfillment of primary needs, and the basic right to self-actualization.

The basic tenets regarding occupational performance are that these tasks are critical and must be performed by the person or by others in order to survive. Through engaging in various occupations the person develops, learns adaptive mechanisms, and meets individual needs. It is important to understand the influence of culture on adaptation. Cultural influences, such as institutions, rules, values, architectural design, art, history, and language affect the ways and the extent to which a person uses adaptive mechanisms.

Conversely, illness, trauma, or injury can cause varying degrees of occupational dysfunction. The individual receiving occupational therapy is most often experiencing permanent, long-term changes in the ability to engage in everyday activities. The continuum between health and illness is dynamic and fluctuating. The individual's state of health or illness can be judged by the ability to engage in activities that meet both immediate and long-range needs, and to assume desired roles. Illness or disability is considered in relationship to its effects on occupational activities and therefore the degree of occupational dysfunction that is experienced.

These precepts are the foundation for the reasoning process described in this book. The combination of these assumptions or beliefs and the occupational performance structure are the frame of reference that provides a unique occupational therapy perspective.

Conditions were chosen for the 13 chapters in this text on the basis of data regarding those most frequently treated by practitioners. The 1986 membership data survey by the AOTA indicated that occupational therapists most often treat individuals with a cerebral vascular accident or a developmental disability. In order of descending frequency the list included cerebral palsy, hand injuries, schizophrenia, mood disorders, traumatic head injury, back pain, organic brain syndrome, spinal cord injury, adjustment disorders, and heart disease. After examining this list, we selected some additional conditions to provide better representation of the various areas of practice, most particularly, mental health and pediatrics.

This book is an instructional tool. It provides an opportunity to examine each condition closely. The reader is urged to use this information as a springboard for further study of the conditions included here and the many other conditions that occupational therapists encounter in practice. The analysis of the impact on occupational performance for a particular condition is dynamic and changing, and the identification of the most important areas of dysfunction and, therefore, treatment will vary from practitioner to practitioner. Of course, factors such as secondary health problems, age, gender, family background, and culture will contribute greatly to the development of a unique occupational performance profile for each individual served.

The occupational performance approach to the identification of dysfunction described in this book can be used to examine the effects of any condition on a person's daily life. This process will enable the therapist to identify and prioritize problems in occupational performance, which, in turn, will serve as the foundation for creating an effective plan of intervention.

REFERENCES

1. American Occupational Therapy Association. Uniform terminology for occupational therapy, 2nd ed. Am J Occup Ther 1989:43:808–815.
2. Reed KL, Sanderson SR. Concepts of occupational therapy. Baltimore: Williams & Wilkins, 1983.

Uniform Terminology for Occupational Therapy
Second Edition

INTRODUCTION

Purpose

Uniform Terminology for Occupational Therapy—Second Edition delineates and defines **OCCUPATIONAL PERFORMANCE AREAS** and **OCCUPATIONAL PERFORMANCE COMPONENTS** that are addressed in occupational therapy direct service. These definitions are provided to facilitate the uniform use of terminology and definitions throughout the profession. The original document, *Occupational Therapy Product Output Reporting System and Uniform Terminology for Reporting Occupational Therapy Services*, which was published in 1979, helped create a base of consistent terminology that was used in many of the official documents of The American Occupational Therapy Association, Inc. (AOTA), in occupational therapy education curricula, and in a variety of occupational therapy practice settings. In order to remain current with practice, the first document (1979) was revised over a period of several years with extensive feedback from the profession. The revisions were completed in 1988. It is recognized and recommended that a document of this nature be updated periodically so that occupational therapy is defined in accordance with current theory and practice.

GUIDELINES FOR USE

Uniform Terminology—Second Edition may be used in a variety of ways. It defines occupational therapy practice, which includes **OCCUPATIONAL PERFORMANCE AREAS** and **OCCUPATIONAL PERFORMANCE COMPONENTS**. In addition, it will be useful to occupational therapists for: a) documentation, b) charge systems, c) education, d) program development, e) marketing, and f) research. Examples of how **OCCUPATIONAL PERFORMANCE AREAS** and **OCCUPATIONAL PERFORMANCE COMPONENTS** translate into practice are provided below. It is not the intent of this document to define specific occupational therapy programs nor specific occupational therapy interventions. Some examples of the differences between **OCCUPATIONAL PERFORMANCE AREAS** and **OCCUPATIONAL PERFORMANCE COMPONENTS** and programs and interventions are:

1. An individual who is injured on the job may be able to return to work, which is an **OCCUPATIONAL PERFORMANCE AREA**. In order to achieve the outcome of returning to work, the individual may need to address specific **PERFORMANCE COMPONENTS** such as strength, endurance, and time management. The occupational therapist, in cooperation with the vocational team, utilizes planned interventions to achieve the desired outcome. These interventions may include activities such as an exercise program, body mechanics instruction and job modification, and may be provided in a work hardening program.

2. An individual with severe physical limitations may need and desire the

opportunity to live within a community-integrated setting, which represents both the **OCCUPATIONAL PERFORMANCE AREAS** of activities of daily living and work. In order to achieve the outcome of community living, the individual may need to address specific **PERFORMANCE COMPONENTS**, such as normalizing muscle tone, gross motor coordination, postural control, and self-management. The occupational therapist, in cooperation with the team, utilizes planned interventions to achieve the desired outcome. Interventions may include neuromuscular facilitation, object manipulation, instruction in use of adaptive equipment, use of environmental control systems, and functional positioning for eating. These interventions may be provided in a community-based independent living program.

3. A child with learning disabilities may need to perform educational activities within a public school setting. Since learning is a student's work, this educational activity would be considered the **OCCUPATIONAL PERFORMANCE AREA** for this individual. In order to achieve the educational outcome of efficient and effective completion of written classroom work, the child may need to address specific **OCCUPATIONAL PERFORMANCE COMPONENTS**, including sensory processing, perceptual skills, postural control, and motor skills. The occupational therapist, in cooperation with the team, utilizes planned interventions to achieve the desired outcome. Interventions may include activities such as adapting the student's seating to improve postural control and stability and practicing motor control and coordination. This program could be provided by school district personnel or through contracted services.

4. An infant with cerebral palsy may need to participate in developmental activities to engage in the **OCCUPATIONAL PERFORMANCE AREAS**

of activities of daily living and play. The developmental outcomes may be achieved by addressing specific **PERFORMANCE COMPONENTS** such as sensory awareness and neuromuscular control. The occupational therapist, in cooperation with the team, utilizes planned interventions to achieve the desired outcomes. Interventions may include activities such as seating and positioning for play, neuromuscular facilitation techniques to enable eating, and parent training. These interventions may be provided in a home-based occupational therapy program.

5. An adult with schizophrenia may need and desire to live independently in the community which represents the **OCCUPATIONAL PERFORMANCE AREAS** of activities of daily living, work activities, and play or leisure activities. The specific **OCCUPATIONAL PERFORMANCE AREAS** may be medication routine, functional mobility, home management, vocational exploration, play or leisure performance, and social skills. In order to achieve the outcome of living alone, the individual may need to address specific **PERFORMANCE COMPONENTS** such as topographical orientation, memory, categorization, problem solving, interests, social conduct, and time management. The occupational therapist, in cooperation with the team, utilizes planned interventions to achieve the desired outcome. Interventions may include activities such as training in the use of public transportation, instruction in budgeting skills, selection and participation of social activities, and instruction in social conduct. These interventions may be provided in a community-based mental health program.

6. An individual who abuses substances may need to reestablish family roles and responsibilities which represent the **OCCUPATIONAL PERFORMANCE AREAS** of activities of daily living and work. In order to achieve the outcome

of family participation, the individual may need to address the **PERFOR- MANCE COMPONENTS** of roles, values, social conduct, self-expression, coping skills, and self-control. The occupational therapist, in cooperation with the team, utilizes planned intervention to achieve the desired outcomes. Interventions may include role and value clarification exercises, role playing, instruction in stress management techniques, and parenting skills. These interventions may be provided in an inpatient acute care unit.

Because of the extensive use of the original document (*Uniform Terminology for Reporting Occupational Therapy Services*, 1979) in official documents, this revision is a second edition and does not completely replace the 1979 version. This follows the practice that other professions, such as physicians, pursue with their documents. Examples are the *Physician's Current Procedural Terminology First— Fourth Editions*, (CPT 1–4) and the *Diagnostic and Statistical Manual First— Third Editions*, (DSM—I—III-R). Therefore, this document is presented as *Uniform Terminology for Occupational Therapy—Second Edition*.

BACKGROUND

Task Force Charge

In 1983, the Representative Assembly of The American Occupational Therapy Association charged the Commission on Practice to form a task force to revise the *Occupational Therapy Product Output Reporting System and Uniform Terminology for Reporting Occupational Therapy Services*. The document had been approved by the Representative Assembly in 1979 and needed to be updated to reflect current practice.

Background Information

The *Occupational Therapy Product Output Reporting System and Uniform Terminology for Reporting Occupational Therapy Services* (hereafter to be referred to as *Product Output Reporting System* or *Uniform Terminology*) document was originally developed in response to Public Law 95-142, the Medicare—Medicaid Anti-Fraud and Abuse Amendments of 1977, which required the Secretary of the Department of Health and Human Services to establish regulations for uniform reporting systems for all departments in hospitals. The AOTA developed the documents to create a uniform reporting system for occupational therapy departments. Although the Department of Health and Human Services never adopted the system because of antitrust concerns relating to price fixing, occupational therapists have used the documents extensively in the profession.

Three states, Maryland, California, and Washington, have used the *Product Output Reporting System* as a basis for statewide reporting systems. AOTA official documents have relied on the definitions to create uniformity. Many occupational therapy schools and departments have used the definitions to guide education and documentation. Although the initial need was for reimbursement reporting systems, the profession has used the documents primarily to facilitate uniformity in definitions.

Task Force Formation

In 1983, Linda Kohlman McGourty, a member of the AOTA Commission on Practice, was appointed by the commission's chair, John Farace, to chair the Uniform Terminology Task Force. Initially, a notice was placed in the *Occupational Therapy Newspaper* for people to submit feedback for the revisions. Many responses were received. Before the task force was appointed in 1984, Maryland, California, and Washington adopted reimbursement systems based on the *Product Output Reporting System*. Therefore, to increase the quantity and quality of input for the revisions, it was decided to postpone the formation of the task force until these states had had an opportunity to use the systems.

In 1985, a second notice was placed in the *Occupational Therapy News* requesting feedback, and a task force was appointed. The following people were selected to serve on the Task Force:

Linda Kohlman McGourty, MOT, OTR, Washington (Chair)
Roger Smith, MOT, OTR, Wisconsin
Jane Marvin, OTR, California
Nancy Mahon Smith, MBA, OTR, Maryland and Arkansas
Mary Foto, OTR, California

These people were selected based on the following criteria:

1. Geographical representation
2. Professional expertise
3. Participation in other current AOTA projects
4. Knowledge of reimbursement systems
5. Interest in serving on the Task Force

Development of the Uniform Terminology—Second Edition

The task force met in 1986 and 1987 to develop drafts of the revisions. A draft from the task force was submitted to the Commission on Practice in May of 1987. Listed below are several decisions that were made in the revision process by the task force and the Commission on Practice.

1. To not replace the original document, (*Uniform Terminology for Reporting Occupational Therapy Services*, 1979), because of the number of official documents based on it and the need to retain a *Product Output Reporting System* as an official document of the AOTA.
2. To limit the revised document to defining **OCCUPATIONAL PERFORMANCE AREAS** and **OCCUPATIONAL PERFORMANCE COMPONENTS** for occupational therapy intervention (i.e., indirect services were deleted and the *Product Output Re-*

porting System was not revised) to make the project manageable.
3. To coordinate the revision process with other current AOTA projects such as the Professional and Technical Role Analysis (PATRA) and the Occupational Therapy Comprehensive Functional Assessment of the American Occupational Therapy Foundation (AOTF).
4. To develop a document that reflects current areas of practice and facilitates uniformity of definitions in the profession.
5. To recommend that the AOTA develop a companion document to define techniques, modalities, and activities used in occupational therapy intervention and a document to define specific programs that are offered by occupational therapy departments. The Commission on Practice subsequently developed education materials to assist in the application of uniform terminology to practice.

Several drafts of the revised *Uniform Terminology—Second Edition* document were reviewed by appropriate AOTA commissions and committees and by a selected review network based on geographical representation, professional expertise, and demonstrated leadership in the field. Excellent responses were received and the feedback was incorporated into the final document by the Commission on Practice.

OCCUPATIONAL THERAPY ASSESSMENT
OCCUPATIONAL THERAPY INTERVENTION

I. OCCUPATIONAL THERAPY PERFORMANCE AREAS
 A. Activities of Daily Living
  1. Grooming
  2. Oral Hygiene
  3. Bathing
  4. Toilet Hygiene
  5. Dressing
  6. Feeding and Eating
  7. Medication Routine

8. Socialization
9. Functional Communication
10. Functional Mobility
11. Sexual Expression
B. Work Activities
   1. Home Management
      a. Clothing Care
      b. Cleaning
      c. Meal Preparation and Cleanup
      d. Shopping
      e. Money Management
      f. Household Maintenance
      g. Safety Procedures
   2. Care of Others
   3. Educational Activities
   4. Vocational Activities
      a. Vocational Exploration
      b. Job Acquisition
      c. Work or Job Performance
      d. Retirement Planning
C. Play or Leisure Activities
   1. Play or Leisure Exploration
   2. Play or Leisure Performance
II. PERFORMANCE COMPONENTS
A. Sensory Motor Component
   1. Sensory Integration
      a. Sensory Awareness
      b. Sensory Processing
         (1) Tactile
         (2) Proprioceptive
         (3) Vestibular
         (4) Visual
         (5) Auditory
         (6) Gustatory
         (7) Olfactory
      c. Perceptual Skills
         (1) Stereognosis
         (2) Kinesthesia
         (3) Body Scheme
         (4) Right-Left Discrimination
         (5) Form Constancy
         (6) Position in Space
         (7) Visual-Closure
         (8) Figure Ground
         (9) Depth Perception
         (10) Topographical Orientation
   2. Neuromuscular
      a. Reflex

b. Range of Motion
c. Muscle Tone
d. Strength
e. Endurance
f. Postural Control
g. Soft Tissue Integrity
   3. Motor
      a. Activity Tolerance
      b. Gross Motor Coordination
      c. Crossing the Midline
      d. Laterality
      e. Bilateral Integration
      f. Praxis
      g. Fine Motor Coordination/Dexterity
      h. Visual-Motor Integration
      i. Oral-Motor Control
B. Cognitive Integration and Cognitive Components
   1. Level of Arousal
   2. Orientation
   3. Recognition
   4. Attention Span
   5. Memory
      a. Short-Term
      b. Long-Term
      c. Remote
      d. Recent
   6. Sequencing
   7. Categorization
   8. Concept Formation
   9. Intellectual Operations in Space
   10. Problem Solving
   11. Generalization of Learning
   12. Integration of Learning
   13. Synthesis of Learning
C. Psychosocial Skills and Psychological Components
   1. Psychological
      a. Roles
      b. Values
      c. Interests
      d. Initiation of Activity
      e. Termination of Activity
      f. Self-Concept
   2. Social
      a. Social Conduct
      b. Conversation
      c. Self-Expression
   3. Self-Management

a. Coping Skills
b. Time Management
c. Self-Control

OCCUPATIONAL THERAPY ASSESSMENT

Assessment is the planned process of obtaining, interpreting, and documenting the functional status of the individual. The purpose of the assessment is to identify the individual's abilities and limitations, including deficits, delays, or maladaptive behavior that can be addressed in occupational therapy intervention. Data can be gathered through a review of records, observation, interview, and the administration of test procedures. Such procedures include, but are not limited to, the use of standardized tests, questionnaires, performance checklists, activities, and tasks designed to evaluate specific performance abilities.

OCCUPATIONAL THERAPY INTERVENTION

Occupational therapy addresses function and uses specific procedures and activities to a) develop, maintain, improve, and/or restore the performance of necessary functions; b) compensate for dysfunction; c) minimize or prevent debilitation; and/or d) promote health and wellness. Categories of function are defined as **OCCUPATIONAL PERFORMANCE AREAS** and **PERFORMANCE COMPONENTS**. **OCCUPATIONAL PERFORMANCE AREAS** include activities of daily living, work activities, and play/leisure activities. Performance components refer to the functional abilities required for occupational performance, including sensory motor, cognitive, and psychological components. Deficits or delays in these **OCCUPATIONAL PERFORMANCE AREAS** may be addressed by occupational therapy intervention.

I. OCCUPATIONAL PERFORMANCE AREAS
   A. Activities of Daily Living

1. *Grooming*—Obtain and use supplies to shave; apply and remove cosmetics; wash, comb, style, and brush hair; care for nails; care for skin; and apply deodorant.
2. *Oral Hygiene*—Obtain and use supplies, clean mouth and teeth; remove, clean, and reinsert dentures.
3. *Bathing*—Obtain and use supplies, soap, rinse, and dry all body parts; maintain bathing position; transfer to and from bathing position.
4. *Toilet Hygiene*—Obtain and use supplies; clean self; transfer to and from, and maintain toileting position on, bedpan, toilet, and/or commode.
5. *Dressing*—Select appropriate clothing, obtain clothing from storage area, dress and undress in a sequential fashion, and fasten and adjust clothing and shoes. Don and doff assistive or adaptive equipment, prostheses, or orthoses.
6. *Feeding and Eating*—Set up food, use appropriate utensils and tableware, bring food or drink to mouth, suck, masticate, cough, and swallow.
7. *Medication Routine*—Obtain medication, open and close containers, and take prescribed quantities as scheduled.
8. *Socialization*—Interact in appropriate contextual and cultural ways.
9. *Functional Communication*—Use equipment or systems to enhance or provide communication, such as writing equipment, telephones, typewriters, communication boards, call lights, emergency systems, braille writers, aug-

mentative communication systems, and computers.

10. *Functional Mobility*—Move from one position or place to another, such as in bed mobility, wheelchair mobility, transfers (bed, car, tub, toilet, chair), and functional ambulation, with or without adaptive aids, driving, and use of public transportation.

11. *Sexual Expression*—Recognize, communicate, and perform desired sexual activities.

B. *Work Activities*

1. *Home Management*

   a. *Clothing Care*—Obtain and use supplies, launder, iron, store, and mend.

   b. *Cleaning*—Obtain and use supplies, pick up, vacuum, sweep, dust, scrub, mop, make bed, and remove trash.

   c. *Meal Preparation and Cleanup*—Plan nutritious meals and prepare food; open and close containers, cabinets and drawers; use kitchen utensils and appliances; clean up and store food.

   d. *Shopping*—Select and purchase items and perform money transactions.

   e. *Money Management*—Budget, pay bills, and use bank systems.

   f. *Household Maintenance*—Maintain home, yard, garden appliances, household items, and/or obtain appropriate assistance.

   g. *Safety Procedures*—Know and perform prevention and emergency procedures to maintain a safe environment and prevent injuries.

2. *Care of Others*—Provide for children, spouse, parents, or others, such as the physical care, nurturance, communication, and use of age appropriate activities.

3. *Educational Activities*—Participate in a school environment and school sponsored activities (such as field trips, work study and extra curricular activities).

4. *Vocational Activities*

   a. *Vocational Exploration*—Determine aptitudes, interests, skills, and appropriate vocational pursuits.

   b. *Job Acquisition*—Identify and select work opportunities and complete application and interview processes.

   c. *Work or Job Performance*—Perform job tasks in a timely and effective manner, incorporating necessary work behaviors such as grooming, interpersonal skills, punctuality, and adherence to safety procedures.

   d. *Retirement Planning*—Determine aptitudes, interests, skills, and identify appropriate avocational pursuits.

C. *Play or Leisure Activities*

1. *Play or Leisure Exploration*—identify interests, skills, opportunities, and appropriate play or leisure activities.

2. *Play or Leisure Performance*—Participate in play or leisure activities, using physical and psychosocial skills.

   a. Maintain a balance of play or leisure activities with work and activities of daily living.

   b. Obtain, utilize, and maintain equipment and supplies.

II. *PERFORMANCE COMPONENTS*

A. *Sensory Motor Component*
1. *Sensory Integration*
   a. *Sensory Awareness*—Receive and differentiate sensory stimuli.
   b. *Sensory Processing*—Interpret sensory stimuli.
      (1) *Tactile*—Interpret light touch, pressure, temperature, pain, vibration, and two-point stimuli through skin contact/receptors.
      (2) *Proprioceptive*—Interpret stimuli originating in muscles, joints, and other internal tissues to give information about the position of one body part in relationship to another.
      (3) *Vestibular*—Interpret stimuli from the inner ear receptors regarding head position and movement.
      (4) *Visual*—Interpret stimuli through the eyes, including peripheral vision and acuity, awareness of color, depth, and figure ground.
      (5) *Auditory*—Interpret sounds, localize sounds, and discriminate background sounds.
      (6) *Gustatory*—Interpret tastes.
      (7) *Olfactory*—Interpret odors.
   c. *Perceptual Skills*
      (1) *Stereognosis*—Identify objects through the sense of touch.
      (2) *Kinesthesia*—Identify the excursion and direction of joint movement.
      (3) *Body Scheme*—Acquire an internal awareness of the body and the relationship of body parts to each other.
      (4) *Right-Left Discrimination*—Differentiate one side of the body from the other.
      (5) *Form Constancy*—Recognize forms and objects as the same in various environments, positions, and sizes.
      (6) *Position in Space*—Determine the spatial relationship of figures and objects to self or other forms and objects.
      (7) *Visual-Closure*—Identify forms or objects from incomplete presentations.
      (8) *Figure Ground*—Differentiate between foreground and background forms and objects.
      (9) *Depth Perception*—Determine the relative distance between objects, figures, or landmarks and the observer.
      (10) *Topographical Orientation*—Determine the location of objects and settings and the route to the location.
2. *Neuromuscular*
   a. *Reflex*—Present an involuntary muscle response elicited by sensory input.
   b. *Range of Motion*—Move body parts through an arc.

c. *Muscle Tone*—Demonstrate a degree of tension or resistance in a muscle.

d. *Strength*—Demonstrate a degree of muscle power when movement is resisted as with weight or gravity.

e. *Endurance*—Sustain cardiac, pulmonary, and musculoskeletal exertion over time.

f. *Postural Control*—Position and maintain head, neck, trunk, and limb alignment with appropriate weight shifting, midline orientation, and righting reactions for function.

g. *Soft Tissue Integrity*—Maintain anatomical and physiological condition of interstitial tissue and skin.

3. *Motor*

a. *Activity Tolerance*—Sustain a purposeful activity over time.

b. *Gross Motor Coordination*—Use large muscle groups for controlled movements.

c. *Crossing the Midline*—Move limbs and eyes across the sagittal plane of the body.

d. *Laterality*—Use a preferred unilateral body part, for activities requiring a high level of skill.

e. *Bilateral Integration*—Interact with both body sides in a coordinated manner during activity.

f. *Praxis*—Conceive and plan a new motor act in response to an environmental demand.

g. *Fine Motor Coordination/Dexterity*—Use small muscle groups for controlled movements, partic-

ularly in object manipulation.

h. *Visual-Motor Integration*—Coordinate the interaction of visual information with body movement during activity.

i. *Oral-Motor Control*—Coordinate oropharyngeal musculature for controlled movements.

B. Cognitive Integration and Cognitive Components

1. *Level of Arousal*—Demonstrate alertness and responsiveness to environmental stimuli.

2. *Orientation*—Identify person, place, time, and situation.

3. *Recognition*—Identify familiar faces, objects, and other previously presented materials.

4. *Attention Span*—Focus on a task over time.

5. *Memory*

a. *Short-Term*—Recall information for brief periods of time.

b. *Long-Term*—Recall information for long periods of time.

c. *Remote*—Recall events from distant past.

d. *Recent*—Recall events from immediate past.

6. *Sequencing*—Place information, concepts, and actions in order.

7. *Categorization*—Identify similarities of and difference between environmental information.

8. *Concept Formation*—Organize a variety of information to form thoughts and ideas.

9. *Intellectual Operations in Space*—Mentally manipulate spatial relationships.

10. *Problem Solving*—Recognize a problem, define a problem, identify alternative plans, se-

lect a plan, organize steps in a plan, implement a plan, and evaluate the outcome.

11. *Generalization of Learning*—Apply previously learned concepts and behaviors to similar situations.
12. *Integration of Learning*—Incorporate previously acquired concepts and behavior into a variety of new situations.
13. *Synthesis of Learning*—Restructure previously learned concepts and behaviors into new patterns.

C. Psychosocial Skills and Psychological Components
  1. Psychological
     a. *Roles*—Identify functions one assumes or acquires in society; e.g., worker, student, parent, church member.
     b. *Values*—Identify ideas or beliefs which are intrinsically important.
     c. *Interests*—Identify mental or physical activities which create pleasure and maintain attention.
     d. *Initiation of Activity*—Engage in a physical or mental activity.
     e. *Termination of Activity*—Stop an activity at an appropriate time.
     f. *Self-Concept*—Develop value of physical and emotional self.
  2. Social
     a. *Social Conduct*—Interact using manners, personal space, eye contact, gestures, active listening, and self-expression appropriate to one's environment.
     b. *Conversation*—Use verbal and nonverbal communication to interact in a variety of settings.
     c. *Self-Expression*—Use a variety of styles and skills to express thoughts, feelings, and needs.
  3. Self-Management
     a. *Coping Skills*—Identify and manage stress and related reactors.
     b. *Time Management*—Plan and participate in a balance of self-care, work, leisure, and rest activities to promote satisfaction and health.
     c. *Self-Control*—Modulate and modify one's own behavior in response to environmental needs, demands, and constraints.

REFERENCES

American Occupational Therapy Association. (1979). *Occupational therapy output reporting system and uniform terminology for reporting occupational therapy services.* Rockville, MD: Author.

American Medical Association. (1966–1988). *Physicians' current procedural terminology first—fourth editions,* (CPT 1–4). Chicago, IL: Author.

American Psychiatric Association. (1952–1987). *Diagnostic and statistical manual of mental disorders—first—third editions,* (DSM—I—III-R). Washington, DC: Author.

Medicare—Medicaid Anti-Fraud and Abuse Amendments (Public Law 95-142) (42 U.S.C. 1305) October 25, 1977.

AUTHORS: The Uniform Terminology Task Force, Linda Kohlman McGourty, MOT, OTR, Chairperson, Mary Foto, OTR, Jane K. Marvin, MA, OTR, CIRS, Nancy Mahan Smith, MBA, OTR, Roger O. Smith, MOT, OTR

The Commission on Practice Members with contributions from Susan Kronsnoble, OTR for The Commission on Practice L. Randy Strickland, EdD, OTR, FAOTA Chairperson.

Approved by the Representative Assembly 4/89.

Reprinted with permission of the American Occupational Therapy Association.
American Occupational Therapy Association.
Uniform terminology for occupational therapy. 2nd ed. Am J Occup Ther 1989;43:808–815.

Cerebrovascular Accident

SUSAN NASSER BIERMAN

Strokes have afflicted mankind since earliest times. Studying the remains of ancient Egyptian mummies has shown that individuals of this era suffered strokes (1). In the past, strokes were referred to as apoplexy, meaning a sudden shock to the senses. Hippocrates, the father of Western medicine, wrote: "it is impossible to remove a strong attack of apoplexy and not easy to remove a weak attack" (2). This bleak statement demonstrates the pessimistic view once held about strokes, but much has changed since Hippocrates' time. Having a stroke does not mean that one should give up all hope and be resigned to a life of disability. Modern medical and surgical techniques, state-of-the-art rehabilitation programs, and knowledge of risk-factor control now make this even more true (3).

The effect that a stroke will have on a person's life depends on many factors that are discussed in this chapter. It is possible to survive, recover, and resume daily activities following a stroke, as is demonstrated by the lives of many famous people. Louis Pasteur, one of our greatest medical and scientific geniuses, experienced a stroke at the age of 46. While still bedridden, he dictated a brilliant bacteriological technique. Later he went on to prove that germs cause disease, founded the science of immunology, and created the basis for all modern aseptic surgery (2). Sir Winston Churchill, despite his stroke at age 79, went on to regain the prime ministry of Great Britain (1). He also subsequently published his four-volume book *A History of the English Speaking Peoples* (2). George Frederick Handel experienced a stroke at the age of 52, but still produced some of his greatest works, including the *Messiah*. Presidents Dwight Eisenhower and Franklin Delano Roosevelt, dancer and choreographer Agnes de Mille, actress Patricia Neal, and Chairman Mao Tse-tung all suffered strokes, and they too went on to lead active lives (2).

ETIOLOGY

A stroke may be defined as an interruption in the blood flow so that an adequate supply of oxygen and nutrients fail to reach portions of the brain. Medical practitioners use the term cerebrovascular accident, often abbreviated as CVA, for stroke. A stroke can occur in any part of the brain—the cerebral hemispheres, the cerebellum, or the brainstem.

Strokes are divided into two main types: hemorrhagic, including intracerebral and subarachnoid hemorrhages, and ischemic, including atherothrombotic, lacunar, and embolic infarctions in that order of frequency (4). Lack of blood supply (ischemia) and leakage of blood outside the normal vessels (hemorrhage) can both cause acute neuronal death. These two groups of strokes can be further differentiated by the location of the insult and

precise causes of the hemorrhage or ischemia (5). In most cases a loss of blood supply is the result of long-standing degeneration of the body's blood vessels. Less
commonly, a CVA occurs because of an
inborn abnormality or weakness of the
brain's vascular supply (6). These two types
of strokes are described in detail following the review of cerebral circulation.

The Brain's Blood Vessels

The blood supply of the brain is extremely important because of the metabolic demands of nervous tissue. The brain
is one of the most metabolically active organs of the body. Although it comprises
only 2% of the body weight, the brain receives approximately 17% of the cardiac
output and consumes about 20% of the
oxygen used by the entire body (7).

In the brain, the arteries of the anterior circulation supply the front, top, and
side portions of the cerebral hemispheres. The brainstem, cerebellum, and
back and under surface of the cerebral
hemispheres is supplied by the posterior
circulation. These two parts of circulation
are further categorized into the extracran-

ial portions (arising from outside the skull
and traveling toward the brain) and the
intracranial portions (arising from within
the skull) (5) (Fig. 2.1).

EXTRACRANIAL VESSELS

The extracranial anterior circulation consists of the two carotid arteries that travel
in the front of the neck on each side of
the trachea and esophagus (6). The word
carotid is derived from the Greek word
karos meaning "deep sleep," indicating
the significance of this main artery in
maintaining consciousness and brain function (8). The right common carotid artery
arises from the innominate artery. The left
common carotid artery originates directly
from the aortic arch. Around the fifth or
sixth vertebrae, these common carotid arteries divide into external carotid arteries
whose branches supply the face and its
structures and the internal carotid arteries, which supply the eyes and the cerebral hemispheres.

The vertebral arteries arise from the
subclavian arteries and make up the extracranial posterior circulation. They remain within the vertebral column for part
of their course from about C6 to C2. The
vertebral arteries enter the cranium
through the foramen magnum (6).

INTRACRANIAL VESSELS

The internal carotid arteries enter the skull
through the carotid canal and form an S-
shaped curve called the carotid siphon (6).
The artery then enters the subarachnoid
space by piercing the dura mater and gives
off the ophthalmic arteries, which supply
the eyes, the posterior communicating arteries, which join with the posterior circulation, and the anterior cerebral arteries, which supply the orbital and medial
surfaces of the frontal lobes and part of
the basal frontal lobe white matter and
caudate nucleus. It also gives off the middle cerebral arteries, which supply almost
the entire lateral surface of the frontal,
parietal, and temporal lobes as well as the
underlying white matter and basal ganglia

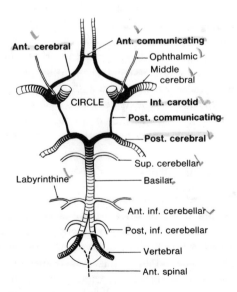

Fig. 2.1. Circle of Willis. (From Moore KL, ed. Clinically oriented anatomy. 2nd ed. Baltimore: Williams &
Wilkins, 1985:880. With permission.)

(6). The middle cerebral artery is the largest of the terminal branches of the internal carotid artery and is the direct continuation of this vessel.

The vertebral arteries enter the cranium within the posterior fossa and travel along the side of the medulla where they give off their longest branch, the posterior inferior cerebellar artery, which supplies the lateral medulla and the back of the undersurface of the cerebellum (6). The two vertebral arteries then join at the junction between the medulla and pons to form the single midline basilar artery (9). The basilar artery gives off penetrating arteries to the base of the pons and two vessels (the anterior inferior and superior cerebellar arteries) that supply the upper and anterior undersurfaces of the cerebellum (6). At the level of the midbrain, the basilar artery bifurcates into the two posterior cerebral arteries (9). As they circle the brainstem, these two arteries give off penetrating branches to the midbrain and thalamus and then divide into branches that supply the occipital lobes as well as the medial and undersurfaces of the temporal lobes (6). One of the branches of the posterior cerebral artery, the calcarine artery, is of special significance since it is the main supplier of the blood for the visual area of cortex (7).

COMMUNICATING ARTERIES

The right and left carotid vessels connect with each other when they enter the brain, by each sending out a small lateral branch meeting in the space between them. These are the anterior communicating arteries. They also branch backward to join with the right and left posterior cerebral arteries, called the posterior communicating arteries. This communicating vascular interchange, the circle of Willis, protects the brain should one of the four major supplying arteries coming up through the neck be blocked (2). The circle of Willis, named for Dr. Thomas Willis, was first described in the mid-17th century. The original diagram of this structure was first drawn for Dr. Willis by Sir Christopher Wren, the architect for St. Paul's Cathedral. Although known primarily for his architectural genius, he was also deeply involved in biology and medicine (2).

Thus we have an arterial circle to provide backup supplies for the essential functions and tissues of the brain. Starting from the midline anteriorly, the circle consists of the anterior communicating, anterior cerebral, internal carotid, posterior communicating, and posterior cerebral arteries, from which it continues to the starting point in reverse order (7). When one major vessel supplying the brain is slowly occluded, either within the circle of Willis or proximal to it, the normally small communicating arteries may slowly enlarge to compensate for the occlusion (9). This system is imperfect, however, and it often fails to prevent strokes for several reasons. In many persons, the same atherosclerotic processes that caused a stroke may also damage communicating arteries. In addition, only about a quarter of strokes are due to a blockage of the major neck vessels (2). Also, approximately half the population have anomalies or deviations in the circle of Willis. The most common defect is the absence of the posterior communicating arteries, so that the two blood supply systems, anterior and posterior, cannot interchange. It is interesting that such anomalies are more common in persons who have strokes than in the general population. Experts feel that such anomalies increase the chances of stroke in persons who also have atherosclerosis (2).

Ischemic Stroke

Cerebral infarction or brain tissue death results from obstruction of circulation to an area of the brain (ischemia) as in thrombotic, embolic, or lacunar strokes. The infarcted area has two components; the tissues that have died as a result of blood supply loss, and the peripheral area in which there may be temporary dysfunction due to edema. Edematous brain tissue sometimes recovers slowly and gradually, resulting in a reappearing of function after a period of 4 to 5 months (13).

The actual physiological events following an ischemic stroke occur in characteristic steps. First, the membrane surrounding each affected neuron leaks potassium (a mineral necessary for producing electrical impulses) and ATP (adenosine triphosphate, an energy-producing biochemical found in the body). Fluid quickly accumulates between the blood vessel and neuron, making it difficult for oxygen and nutrients to pass from the bloodstream into the damaged neuron. The initial injury produces a vicious circle in which more cellular injury results. Irreversible cell death will occur in 5 to 10 minutes if oxygen and nutrients are unable to pass to them from the bloodstream, or in a slightly longer period of time if blood flow is only partially interrupted. These dead cells form a zone of infarction that is dead tissue that will not regenerate.

Downstream from the infarcted zone is a zone of injury (penumbra). This area may be served by collateral blood vessels and is capable of returning to normal functioning. A third area that is reacting quite differently to the stroke process may also exist. In this area of hyperemia, the blood vessels are congested and swollen and may also have the potential for recovery.

The presence of these two zones, the regions of penumbra and hyperemia may serve to minimize the total area of infarction. However, they do present problems for treatment, since interventions that are beneficial to one region are not for the other (1).

THROMBOSIS

Cerebral thrombosis occurs when a blood clot forms in one of the arteries supplying the brain, causing vascular obstruction at the point of its formation. The size and location of the infarct depends on which vessel is occluded and the amount of col-

lateral circulation. Thrombosis occurs most frequently in blood vessels that have already been damaged by atherosclerosis (1) (Fig. 2.2).

Atherosclerosis is a gradual degenerative vessel-wall disease that is pathological and not a normal aspect of human aging (1). It appears as rough, irregular fatty deposits formed within the intima and inner media of the arteries. Large vessel atherosclerosis accounts for 60% of ischemic stroke. In nearly all cases, this atherosclerosis leads to the occurrence of stroke via the generation of a thrombus. Only rarely does stenosis alone cause stroke (10). The body's blood vessels have a significant reserve capacity so atherosclerosis does not usually occur until the vessel is two-thirds blocked (1).

To understand the process for producing a mass of degenerated, thickened material (plaque) called atheromas, imagine a glue bottle that has been allowed to collect the residuals of dried glue. The more clogged the cap of the bottle becomes, the more difficult it is for the glue to flow through it. Squeezing the glue through the opening can push already dried glue more firmly against the opening. The opening will become smaller and smaller until it closes completely or bursts from the increased pressure.

In the cerebral circulation, atherosclerosis and thrombus formation are most

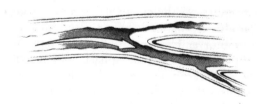

Fig. 2.2. Atherosclerosis is an abnormal condition of the arteries in which a thick, rough deposit forms on the inner wall of the arteries and gradually narrows the passageway so that the blood flow is slowed. (Reproduced with permission from "Strokes: a guide for the family," 1989. Copyright American Heart Association.)

likely to occur in areas where blood vessels turn or divide, such as the origins of the internal carotid artery and the middle cerebral artery and the junction of the vertebral and basilar arteries (1, 11).

Cerebral thrombosis often causes stuttering or progressive symptoms that occur over several hours or sometimes days. Onset during sleep is common. Often a patient notices mild arm numbness at night and then awakens the next morning with paralysis. Transient ischemic attacks precede actual infarction about half the time (4).

LACUNAR STROKES

Lacunar strokes were first described by the French physician, Pierre Marie, at the beginning of the 20th century (1). These are small infarcts usually lying in the deep noncortical parts of the cerebrum and brainstem including the basal ganglia, thalamus, pons, internal capsule, and deep white matter (11, 12). Within a few months of onset of a lacunar stroke, a small cavity (lacune in French) is left (1).

Lacunar strokes result from an occlusion of small branches of larger cerebral arteries—middle cerebral, posterior cerebral, basilar, and to a lesser extent, anterior cerebral and vertebral arteries (12). Lacunar infarcts range in size from 2 to 15 mm (11). Due to their small size, usually only minimal neurological symptoms result, and many go undetected.

Commonly, lacunar strokes produce purely motor deficits (weakness or ataxia), purely sensory deficits, or a combination of motor and sensory deficits. Symptoms usually do not include aphasia, changes in mental activity or personality, loss of consciousness, homonymous hemianopsia, or seizures (12).

Causes of vascular occlusion in lacunar infarcts include atheroma in a small vessel, an embolic particle of a thrombus lodging in a small vessel, or lipohyalinosis in which hypertension reduces the wall of the artery to connective tissue shreds (12). Hypertension is the most consistently

identified risk factor for lacunar infarction, so treatment is aimed at controlling it (11). Prognosis for recovery following a lacunar stroke is excellent (12).

EMBOLISM

Embolism occurs when a clot that has been formed elsewhere (thrombus) breaks off (embolus) and travels up the bloodstream until it reaches an artery that is too small for it to pass, and it blocks the artery (5) (Fig. 2.3). At this point its effects are similar to those produced by thrombosis. Approximately 5 to 14% of strokes appear to be the result of this process (1).

Embolic materials that travel to the arteries of the brain can originate from many sources, including the aortic arch and arteries arising from it, the extracranial carotid and vertebral arteries, and thrombi in the heart. Cardiac source emboli are common and are referred to as cardiogenic. Many cardiac abnormalities can give rise to a cerebral embolism, includ-

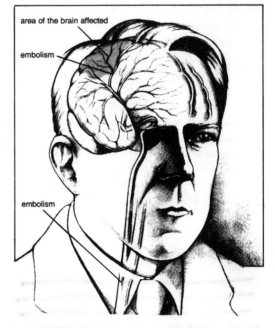

Fig. 2.3. Embolism. (Reproduced with permission from "1991 Heart and stroke facts," 1990. Copyright American Heart Association.)

ing atrial fibrillation, coronary artery disease, valvular heart disease, and arrythmias. The middle cerebral artery is by far the most common destination of cardiac emboli, followed by the posterior cerebral artery (6).

In contrast to thrombotic strokes, embolic strokes typically occur during daytime activity. The embolism can be precipitated by a sudden movement or even a sneeze. Clinical symptoms are usually maximal at onset, but in some cases the neurological symptoms improve or stabilize somewhat, then worsen as the embolus moves and blocks a more distal artery. A history of transient ischemic attacks is rare. Seizures are often associated with embolic strokes (6).

Hemorrhagic Stroke

Hemorrhagic strokes are caused by a rupture in a blood vessel or an aneurysm with resultant bleeding into or around cerebral tissue (Fig. 2.4). These types of strokes have a much higher fatality rate than those caused by clots. An aneurysm is a bulging or out-pouching of a wall of an artery due to weakness in the vessel wall, and it is prone to rupture at any time (Fig. 2.5). Aneurysms are often seen in young persons, and hemorrhagic strokes are more common in young people than are in-

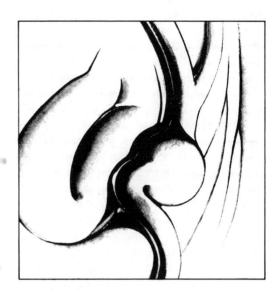

Fig. 2.5. Aneurysms are blood-filled pouches that balloon out from weak spots on the artery wall. (Reproduced with permission from "1991 Heart and stroke facts," 1990. Copyright American Heart Association.)

farcts. The vessel wall anomaly is often congenital. There are two types of hemorrhagic strokes. An intracerebral hemorrhage refers to bleeding directly into brain substance, while a subarachnoid hemorrhage is bleeding occurring within the brain's surrounding membranes and cerebrospinal fluid (10). These two types of hemorrhage differ not only in incidence, but also in etiology, clinical signs, and treatment.

SUBARACHNOID HEMORRHAGES

Subarachnoid hemorrhages account for about 7% of all strokes (5). Their most common cause is leakage of blood from aneurysms. A combination of congenital and degenerative factors, usually at the points of origin or bifurcations of arteries, can precipitate formation of an aneurysm. Blood may break through the weak point of the aneurysm at any time and because of the force of arterial pressure spread quickly into the cerebrospinal fluid surrounding the brain. A subarachnoid hemorrhage may also be caused by bleeding

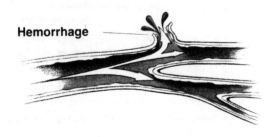

Hemorrhage

Fig. 2.4. Blood flowing into brain tissue through a ruptured arterial wall destroys brain tissue directly or indirectly by compression. (Reproduced with permission from "Strokes: a guide for the family," 1989. Copyright American Heart Association.)

from an arteriovenous malformation, which is an abnormal collection of vessels near the surface of the brain. Other less common causes of subarachnoid hemorrhages are hemophilia, excessive anticoagulation therapy, and trauma to the skull and brain (6).

Extravasated blood irritates the meninges, and intracranial pressure is increased due to extra fluid in the closed cranial cavity. This can lead to headache, vomiting, and altered state of consciousness. Sleepiness, stupor, agitation, restlessness, and actual coma are various manifestations of reduced consciousness. Headaches are usually severe and are described as the worst in the patient's life. Since the bleeding takes place around the brain and not in the actual brain substance, motor, sensory, or visual abnormalities on one side of the body are usually not seen. Lumbar puncture with analysis of the cerebrospinal fluid is the most reliable method of diagnosing subarachnoid hemorrhage (6).

INTRACEREBRAL HEMORRHAGES

Intracerebral hemorrhage usually begins with bleeding from small, deep penetrating vessels under arteriolar or capillary pressure as opposed to arterial pressure as with a subarachnoid hemorrhage. Therefore, onset of symptoms from intracerebral hemorrhages develop gradually over minutes, hours, or sometimes days. Release of blood into brain tissue and surrounding edema will then disrupt the function of that particular brain region (6). Hypertension is the most common cause of bleeding into the brain. Less common causes are arteriovenous malformations, aneurysms, drugs (especially methamphetamines and cocaine), use of anticoagulants, and trauma (14).

Clinical signs of intracerebral hemorrhage are usually focal at first and depend on the location of the bleeding. There are also some general symptoms regardless of the location, and extremely small hemorrhages may go undetected. A large hematoma causes headache, vomiting, convulsions, and decreased levels of alertness (14).

Stupor and coma are common signs of very large hemorrhages and carry a poor prognosis. Nevertheless, recovery is possible. Agnes de Mille's book *Reprieve— A Memoire* is a story of cerebral hemorrhage and subsequent recovery (1).

Cerebral injury due to intracerebral bleeding results from the damaging effect that the abnormal presence of blood has on the neurons. Abnormal pressure on neurons distorts their normal architecture. It also prevents oxygen and nutrients from passing to the cells from the bloodstream. Eventually, bleeding will stop and a hard clot will be formed. Over a period of months, the clot slowly recedes, breaks down, and is absorbed by the body's white blood cells (1).

INCIDENCE AND PREVALENCE

Strokes are the third leading cause of death in the United States, surpassed only by heart disease and cancer (3). It is the most common diagnosis among clients seen by occupational therapists for the treatment of physically disabled adults. At least 500,000 people suffer an episode each year. Of the two million persons in this country who have experienced a stroke and who are alive at any one time, 10% will fully recover, 40% will be left with a mild disability, and 50% will be severely disabled and may require institutional care (3). Of the two main types, hemorrhagic strokes occur much less frequently (20% of all strokes) than ischemic strokes, which account for about 80% of all strokes (6). Approximately 10% of all strokes result from intracerebral hemorrhage (5), and approximately 18% are lacunar (15).

Despite these grim statistics, there is some good news. With the exception of subarachnoid hemorrhage, all types of strokes have shown a significantly decreased incidence in the last 4 to 5 decades. This may be partly due to increased control of risk factors such as hypertension, diabetes mellitus, and heart disease and the fact that individuals are trying to lead healthier lifestyles (16). Individuals who have had a stroke are now living almost twice as long (4). While debate continues as to whether this decline is due to fewer strokes occurring or to better medical treatment, fewer people now die of stroke (5).

SIGNS AND SYMPTOMS

Stroke Warning Signs

To educate the public, the American Heart Association has published several pamphlets listing signs that are considered preliminary warnings of an impending serious stroke. These include sudden weakness or numbness of the face, arm, and leg on one side of the body; loss of speech or trouble talking or understanding speech; dimness or loss of vision, particularly in only one eye; and/or unexplained dizziness, unsteadiness, or sudden falls (1).

Some general medical symptoms related to *type* of stroke were discussed under Etiology. The outward signs and symptoms also depend on the size and location of the injury (Fig. 2.6), and neurologists can often predict location by the symptoms with which the individual presents (Fig. 2.7). However, it is important to remember that a stroke is complex and manifested symptoms are as variable as each individual. Any reliance on stereotyped models of stroke leads to generalized and often inappropriate therapy.

Symptoms that result from a partial reduction or temporary change in the blood flow to the brain are extremely important warning signs for stroke (16). Several of these conditions are discussed below.

TRANSIENT ISCHEMIC ATTACKS

Transient ischemic attacks, or TIAs, result from a temporary interference with blood supply to the brain. The symptoms occur rapidly and last for about 1 minute up to but not exceeding 24 hours. The specific signs and symptoms depend on the portion of the brain affected, but may include fleeting blindness in one eye, hemiparesis, hemiplegia, aphasia, dizziness, double vision, and staggering. Carotid artery disease and vertebral basilar artery disease may lead to TIAs (1). The

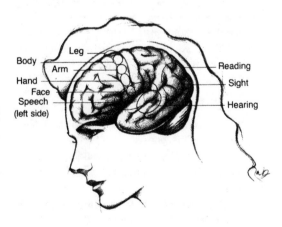

Fig. 2.6. Control zones of the brain. Different areas of the brain control bodily functions. (Reproduced with permission from "Strokes: a guide for the family," 1989. Copyright American Heart Association.)

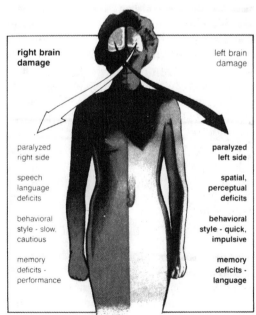

Fig. 2.7. Symptoms of brain damage. (Reproduced with permission from "1991 Heart and stroke facts," 1990. Copyright American Heart Association.)

main distinction between TIAs and stroke is the short duration of the symptoms and the lack of permanent neurological damage. People who have had TIAs are nine and one-half times more likely to have a stroke than people of the same age and sex who have never had a TIA (16).

SMALL STROKES

In some cases, the symptoms of a TIA may last longer than 24 hours. If they last a day or more and then completely resolve or leave only minor neurological deficits, they are called "small strokes." Often, the remaining neurological deficits are barely noticeable. Like TIAs however, these small strokes are important warning signs that a more serious cerebrovascular accident may occur (1).

A small stroke that completely resolves is called a reversible ischemic neurological deficit (RIND). An episode that lasts more than 72 hours and leaves some minor neurological impairments is called a partially reversible ischemic neurological deficit (PRIND). The mechanism of injury in RIND and PRIND is the same as that for a stroke or TIA. Blood flow to the brain is reduced below the critical level needed for normal neurological activity (1).

Many small strokes are not reported to a medical practitioner, which makes the exact frequency of occurrence of these strokes difficult to determine. However, the occurrence of a small stroke increases the risk of a serious stroke by as much as tenfold (1). It is important to recognize the symptoms of a small stroke so that it can be treated early, reducing the risk of more permanent injury.

SUBCLAVIAN STEAL SYNDROME

This is a rare condition in which there is a narrowing of the subclavian artery that runs under the clavicle. Symptoms occur when the arm on the side of the narrowed vessel is exercised. Usually movement of the arm produces light-headedness, numbness, and weakness. Other neurological symptoms may also be pres-

ent. In this syndrome, blood is "stolen" from the brain and instead is delivered to the exercised arm. It is a warning sign that advanced atherosclerosis may be present in the arteries throughout the body, including the cerebral arteries (1).

Neurological Effects of Stroke

An occlusion causing a serious stroke can occur anywhere in the extracranial or intracranial system, but the most common site is in the distribution of the middle cerebral artery and its branches in the cerebrum. The majority of cerebral strokes occur in one or the other cerebral hemisphere, but not both (1). It is important to note that even in individuals with the same neurological deficit, the impact of disability is different and often dependent on the individual's life situation.

LEFT-SIDED CEREBRAL INJURIES— MIDDLE CEREBRAL ARTERY

The left cerebral hemisphere controls most functions on the right side of the body because of the decussation of motor fibers (decussation of the pyramids) in the medulla. These fibers that cross, or decussate to the opposite side, form the lateral corticospinal tract. The rest of the fibers descend ipsilaterally, forming the anterior corticospinal tract (17). The proportion of crossing fibers varies from person to person, with an average of about 85% (7). The following story written by a man who suffered a stroke is an example of a left cerebral injury and illustrates some of the deficits that may result.

Wednesday, January 31st, began as a normal day. This consisted of getting up for work at 4:45 AM, having breakfast and arriving at Buick Engine Plant to begin my work shift of 6:00 AM to 2:30 PM.

After spending 8 hours made up of 50% desk work and 50% floor work, I arrived back home feeling exceptionally fatigued. After a usual greeting and reading the mail, I proceeded to the couch for a nap. My wife woke me for dinner around 5:00 PM.

Within a couple of hours I returned to the couch still feeling the need for more rest. Waking up in time for the 11:00 PM news, I felt more refreshed and rested.

Just prior to retiring to the bedroom about midnight, I felt a "tingling" in my head lasting for no more than a couple of minutes. Fifteen to 20 minutes later, the "tingling" returned, accompanied by the inability to move the limbs on my right side. Movement returned and the "tingling" ceased after about 10 minutes. Within another 15 minutes the sensation returned, along with a slurring of speech.

After noting the happenings to my wife, she called 911 and within a short time both a local ambulance and a sheriffs' paramedic arrived at our home. Noting the pattern that each time the "tingling" returned the loss of limb movement and slurred speech occurred, the paramedics decided I needed medical attention immediately.

While in the emergency room for a period of 4 to 5 hours, the sensation returned several times. During this time they performed x-rays, ECG, blood pressure, and other tests. Emergency personnel later told me that the CVA was "evolving" with each recurrence of the symptoms. At about 5:00 AM, I was admitted to the hospital.

After being settled in a room, I became aware that I was there for more than a long weekend with hopes of returning to work on Monday. The next 2 days consisted of a series of tests, accompanied by a "state of confusion," being scared, questioning why and what the future held.

By late Friday afternoon, February 2nd, they had determined what had happened and why. I had suffered a cerebral hemorrhage on the left side of my brain. I was then transferred to the rehab floor. Saturday and Sunday consisted of evaluating my abilities, or lack of abilities of speech and limb movement. Therapy then began on Monday, February 5th. Therapy consisted of physical, occupational, and speech. Speech therapy ended after 1 week, but I was advised to practice fundamentals.

During my stay of 4 weeks at McLaren Regional Medical Center, I began the journey to good health. Along with scheduled therapies, a bonus of mental therapy came about from the camaraderie with fellow rehab patients. I was not alone! All at once the usual routine of earning a wage and maintaining a home was ended. The roles my wife and I previously played were now changed. She now became financial secretary, part-time mechanic, snow-shoveler, and chauffeur in addition to spending several hours each day at the hospital.

As a result of my affliction, values of certain things such as good health, relationships of family and friends, and a closeness to God are no longer taken for granted. Only with hope and a firm determination to improve will my full recovery come about.

A cerebrovascular accident in the region of the middle cerebral artery in the left cerebral hemisphere may produce the following symptoms:

1. Loss of voluntary movement and coordination on the right side of the face, trunk, and extremities.
2. Impaired sensation including temperature discrimination, pain, and proprioception on the right side (hemianesthesia).
3. Language deficits, called aphasia, in which the patient may be unable to speak and/or understand speech, writing, and gestures. The breakdown of language function is complex, and there are many types of aphasia which will be discussed later in this chapter.
4. Produce problems with articulation of speech because of disturbances in muscle control of the lips, mouth, tongue, and vocal cords (dysarthria).
5. Create blind spots in the visual field, usually on the right side.
6. Produce a slow and cautious personality.
7. Produce memory deficits for recent and/or past events (1).

RIGHT-SIDED CEREBRAL INJURIES— MIDDLE CEREBRAL ARTERY

The right cerebral hemisphere controls most of the functions on the left side of the body. The right cerebral hemisphere is also responsible for spatial sensation, perception, and judgement. The following story written by a nurse who suffered a stroke describes a person with a stroke in the right cerebral hemisphere.

> On February 16th, I underwent surgery for a right endarterectomy due to complete blockage of the carotid artery. As in any major surgery there are certain risks involved. With this surgery it was the possibility of a stroke. Six hours later while I was in ICU, I suffered a stroke, with left hemiplegia. I was still somewhat anesthetized, but I vaguely remember I was surrounded by a team of doctors and they were asking me to lift my left arm and leg, wiggle my toes, lift my brow, and smile. I was unable to perform these simple functions satisfactorily, and I was extremely frightened as I became aware of what happened. I was repeatedly asked to perform these tasks, and each time I failed. This resulted in feelings of fear, anger, helplessness, and above all frustration. My speech was slow and hesitant, and my memory confused. The following day I realized I had lost my peripheral vision on the left and I had to turn my head to the left to compensate for this visual loss.
>
> I had always been an independent woman, and spent many sleepless hours wondering what was going to happen to my life. I was determined to fight this illness so I could return to my normal lifestyle. Rehabilitation started, and with the help of wonderful therapists, supportive family and friends, a lot of hard work and determination on my part, and with God's guidance, today two and one-half years later, I am once again enjoying a full life.

Injury to the middle cerebral artery of the right cerebral hemisphere may produce a combination of the following deficits:

1. Weakness (hemiparesis) or paralysis (hemiplegia) on the left side of the body (face, arm, trunk, and leg);

2. Impairment of sensation (touch, pain, temperature, and proprioception) on the left side of the body;
3. Spatial and perceptual deficits;
4. Unilateral neglect, in which the patient neglects the left side of the body and/or the left side of the environment;
5. Dressing apraxia, in which the patient is unable to relate the articles of clothes to the body (18);
6. Defective vision in the left halves of visual fields or left homonymous hemianopsia in which there is defective vision in each eye (the temporal half of the left eye and the nasal half of the right eye);
7. Impulsive behavior, quick and imprecise movements, and errors of judgement (1).

ANTERIOR CEREBRAL ARTERY STROKE

The territory of the anterior cerebral artery is rarely infarcted because of the side-to-side communication provided by the anterior communicating artery in the circle of Willis (15). Symptoms of an anterior cerebral artery stroke include:

1. Paralysis of the lower extremity, usually more severe than the upper extremity, contralateral to the occluded vessel;
2. Loss of sensation in the contralateral toes, foot, and leg;
3. Loss of conscious control of bowel and/or bladder;
4. Balance problems in sitting, standing, and walking;
5. Lack of spontaneity of emotion, whispered speech, or loss of all communication;
6. Memory impairment or loss (1).

VERTEBROBASILAR STROKE

The vertebrobasilar system of arteries supplies blood primarily to the posterior portions of the brain including the brainstem, cerebellum, thalamus, and parts of the occipital and temporal lobes. This posterior circulation is not divided into right and left halves as in the anterior circulation. An occlusion here might produce:

1. A variety of visual disturbances, including impaired coordination of the eyes;
2. Impaired temperature sensation;
3. Impaired ability to read and/or name objects;
4. Vertigo, dizziness;
5. Disturbances in balance when standing or walking (ataxia);
6. Paralysis of the face, limbs, or tongue;
7. Clumsy movements of the hands;
8. Difficulty judging distance when trying to coordinate limb movements (dysmetria);
9. Drooling and difficulty swallowing (dysphagia);
10. Localized numbness;
11. Loss of memory;
12. Drop attacks where there is a sudden loss of motor and postural control resulting in collapse, but the individual remains conscious (1).

TIAs in this area are common in the elderly. The vertebral arteries travel up to the brainstem through a bony channel in the cervical vertebrae. In older persons, osteoarthritis may develop in cervical bones, causing narrowing of the cervical canal, especially when the head is extended or rotated.

WALLENBURG'S SYNDROME

Wallenburg's syndrome is a classic brainstem stroke and is also referred to as the lateral medullary syndrome (15). It occurs as the result of an occlusion of the posterior inferior cerebellar artery or one of its branches supplying the lower portion of the brainstem (1). It is located in an area of the brainstem that both relays nerve fibers from the spinal cord and regulates many vital senses (1). Strokes in this area may produce contralateral pain and temperature loss, ipsilateral Horner's syndrome (sinking of the eyeball, ptosis of

the upper eyelid, and a dry cool face on the affected side), ataxia, and facial sensory loss. Ischemia to ipsilateral cranial nerve fibers 8, 9, and 10 result in palatal paralysis, hoarseness, dysphagia, and vertigo. There is no significant weakness in this syndrome (15).

Brainstem strokes can often result in coma because of damage to the centers involved with alertness and wakefulness (reticular system) (15). A hemorrhage into the brainstem area is rare, quickly accompanied by loss of consciousness, and usually fatal. In patients surviving brainstem stroke, however, recovery is often good.

PROGRESSION AND PROGNOSIS

Strokes cause anoxic damage to nervous tissue that causes various neurological deficits depending on where the blood supply was lost. If neuronal cell death occurs, it is considered irreparable and permanent, as no way has yet been found to regenerate nerve cells (2). However, the nervous system has a high level of plasticity, especially during early development, and individual differences in neural connections and learned behaviors play a major role in functional recovery. No two brains can be expected to be structurally or functionally identical (19). Spontaneous recovery may occur as edema subsides or viable neurons reactivate. Recovery may also occur with physiological reorganization of neural connections and/or developmental strategies. Any injury brings different factors into play, affecting axonal and dendritic sprouting or collateral rearrangement, synaptic formation, the excitability of neurons, "substitution of parallel channels," and "mobilization of redundant capacity". (20).

Accuracy in the prediction of function or rate of return in a given stroke patient is difficult because of individual variability of anatomy and extent of brain damage, as well as differences in types of CVA, learning ability, premorbid personality and intelligence, and motivation (21). However, generally, prognosis for recovery of function is greater in young clients, possibly because the young brain is more plastic and/or because the young are generally in better physical condition.

Secondary complications are important to recovery and rehabilitation and may actually be more disabling than the stroke itself (13). These complications are discussed in detail in this chapter and include depression, seizures, infection, bowel/bladder incontinence, thromboembolism, shoulder subluxation, painful shoulder, shoulder-hand syndrome, abnormal muscle tone, and associated reactions and movements.

Individuals with good sensation, minimal spasticity, some selective motor control, and no fixed contractures seem to make the greatest improvements in functional abilities. If an individual does not have any concept of the affected side and cannot localize stimuli to the affected side or has fecal or urinary incontinence, the outlook for independence is generally poor. Some individuals may continue to have strokes, complicating recovery. (21).

Medications and surgery may make a difference in the prognosis of an individual at risk or having had a CVA.

DIAGNOSTICS, MEDICATIONS, AND SURGERY

Diagnosis

There are preventive treatments, surgical interventions, and general lifestyle changes that can reduce the likelihood or severity of stroke (1). The best way to prevent a stroke from occurring is to control risk factors and be aware of warning signs and symptoms. The diagnosis of stroke requires a knowledge of the incidence of the different types of stroke as well as the presence of these risk factors. These symptoms must be carefully obtained from either the patient or the family if the patient is too ill, frightened, or confused (6). Neurologists, neurosurgeons, and some internists are the specialists usually involved in this acute diagnostic phase of treatment (13).

The physical examination of the patient with a suspected stroke or TIA includes a search for possible cardiac sources of emboli by listening to the heart and arteries of the neck. Also useful in the determination of cardiac source emboli are electrocardiography (ECG), echocardiography, and monitoring for arrhythmias. A neurological examination assists in determining the neurological disability and usually includes evaluation of higher cortical function (memory and language), level of alertness, visual and oculomotor system, behavior, and gait (6).

Laboratory and other diagnostic procedures are carefully selected to test, confirm, and elaborate on the hypothesis of the mechanism and location of the stroke suggested (6). Blood studies are essential and very useful in the diagnosis. Other diagnostic techniques include neuroimaging techniques, noninvasive studies of blood vessels and invasive techniques (Fig. 2.8).

NEUROIMAGING TECHNIQUES

Computed tomography (CT) and magnetic resonance imaging (MRI) are invalu-

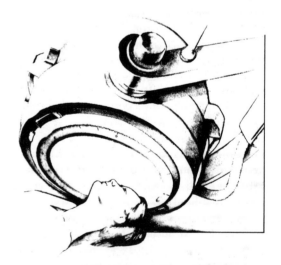

Fig. 2.8. Many nonsurgical techniques can be used to measure blood flow and detect artery blockages in the brain. (Reproduced with permission from "1991 Heart and stroke facts," 1990. Copyright American Heart Association.)

able noninvasive tools that depict patho-logical changes in the brain in patients with stroke (6). One or the other of these is almost always used at some point for every patient with a suspected stroke.

COMPUTED TOMOGRAPHY

Computed tomography, or CT scan, is a type of x-ray examination allowing accurate analysis of cerebral injury (1). One important distinction that a CT scan can make is the difference between a hemorrhagic stroke and an ischemic stroke. It is useful in clarifying not only the location but also the mechanism and severity of stroke. It can also determine associated changes such as edema, shift of brain contents, hematomas, and infarcts due to ischemia. It is most useful in the diagnosis of stroke due to hemorrhage and may even be normal in patients with recent infarction. It is often not diagnostic in patients with TIAs and is also not useful for imaging brainstem infarcts (6).

MAGNETIC RESONANCE IMAGING

Magnetic resonance imaging, or MRI, is more sensitive than a CT scan and requires no radiation from x-rays. It provides detailed pictures of the brain by using a magnetic field. MRI is particularly helpful in revealing arteriovenous malformations (AVMs) (6). It is superior to the CT in imaging the cerebellum, brainstem, thalamus, and spinal cord. MRI also provides better anatomic definition of the injury, but it does not distinguish hemorrhage, tumor, and infarction as well as CT.

POSITRON EMISSION TOMOGRAPHY

Positron emission tomography, or PET scan, is currently being used experimentally. This scan shows how the brain uses oxygen, glucose, and other nutrients. With PET scan, weakened or damaged areas can be identified (1).

NONINVASIVE STUDIES OF BLOOD VESSELS

Two noninvasive procedures used to evaluate both extracranial and intracranial blood flow are duplex scanning and transcranial doppler ultrasound. These techniques can localize and determine the approximate size of the lesions within the arteries (6).

Duplex scanning is useful in detecting the presence and severity of disease in the common and internal carotid arteries and in the subclavian and vertebral arteries in the neck. This scan can reliably differentiate between minor plaque disease, stenosis, and occlusive lesions. It is an excellent method of monitoring the progression or regression of atherosclerotic disease in the neck (6).

Transcranial Doppler ultrasound gives information about pressure and flow in the intracranial arteries. A probe is placed on the head and is attached to a computer. This procedure is useful in monitoring changes in arterial flow later in the course of the patient's disease (6).

INVASIVE TECHNIQUES

Cerebral angiography involves radiography of the vascular system of the brain following injection of a dye or other contrast medium into the arterial blood system. The entire visible length of cerebral arteries can be defined as well as the nature, location, and extent of pathological changes. This technique is now safer than ever before (less than 1% incidence of mortality and serious morbidity) (6).

Analysis of cerebrospinal fluid is helpful in diagnosing subarachnoid hemorrhage. In a lumbar puncture, the subarachnoid space (usually between the third and fourth lumbar vertebrae) is tapped, and cerebrospinal fluid is withdrawn. Analysis of the pigments in the spinal fluid can also help in estimating the age of the hemorrhage and detecting rebleeding (6).

OTHER TECHNIQUES

Other diagnostic techniques used for stroke include electroencephalography (EEG), single photon emission tomography (SPET), and special cardiac and coagulation tests that are useful in detecting unusual heart and blood disorders that can bring on a stroke (6). Following this diagnostic phase of evaluation, the patient is then usually seen by the physiatrist who evaluates the brain-damaged person's ability to function. Rehabilitation will often begin at that point to return the patient to the highest level of independent functioning possible.

Medications

At present, the treatment of acute stroke is limited to management of the results of the primary event and preventative measures against further injury or occurrence (22). There remains much controversy about the routine use of agents to reverse the cause or decrease the effects of stroke. The value of secondary preventative measures is also far from clear (22). However, many treatments have been tried with acute stroke. Before the stroke can be treated, it must be accurately identified as either cerebral infarction or cerebral hemorrhage (22). Medications that are of benefit with one of these types of stroke may be potentially dangerous to the other. Therefore, careful and exact diagnosis must be made first.

CEREBRAL INFARCTION

Some common categories of drugs used for cerebral infarction are:

Anticoagulants. These drugs inhibit clotting by interfering with the activity of chemicals in the liquid portion of blood that are essential for the coagulation process (1). One of the most commonly used drugs is heparin, although recent studies fail to support its use in completed cerebral infarct unless a cardiac source of emboli is likely (22). Nevertheless, 70% of neurologists questioned in one survey felt that prevention of stroke progression was a potential indication for the use of heparin (23). Subcutaneous heparin has also been found to dramatically reduce

DVT formation—a serious complication of stroke.

Antiplatelet therapy. Aspirin and ticlopidine are two commonly used antiplatelet agents that can reduce the risk of stroke recurrence. The use of aspirin in TIAs can result in a 30% reduction in the development of full stroke (22). It also benefits patients with a mild stroke but is not as effective in those with moderate or severe strokes (24). Aspirin is clearly not suitable for patients with cerebral hemorrhage or those at risk of bleeding. It is less successful when used by women, as compared with men. Aspirin is relatively safe and inexpensive. Recently published studies have recommended a lower dose of aspirin to reduce harmful side effects (24, 25).

Ticlopidine is a new drug that is being tested and may be better than aspirin in preventing the formation of clots. Based on early studies, ticlopidine has been found to be just as effective for women as men (1).

Thrombolysis. Thrombolysis, the dissolution of an occluding thrombus, is used frequently in the acute treatment of myocardial infarction. When used within the first few hours following cerebral infarction, substantial tissue recovery results. This must be weighed against reperfusion damage, a bleeding tendency, and the possibility of reocclusion. Some commonly used thrombolytics are streptokinase, urokinase, and acetylated plasminogen-streptokinase complex or APSAC (22).

CEREBRAL HEMORRHAGE

Very little work has been done on the specific treatment of cerebral hemorrhage with medication. Some promising studies have been done on the use of calcium antagonists for prevention or reduction of poor neurologic outcome due to vasospasm. Nimodipine, one of these calcium antagonists, has been tested in several clinical trials and has been shown to have some positive benefits in aneurysmal subarachnoid hemorrhage. It limits the flow of calcium into the cells. Nimodipine dilates the blood vessels, allowing more blood to flow to the brain. (Please see Appendix 2.2 for a detailed chart of medications.)

POST-CVA

Following cerebrovascular accident, there are specific pathophysiological sequelae. It is these secondary effects of stroke to which important treatment is aimed. Two of the cerebral effects of stroke are edema and ischemia. Some treatments that have been tried for ischemia are oxygen therapy to reduce hypoxia, vasodilation in attempt to improve blood flow through ischemic areas, therapeutic hypertension, and hemodilution therapy. Hemodilution results in a significant rise in cerebral blood flow and increased oxygen transfer (22).

Edema often complicates ischemic strokes and must be controlled, since most deaths during the first week after a massive stroke are due to extensive cerebral edema and increased intracranial pressure. This can displace the cerebrum downward and interfere with the functioning of the midbrain and lower brainstem, which control basic vital functions such as respiration and heart action (2).

Corticosteroid therapy can cause a significant reduction in the interstitial cerebral edema. Osmotic agents such as mannitol and glycerol can reduce both intracellular and interstitial edema. It appears logical that elevation of the patient's head might reduce edema formation, but this upright posture could also reduce cerebral blood flow. Formal studies have not been performed (22).

Surgery

In some cases, surgical treatment may be the best choice for the patient. The neurosurgeon must carefully consider many factors before surgery is performed. One of the most commonly performed vascular surgeries in the United States is the carotid endarterectomy. During this type of surgery, the diseased vessel is opened, the clot is removed, and an artificial graft is put in its place (1). This surgery is currently considered in patients with greater than 50% stenosis of the carotid artery ipsilateral to the affected hemisphere (10).

Subarachnoid hemorrhages are often brought on by ruptured aneurysms or arteriovenous malformations. Surgical clipping or removal of the lesions is the most effective treatment of these anomalies. If the patient survives the initial bleeding, the goal of surgery is to correct the problem before it bleeds again. In intracerebral hemorrhage, small hematomas often resolve spontaneously. Large hematomas, however, often produce death. Some lesions may expand, causing gradually increasing neurological signs. These expanding lesions can be drained surgically if they are near the surface of the brain, especially in the cerebral or cerebellar white matter. Generally, hemorrhages are evacuated only if they are large and life threatening or when surgery is necessary to treat an aneurysm, tumor, or arteriovenous malformation (6).

Superficial temporal artery bypass is a new, more delicate surgical therapy for preventing future strokes (1). Beginning with craniotomy to expose the brain, microsurgery is used to connect a scalp artery to an intracranial artery. This operation is trickier and less often performed than the carotid endarterectomy. Those practicing this type of surgery are enthusiastic about their results and claim that it revascularizes the brain better than the endarterectomies (2).

[*Editors'* note: The author of this chapter elected to use a different method of presentation for this section and to use definitions of terms that are different from the AOTA's Uniform Terminology.]

IMPACT OF CONDITION ON PERFORMANCE

Sensory motor, cognitive, and psychosocial components are almost always affected by a cerebrovascular accident.

Deficits in these areas and any secondary complications profoundly affect an individual's occupational performance in work, leisure, and activities of daily living.

Sensorimotor

Almost all individuals with cerebral or brainstem strokes initially develop some physical disability affecting skills in eating, dressing, personal hygiene, and functional mobility (e.g., transfers and ambulation). This may include weakness (hemiparesis) or loss of movement (hemiplegia), usually on one side of the body, incoordination, abnormal muscle tone, and/or balance problems.

Motor dysfunction following a stroke usually results in initial hypotonicity (flaccid hemiplegia) followed by increasing hypertonicity (spastic hemiplegia). The spasticity makes it difficult to dissociate gross motor movements and interferes with efficient completion of most tasks. Occasionally the person will progress into a final stage of normal movement patterns.

Somatosensory dysfunction includes both disorders of sensation and perception, although it is often difficult to differentiate between the two. Sensation involves distortion of information from self and the environment, and perception is a dysfunction in understanding and interpreting information from self and the environment. Sensory loss seldom occurs in isolation but goes along with motor loss and compounds the loss of functional activity.

Proprioception is a sensory awareness of the position of body parts. Individuals with dysfunction in this area may show asymmetrical posture, have difficulty maintaining balance, appear to forget affected body parts, be unable to describe position or movement of limbs, and be susceptible to joint damage. Individuals with a loss of tactile sensation may demonstrate a lack of awareness of body parts simply because they forget what they cannot feel. They are also susceptible to damage of affected body parts, particularly to skin breakdown. Astereognosis affects functional use of the affected hand whenever vision is occluded, so that tasks such as finding keys or coins in a pocket or a glass on a bedside table when it is dark may be difficult. Asomatognosia, in which an individual does not have an awareness of his/her own body and its condition, is commonly seen in right parietal lobe lesions. Deficits that result from right cerebral injuries often cause unilateral perceptual problems of the left body side and space, such as unilateral neglect, while lesions in the left cerebral hemisphere cause bilateral problems, such as right/left discrimination (18).

Orofacial weakness may cause difficulties in expression, speech (dysarthria), mastication, and swallowing (dysphagia).

Impaired balance may cause difficulties in assuming and maintaining a vertical posture and in automatic adjustments to changes of position and antigravity movement. As a result, individuals demonstrate an asymmetrical posture at rest, leaning or falling to the hemiplegic side during mobility, or fail to use normal protective reactions when falling.

Impairment of the left parietal lobe results in apraxia, where individuals are unable to adjust movement of their own body parts, while impairment of the right parietal lobe results in an inability to adjust the position of external objects. Lesions of frontal lobes result in apraxia, in which sequencing of movement is a major difficulty. Individuals may be unable to carry out a verbal request (such as a simple task like combing the hair), although they can often perform such tasks automatically; they may perseverate in purposeless movement, be unable to complete a required sequence of acts, be unable to copy gesture, drawings, or simple spatial constructional tasks.

Bladder or bowel incontinence may result from a communication disorder or be due to disruption of normal routine and diet, lack of awareness of body function, or emotional disorder (13).

Cognitive and Perceptual

Visual field defects may impair reading, even in the absence of language dysfunction. Reading may also be impaired by right cerebral lesions because the visuospatial deficits result in poor tracking across the printed page. Individuals with homonymous hemianopsia of either side demonstrate a lack of response to people, objects, or the environment on the affected side so may bump into objects or be startled by their sudden appearance. With visual inattention, individuals have difficulty scanning and shifting their gaze, particularly toward the affected side. Visual agnosias and visuospatial agnosia, or difficulty in understanding the relationship between objects and between self and objects, are also present. Individuals lose their way in a familiar environment, cannot trace a route on a map, cannot pick out objects from a cluttered environment, cannot copy drawings or simple construction, and may have difficulty in functional (spatial) tasks such as dressing and reading a newspaper. Agnosia for sounds may also occur, characterized by not understanding or confusing nonverbal sounds (18).

Cognitive disturbance is often associated with more severe strokes (25) with potential deficits in learning and judgment. There can also be impaired powers of concentration, reduced initiative, and poor short-term memory.

Perceptual and cognitive problems are described more thoroughly in other texts, and the reader is referred to *Perceptual and Cognitive Dysfunction in the Adult Stroke Patient* by Siev, Freishtat, and Zoltan for an excellent review of these deficits (18).

Language and Aphasia

The left cerebral hemisphere controls language in about 99% of all right-handed persons and in approximately 50% of individuals who are left-handed (1, 17). In a small percentage of the population, neither the right nor the left cerebral hemisphere is dominant for language, which often afflicts these individuals with a variety of speech and language problems. In his book *The Brain: The Last Frontier*, Richard Restak writes about an interesting way to distinguish left-handers whose right cerebral hemisphere is dominant for language from left-handers whose left cerebral hemisphere is dominant for language. He states that the inverted hand position in writing is a biological marker dividing these two groups. Many left-handers (60%) write with their hand inverted, that is, with the greater part of the hand above the line of print and pointing toward the bottom of the paper. In these people, the language hemisphere is the left cerebral hemisphere. In left-handed people who write in a non-inverted manner which is the hand position used by most right-handers, the area of language specialization is right cerebral hemisphere (26).

The word aphasia means "speechlessness" but entails much more than just loss of speech. Other language components that may be affected in aphasia include listening, understanding, reading, writing, gesturing, and thinking. Thinking has been hypothesized as silent speech, and certain investigations have shown that people actually talk to themselves without making sounds while thinking (2). Aphasia is a particularly tragic consequence of stroke. It affects the human being's unique ability to speak and communicate with his fellow man (2).

April Oursler Armstrong's book *Cry Babel* is a story of an aphasic woman's struggle to recover and rebuild her life. She had been a college professor, with a doctorate in theology, and a well-known author when her life was abruptly changed by a cerebral hemorrhage on the left side of her brain leaving her globally aphasic. Her book, written during the long recovery process, gives the reader an excellent insight into what it is like to be aphasic (27).

In normal speech, the selection of desired words and their sequence begins in

Wernicke's area. This information is transferred to Broca's area through a connective bundle of fibers, the arcuate fasciculus, where a detailed and coordinated program for expression of language is created (28). This information is then passed to the motor cortex and language is either spoken or written.

Broca's aphasia results from injury to the left inferior frontal lobe. It was first described by the French neurologist, Paul Broca in 1861, when he found that his 51-year-old patient could understand anything that was said to him, yet his speech was poor. When the patient died, a post-mortem examination found the site of injury to be a specific localized area lying roughly in front of the ear. Paul Broca later showed that this was limited to the left side, for if the same area on the right side of the brain were damaged, aphasia was not present (2).

In Broca's aphasia, speech production is limited and requires great effort, but it accurately conveys the patient's thought. It is often called expressive or nonfluent aphasia. The choice of words is usually correct, but output is often limited to nouns and verbs without grammatical words that are used in the normal flow of speech (2, 15). Broca's area is a true language area, demonstrated by the fact that injury in this area limits writing and sign language as well as verbalizations. Broca's aphasia is a specific, localized syndrome often accompanied by a right hemiplegia (2).

Slurred speech with poor articulation (dysarthria) often accompanies Broca's aphasia because of weakness of the right side of the face, jaw, mouth, and throat. This dysarthria is also produced on the left side of the face if a right cerebral injury occurs, however, there is no aphasia (2). Dysarthria reflects motor weakness or poor coordination of the muscles of articulation. It can be the result of a variety of lesions, does not represent a language disorder, and is not localized (15).

Damage to Wernicke's area produces an entirely different kind of aphasia. Its most outstanding characteristic is the inability to understand language (4). This kind of aphasia is named after Dr. Karl Wernicke, a famous German neurologist. He found that there was a separate region of the brain, the left superior temporal gyrus, devoted to the understanding of language (reading, listening to speech, and understanding gestures). These are called receptive language functions. If Broca's area remains intact, words may be spoken in sentences with ease, but they have no meaning. Even simple commands are not understandable. These patients are often inconsistent in answering even simple yes-and-no questions. Sometimes they can follow one-step commands, such as "turn on the water," but have difficulty with more complex directions like "turn on the water and fill up the pan." As mentioned before, the structure of what is said begins in Wernicke's area, so although fluent, the speech will be contaminated with words that are not correct. For example, the patient might say nook when meaning book, or police when meaning doctor. These are called paraphasic errors. The patient may also create new words that have no meaning such as "snid" or "dasker." These are called neologisms. Since these patients do not understand speech, they do not monitor what they are saying and are unaware of their errors. Their speech is sometimes described as word salad. In some situations, these patients may be thought of as confused, disoriented, or mentally ill, when actually their behavior is the sign of a specific cerebral injury (2).

If there is isolated injury to the connecting bundle, the arcuate fasciculus, fluent speech and intact comprehension remain. There are many paraphasic errors, however, since Wernicke's area is unable to transmit the correct semantic information to Broca's area. The patients can hear their errors, and are frustrated by not saying what they are thinking. This is called conduction aphasia.

Most aphasias are a mixture of all of the symptoms described. Frequently in strokes that result from an occlusion of the internal carotid or middle cerebral artery, there is global aphasia (15). In global aphasia, there are both expressive and receptive deficits.

Communicating is a highly complex and specialized activity of the human brain, which has developed over millions of years of evolution (1). This highly specialized and important ability may be quickly taken away by a large vessel anterior circulation injury, almost always on the left side (6).

Psychosocial

Stroke patients may experience a number of psychological changes including depression, which are often a major cause of concern to relatives and the individual (e.g., irritability due to loss of interest and depression of mood, an inability to withstand stressful situations, fear and anxiety, anger, frustration, swearing, emotional lability, and catastrophic reactions).

Significant depression has been recorded in 30 to 50% of stroke survivors (29). This depression is often viewed by family and medical practitioners as a natural and understandable consequence of reduced function caused by stroke. However, appropriate attention to depression can result in observable improvement. Depression has been found to be more frequent and severe with lesions in the left hemisphere, as compared with right hemisphere or brainstem strokes (29, 30). Both organic and psychological factors are probably involved in poststroke depression. These patients usually respond well to antidepressants, and psychological support, and encouragement (6).

Emotional lability may appear mostly through a release of inhibition. The individual may switch from laughing to crying without apparent reason. Excessive crying is the most common problem and is frequently due to organic emotional lability rather than to depression or sadness over perceived losses. Organic emotional lability is characterized by little or no obvious relation between the start of emotional expression and what is happening around the person.

Catastrophic reactions are outbursts in which frustration, anger, and depression are combined. When individuals cannot perform tasks that used to be very easy, they may be unable to inhibit emotional expression and break into sobbing, expressing a sense of hopelessness.

Outbursts and emotional difficulties are "normal" after stroke. Relatives and families should be told that a tendency to cry easily or get upset will improve with time. Families and therapists need to develop a positive, understanding attitude if the individual is to overcome psychological sequelae.

OTHER COMPLICATIONS OF STROKE

In addition to these deficits, secondary conditions may occur. These are important manifestations to consider in regard to the patient's recovery and rehabilitation and may actually be more disabling than the stroke itself (13). It is important to be aware of these complications so that they may possibly be prevented.

Seizures. Brain scars due to stroke may irritate the cortex and cause a spontaneous discharge of nerve impulses that may generalize to a full grand mal convulsion (13). Seizures develop in up to 10% of stroke patients (6). They are more common with embolic than thrombotic infarcts (31). Anticonvulsant drugs are sometimes used in patients with early seizures, but their use is controversial. Some studies have shown that seizures usually resolve spontaneously (31).

Infection. Alteration of swallowing function, aspiration, hypoventilation, and immobility in the stroke patient often lead to pneumonia. Changes in bladder function may lead to bladder distention and urinary tract infection (6). Impaired sensation and inadequate position changes may result in pressure sores (decubiti) and consequent infection of these areas.

Thromboembolism. Immobility of the legs and bed rest often lead to thrombosis of dependent leg veins. In deep vein thrombosis (DVT), local pain and tenderness may develop in the calf, with some swelling and a slight increase in temperature. The risk of venous thrombosis occurring in a paralyzed leg approaches 60% (32). If the thrombosis is confined to the calf, it may not be serious, but if the thrombosis spreads up toward the groin to involve the veins in the pelvis, then there is a very real possibility of a clot breaking off into the bloodstream. The clot will then travel through the right side of the heart and enter the lungs through the pulmonary arteries, resulting in sudden collapse and death due to obstruction of the pulmonary arteries (32). Early mobilization of the patient is of utmost importance in preventing deep vein thrombosis and subsequent pulmonary embolism.

Shoulder Subluxation. A common concern related to motor function involves the shoulder. Common problems include shoulder subluxation, pain, and immobility. The causative factors in shoulder subluxation following stroke are related to changes in muscle tone and movement, the position of the scapula, and joint capsule stability. Shoulder subluxation at the glenohumeral joint occurs when the weight of the arm and pull of gravity draws the head of the humerus out of the glenoid fossa of the scapula. Two-thirds of the humeral head is not covered by the glenoid fossa. This lack of stability is partly compensated for by a strong surrounding musculature. In the normal orientation of the scapula, there is an upward slope of the glenoid fossa which plays an important role in preventing downward dislocation of the humerus. The humeral head would have to move laterally in order to move downward. When the arm is adducted, the superior part of the capsule and the coracohumeral ligament are taut, which prevents lateral movement of the humeral head. This safeguards against downward displacement. The supraspinatus muscle reinforces the horizontal tension of the capsule. The infraspinatus and posterior portion of the deltoid also

play an important role in preventing subluxation, because of their horizontal fibers. When the humerus is abducted sideways or flexed forward, the superior capsule becomes lax, eliminating the support, and joint stability must then be provided by muscle contraction. The integrity of the joint then depends almost exclusively on the rotator cuff muscles. In hemiplegia, patients have lost the voluntary movement in relative muscles. These include the supraspinatus, infraspinatus, and posterior fibers of the deltoid. In addition, the muscles that support the scapula in its normal alignment are affected, allowing a change in angulation of the glenoid fossa. Subluxation is therefore inevitable (33).

The Painful Shoulder. The painful shoulder may develop quickly following a stroke or can develop at a much later stage. It can present with flaccid or spastic muscle tone and with or without subluxation. In hemiplegia, the normal, coordinated, and timed movement of the scapula and humerus (scapulohumeral rhythm) has been disturbed by abnormal and unbalanced muscle tone. The typical hemiplegic postural components of depression and retraction of the scapula and internal rotation of the humerus are of particular relevance to the mechanism of pain. Fear of pain upon passive movement of a painful arm will further increase abnormal flexor tone, which can become a vicious circle (33).

Shoulder-Hand Syndrome. A chronically painful shoulder can lead to shoulder-hand syndrome. This is a complex condition producing severe pain, edema of the hand, and limitations in range of motion on the involved side (13).

Abnormal Muscle Tone. The person with an intact central nervous system, has a wide range of muscle tone. Muscle tone can be changed according to the activity that is to be performed. Normal muscle tone is high enough to stabilize and maintain a person through an activity, while at the same time, low enough to allow ease of movement. There is a mix of tone that allows mobility to be superimposed on stability (34).

Upon passive movement of an extremity, abnormal muscle tone can often be felt. Normal tone is felt as an appropriate amount of resistance, allowing the movement to proceed smoothly. Hypotonus, or flaccidity, is felt as too little resistance or floppiness. When released, the extremity will drop into the direction of gravity.

Hypertonus, or spasticity, is felt as too much resistance as a result of hyperactive reflexes and loss of moderating or inhibiting influences from higher brain centers (33). Spasticity is often enhanced by pain, emotional upset, or trying to hurry (13).

Spasticity is never isolated to one muscle group. It is always a part of extensor or flexor synergy or grouping of stereotypical movements. These usually involve a flexion pattern in the arm (scapular retraction and depression, shoulder adduction and internal rotation, elbow flexion, forearm pronation, wrist flexion, finger and thumb flexion and adduction) and an extension pattern in the leg (pelvis rotated back and internal rotation, knee extension, foot planter flexion and inversion, toe flexion and adduction). In addition to the extremities, abnormal tone is also manifested in the head and trunk. The head is usually flexed toward the hemiplegic side and rotated so that the face is toward the unaffected side. The trunk is rotated back on the hemiplegic side with side flexion of the hemiplegic side (33). These typical patterns of spasticity interfere with the normal, smooth, efficient, and coordinated movement the patient has relied upon for locomotion in and manipulation of the environment. If untreated, this spasticity may lead to contractures.

Associated Reactions and Associated Movements. Associated reactions in hemiplegia are abnormal reflex movements of the affected side and duplicate the synergy patterns of the arm and leg. They are observed when the patient moves with effort, is trying to maintain balance, or is afraid of falling (33). A flexor pattern of involuntary movement in the arm is often seen with a yawn, cough, or sneeze. Associated reactions are also seen when new activities such as running or putting on socks after a stroke are attempted. They are stereotyped reactions and may occur even if no active movement is present in the limb. The patient is unable to relax them voluntarily. The limb returns to its normal position only after cessation of the stimulus, and usually does so gradually (33).

Associated movements accompany voluntary movements and are normal automatic postural adjustments. They reinforce precise movements of other parts of the body or occur when a great amount of strength is required. They are not pathological and can be stopped at will, as opposed to associated reactions. Associated movements can often be observed in stroke patients' unaffected extremities when they are trying a new activity.

RISK FACTORS

The best way to prevent a stroke from occurring is to control the risk factors that can cause a stroke. Regular visits to a family physician are important and modifications in lifestyle and diet are best made early in life. Risk factors for stroke are similar to those for heart attacks, since atherosclerosis is a common underlying cause for both. The following profile exemplifies a person who may be at risk for a stroke or heart attack.

J.S., a 50-year-old black man, was born and raised in a small farming community in Alabama. His father worked long hard hours on the family farm and died of a stroke at the age of 52. J.S. decided at a young age that farming was not for him, and went to college to earn a degree in management. His current position as director of hourly employees in a large industrial firm is a highly stressful one, and he often puts in long hours. He smokes about a pack of cigarettes every day, is moderately overweight, and does not have time for exercise. His blood pressure, when last checked 2 years ago by his family physician, was at the upper limit of normal. Yesterday, J.S. went to work earlier than usual, to catch up on some desk work, when he noticed that he had difficulty seeing out of his right eye and was unable to control his pen when writing. However, after resting his head on his desk for a few minutes, these symptoms disappeared. J.S. attributed them to lack of sleep, and forgot about them quickly.

J.S. has many risk factors for stroke. They include:

1. Race—Black Americans are 50% more likely to have hypertension than white Americans, and they suffer strokes more often and at a younger age (2). According to one study, black men aged 35 to 74 were two to five times more likely than whites to die of stroke (35).
2. Age—In the Framingham Heart Study, it was reported that 45- to 64-year-old men had a 25.4% incidence rate of first stroke, compared with only 5.5% in the 30- to 44-year-old age range. Approximately 29% of people who suffer a stroke in a given year are under the age of 65 (5).
3. Heredity—J.S.'s father died of a stroke at a young age, and this family history of stroke increases J.S.'s risk.
4. Obesity—Being overweight is known to be a risk factor for hypertension and diabetes mellitus and is also associated with stroke. Many overweight persons have hyperlipidemia (raised levels of cholesterol and triglycerides in the blood) (1). The Framingham Study found that in men between the ages of 30 and 62, cholesterol levels of 250 carried about three times the risk of heart attack and stroke as did cholesterol levels that were under 194 (2).
5. Hypertension—It has long been known that hypertension is the major risk factor for stroke. It is, however, a risk that can be controlled through antihypertensive drug therapy, stress reduction, dietary control, and regular exercise. Chronically elevated blood pressure exerts pressure on intracranial and extracranial cerebral vessels, often resulting in lacunar infarctions or intracerebral hemorrhage. It has also been implicated in the atherosclerotic process by driving fatty substances into the walls of arteries making them brittle, narrowed, and hardened (1). Hypertension has often been called the silent disease because there are often no symptoms (1). An occasional headache, dizziness, or light-headedness, which are all symptoms of hypertension, can easily be attributed to other factors. High blood pressure that continues over several years can also damage the heart. If a person has a stroke, the already damaged heart will be less capable of delivering needed blood to the brain tissues. This may influence the severity of the episode (1). It is important to have regular blood pressure checks and to follow the drug treatment and recommendations prescribed by a physician to control this major risk factor. J.S.'s lack of exercise, extra weight, and stressful job all contributed to his elevated blood pressure. In addition, he has not had a regular check-up in 2 years.
6. Smoking—There is strong evidence for a relationship between smoking and increased risk of stroke (8). Quitting smoking reduces that likelihood of stroke, even in a long-term smoker.
7. Transient ischemic attacks—J.S. did not even realize that the impaired vision and clumsy right hand he experienced while doing his desk work were probably symptoms of a transient ischemic attack. Most medical professionals consider a TIA to be an important risk factor for an impending stroke. Approximately 30% of all patients who have had a TIA are at risk of having a stroke within 2 years. This risk is greatest in the first month, so it is extremely important to seek medical intervention quickly (1).
8. Geographic location—The number of deaths from strokes in the United States are greatest in North and South Carolina, Georgia, northern Florida, Alabama, Mississippi, and Tennessee. There are also specific pockets of high death rates in Texas, Oklahoma, and

all of the Hawaiian islands. This geographical strip, often termed the "stroke belt," is the source of numerous studies on environmental, cultural, or other geographically determined risk factors. A person who grows up in a high-risk area and then moves to a lower-risk area as an adult continues to carry a greater likelihood of having a stroke. This had led to speculation that the causes may be diet-related, cultural, or even possibly related to water supply or altitude (2).

J.S. is at high risk for a stroke; however, he can learn to control many of his own risk factors and he can receive help from his physician. Other common risk factors for stroke include:

9. Diabetes mellitus—This disease is more common in stroke patients than in a normal population of similar age. However, since diabetes is associated with hypertension, obesity, and hyperlipidemia, it is difficult to be certain of a relationship with stroke when these other conditions are also present (2). Persons with diabetes mellitus are two to four times more likely to have a stroke, and this is even more true for women than for men (5, 36).

10. Oral contraceptives—Women who have taken birth control pills, especially those with a high estrogen content, become increasingly at risk for having a stroke as they become older. Smoking while taking the pill further increases the risk (1).

11. Polycythemia—Increased blood viscosity (polycythemia) causes blood to flow sluggishly. This increases the likelihood of thrombosis and embolism and therefore heart attacks and to a lesser extent, stroke (1).

12. Asymptomatic carotid bruits—A bruit is an abnormal sound or murmur heard when a stethoscope is placed over the carotid artery. This slushing noise indicates turbulent blood, often caused by a significant degree of stenosis. Carotid bruit clearly indicates increased stroke risk. Complete occlusion of the carotid artery sometimes follows, resulting in stroke (16).

13. Prior stroke—The risk of stroke for a person who has already suffered a stroke is increased four to eight times (32).

14. Heart disease—A diseased heart (whether it be chronic disease, acute heart attacks, or prosthetic heart valves) increases the risk of stroke. Independent of hypertension, people with heart disease have more than twice the risk of stroke than people with normally functioning hearts (5).

15. Alcoholism—In 1984, the Stroke Council's Subcommittee on Risk Factors and Stroke stated that alcohol was a "less well-documented" risk factor for stroke (37).

Of these many risk factors, several can be controlled by changes in lifestyle, including elevated blood cholesterol and lipids, cigarette smoking, use of oral contraceptives, excessive drinking of alcohol, and obesity. Some can be controlled by medical intervention, such as hypertension, heart disease, TIAs, carotid bruits, and polycythemia. Factors that cannot be changed are age, sex, race, family history, diabetes mellitus, and a prior stroke. The potential benefits of all medical and surgical interventions currently available for cerebrovascular disease pale in comparison to what can be achieved through risk factor control. Understanding and awareness of these risk factors for stroke is an important first step in reducing the likelihood of having stroke.

CASE STUDY

D.B., a 52-year-old male, left work and went to his doctor's office complaining of slurred speech and weakness in his left arm and leg. He was admitted to a local hospital, where a CT scan revealed infarction in the territory of the right middle cerebral artery of embolic origin. After 5 days, D.B. was transferred to another hospital's rehabilitation unit, where he began an intensive inpatient therapy program. D.B.'s previous medical history includes diabetes mellitus for 12

Table 2.1.
Occupational Performance Profile[a]

			Performance			
			Work Activities			
			Vocation	Education	Home Management	Care of Others
PERFORMANCE COMPONENTS	SENSORIMOTOR	**SENSORY INTEGRATION**				
		NEURO-MUSCULAR Hemi-paresis with increased spasticity in left extremities. Wears antispasticity ball splint at night				
		MOTOR	Abnormal reflexes in left UE		Unable to physically perform chores	
	COGNITIVE	**COGNITIVE** Intact				
	PSYCHOSOCIAL	**PSYCHOLOGICAL**	Impulsive, denial of illness			
		SOCIAL				
		SELF-MANAGEMENT	Good employment record; unable to answer questions about plans for future if unable to return to job		Requires assistance from wife in money management, paying bills	

EXTERNAL FACTORS WHICH INFLUENCE PERFORMANCE

CULTURE, ECONOMY, ENVIRONMENT	Previous medical history includes: diabetes mellitus (past 12 years); coronary spasm (past 10 years); hypertension; bursitis (right shoulder); arthritis (both knee joints); smoker; moderately overweight.

Grid adapted from Uniform Terminology (2nd ed.) Developed by the occupational therapy faculty at Eastern Michigan University.

Client initials: D.B.
Diagnosis: CVA—Left hemiparesis
Age: 52

Areas

| Play or Leisure Activities | | Activities of Daily Living | | | | |
Exploration	Performance	Self-Care	Socialization	Functional Communication	Functional Mobility	Sexual Expression
		Independent with compensatory techniques				
	Uses card-holding device			Slurred speech	Walks independently with a straight cane; uses ankle-foot orthosis (AFO) on left to prevent "toe-drag"	
		Right-handed; uses left UE as gross assist in some activities				
	Good leisure performance in the past	Unable to answer questions about cause of stroke and risk factor control				
	Continues to play cards with friends		Congenial, enjoys time with family & friends			
		Left unilateral neglect poses safety problems				

years, coronary spasm 10 years previous to this admission, hypertension, bursitis in the right shoulder (at present), and arthritis in both knees. D.B. is a smoker and is moderately overweight.

D.B. is married, with two grown children and two grandchildren. He had been employed as a pharmacist for 27 years at a local drugstore, and he enjoyed his job. His hobbies before his stroke included yard work, general handyman jobs around the house, playing cards, traveling, and helping his wife babysit the grandchildren. D.B. is an easygoing, friendly person who appears to have a positive attitude about his stroke and expected recovery. However, he is unable to answer questions about the cause of his stroke, and risk factor control and does not have a plan for the future if he is unable to return to his job.

Some of the general symptoms that D.B. now exhibits 4 months poststroke are hemiparesis and abnormal muscle tone in the left extremities, mild left unilateral neglect, decreased sensation in the left extremities, and impulsive behavior. D.B. can walk independently with a straight cane. He is fitted with an ankle-foot orthosis to maintain his ankle in a neutral position and prevent "toe-drag" during ambulation. He is right-handed and is now using the left upper extremity as a gross assist in some activities. The abnormal flexor tone in his hand interferes with function, so at night D.B. wears an antispasticity ball splint issued by the O.T. to control this hypertonicity. D.B.'s left unilateral neglect is most apparent while moving. He sometimes bumps into the left side of the doorway and is unable to find road signs while riding in the car with his wife. He often tries to get up from a chair before checking to be sure that his left foot is flat on the floor. D.B. also occasionally quickly slides his chair back from a table, letting his left arm fall to his side. D.B.'s CVA results in many occupational performance deficits (See Table 2.1).

D.B. is currently able to perform all self-care activities independently. He has been very resourceful and creative in coming up with new strategies to maintain his independence. He uses a tub bench, grab bar, and a hand-held shower for bathing. He is anxious to resume driving, but has been advised by his doctor and therapists to refrain from driving at present because of his impulsiveness and unilateral neglect. D.B. has had some difficulty adjusting to the amount of time he now spends at home. He has found that he is physically unable to perform many household repairs and maintenance such as cutting the grass, sweeping the driveway, painting the trim around windows. He now requires assistance from his wife for money management and paying bills. D.B. and his family or occasionally some friends get together to play cards. D.B. uses a card-holding device that was recommended by O.T. and recreational therapy to hold his cards. He enjoys this activity and the socialization that goes with it. He and his family just returned from a 1-week vacation near a lake, which he thoroughly enjoyed. Considering the extent of his disability, D.B. appears to be making an excellent adjustment to his stroke, and in fact, appears to deny the illness. He believes that soon everything will return to normal, that he will regain his physical abilities and will be able to return to work.

ACKNOWLEDGMENTS

I would like to sincerely thank my friend and sister, Lorie Smith, for typing this manuscript, my wonderful husband, James Bierman, for his assistance and support, all of my colleagues, and all of the stroke patients that I have had the pleasure of working with and learning from, especially Marge Wren and Robert Ringlein.

REFERENCES

1. Foley C, Pizer HF. The stroke fact book. Golden Valley: Courage Press, 1990.
2. Freese A. Stroke—the new hope and the new help. New York: Random House, 1980.
3. Doolittle ND. Stroke recovery: review of the literature and suggestions for future research. J Neurosci Nurs 1988;20:169–173.
4. Miller VT. Diagnosis and initial management of stroke. Neuropsychiatry 1988;14(7):57–65.
5. Anonymous. 1988 stroke facts. Dallas: American Heart Association.
6. Caplan LR. Stroke. Clin Symp 1988;40(4):1–32.
7. Barr ML. The human nervous system, 2nd ed. Hagerstown: Harper & Row, 1974.
8. Sherman DG. The carotid artery and stroke. Am Fam Physician 1989;40(5):415–495.
9. Nolte J. The human brain. St. Louis: CV Mosby, 1981.
10. Nadeau SE. Stroke. Med Clin North Am 1989;73(6):1351–1369.
11. Gorelick PB. Etiology and management of ischemic stroke. Compr Ther 1989;15(3):60–65.
12. Fisher CM. Lacunar strokes and infarcts: a review. Neurology 1982;32:871–876.
13. Anderson TP. Stroke and cerebral trauma: medical aspects. In: Stolov WC, Clowers MR, eds. Handbook of severe disability. Seattle: University of Washington, 1981:119–126.
14. Caplan LR, Stein RW. Intracerebral hemorrhage. In: Stroke—a clinical approach. Austin: Butterworth, 1986:261–292.
15. Kawalick M, Lerer A. Stroke syndromes. In: Erickson RV, ed. Medical management of the elderly stroke patient. Philadelphia: Hanley & Belfus, 1989:469–477.
16. Anonymous. Facts about strokes. Dallas: American Heart Association.
17. Afifi AK, Bergman RA. Basic neuroscience. Baltimore: Urban & Schwarzenberg, 1986.
18. Siev E, Freishtat B, Zoltan B. Perceptual and cognitive dysfunction in the adult stroke patient. Thorofare, NJ: Slack, 1986.

19. Moore JC. Recovery potentials following CNS lesions: a brief historical perspective in relationship to modern research data on neuroplasticity. Am J Occ Ther 1986; 40(7):459–463.

20. Devor M. Plasticity in the adult nervous system. In Illis L. S., Sedgewick EM, Glanville HJ, eds. Rehabilitation of the neurological patient. Oxford: Blackwell Scientific, 1982:44–84.

21. Trombly C. Occupational therapy for physical dysfunction. Baltimore: Williams & Wilkins, 1989.

22. Harper GD, Castleden CM. Drug therapy in patients with recent stroke. Br Med Bull 1990;46(1):181–199.

23. Utley J. Adult hemiplegia NDT certification course. Flint, MI: McLaren Regional Medical Center, 1989.

24. Davies PM. Steps to follow. Berlin: Springer-Verlag, 1985.

25. Restak RM. The brain: the last frontier. New York: Warner Books, 1979.

26. Armstrong AO. Cry babel. Garden City: Doubleday, 1979.

27. Grotta JC. Post-stroke management concerns and outcomes. Geriatrics 1988;43(7):40–48.

28. Starkstein SE, Robinson RG, Price TR. Comparison of patients with and without post-stroke major depression matched for size and location of lesion. Arch Gen Psychiatry 1988;45:247–252.

29. Kilpatrick CJ, Davis SM, Tress BM, Rossiter SC, Hopper JL, Vanpendriesen ML. Epileptic seizures in acute stroke. Arch Neurol 1990; 47:157–160.

30. Rose FC, Capileo R. Stroke. Oxford: Oxford University Press, 1981.

31. Gillum RF. Strokes in blacks. Stroke 1988;19(1):19.

32. Dobkin BH. Management of geriatric TIA and stroke. Geriatrics 1988;43(11):27–34.

33. Gorelick PB. The status of alcohol as a risk factor for stroke. Stroke 1989;20(12):1607–1610.

Glossary

Aneurysm: A sac formed by the localized dilation of the wall of an artery or vein or the heart; an actual bulging or out-pouching of the weakened wall of the artery is evident. Atherosclerosis is responsible for most arterial aneurysms, although any injury to the middle or muscular layer of the arterial wall (tunica media) can predispose the vessel to stretching of the inner and outer layers of the artery and the formation of a sac. Other diseases that can lead to aneurysm include syphilis, cystic medionecrosis, certain nonspecific inflammations, and congenital defects.

Anomaly: Marked deviation from normal.

Aphasia: Defect or loss of the power of expression by speech, writing, or signs (e.g., gestures), or of comprehension of spoken or written languages, due to disease or injury of the brain centers. Broca's aphasia: Expressive aphasia in which the patient understands written and spoken words and knows what he wants to say, but speech production is limited or absent, usually due to damage of the left inferior frontal lobe. Also called apraxia of speech, motor aphasia, and nonfluent aphasia. Conduction dysphasia: Impairment of speech consisting of lack of co-ordination and failure to arrange words in their proper order possibly due to a lesion of the pathway between the sensory and motor speech centers (arcuate fasciculus). Wernicke's aphasia: Receptive aphasia in which a patient is unable to understand written, spoken, or tactile speech symbols, usually due to damage of the left superior-temporal gyrus; also called

sensory aphasia. Global aphasia: Both expressive and receptive deficits, usually due to an occlusion of the internal carotid or middle cerebral artery.

Apoplexy: Copious extravasation of blood into an organ; often used alone to designate extravasations into the brain (cerebral apoplexy) after rupture of an intracranial blood vessel; synonymous with stroke, the term is extended by some to include occlusive cerebrovascular lesions.

Apraxia: Loss of ability to carry out familiar purposeful movements in the absence of sensory or motor impairment, especially impairment of the ability to use objects correctly. Motor apraxia: loss of ability to make proper use of an object, although its proper nature is recognized. Sensory apraxia: loss of ability due to lack of perception of an object's purpose.

Arcuate fasciculus: The bundle of fibers in the brain that connect Wernicke's area to Broca's area. The pattern of normal speech starts with the selection of desired words and their sequence in Wernicke's area; this information is transferred through the arcuate fasciculus to Broca's area, where a detailed and coordinated program for expression of language is created. Finally, the information is passed to the motor cortex, and language is either spoken or written.

Arrhythmia: Variation from the normal rhythm, especially of the heartbeat.

Arteriovenous: Pertaining to both artery and vein. Arteriovenous malformation: A congenital malformation in which there is an abnormal collection of blood vessels near the surface of the brain that can cause a subarachnoid hemorrhage.

Associated reactions: Involuntary movements or reflexive increases of tone of the affected side of individuals with hemiplegia; movements duplicate synergy patterns and are often seen during stressful or new activities. For example, resisted grasp by the noninvolved hand causes a grasp reaction in the involved hand.

Ataxia: Incoordination occurring in the absence of apraxia, paresis, rigidity, spasticity, or involuntary movement manifested when voluntary muscular movements are attempted. In posterior column damage of the spinal cord, there is a loss of proprioception and incoordination due to misjudgement of limb position with balance problems. Cerebellar ataxia produces a reeling, wide-based gait.

Atheroma: An abnormal mass of fatty or lipid material with a fibrous covering, existing as a discrete, raised plaque within the intima of an artery.

Atherosclerosis: An extremely common form of arteriosclerosis in which deposits of yellowing plaques (atheromas) containing cholesterol, other lipid material, and lipophages are formed within the intima of large and medium-sized arteries.

Bruit: An abnormal sound or murmur heard in auscultation. When a stethoscope is placed over an artery, a slushing noise indicative of turbulent blood flow may indicate a significant degree of stenosis. Aneurysmal bruit: a blowing sound heard over an aneurysm. Asymptomatic carotid bruit: A bruit heard over the carotid artery.

Cerebral vascular accident (stroke): A disorder of the blood vessels serving the cerebrum, resulting from an impaired blood supply to, and ischemia in, parts of the brain. There are five neurologic events associated with cerebral vascular accident: (*a*) Transient ischemic attack (TIA) due to temporary interference in blood supply lasts only a few minutes and no longer

than 24 hours. (*b*) Small strokes last a day or more and completely resolve or leave only minor neurologic deficits. Reversible ischemic neurologic deficits (RIND) are small strokes that resolve completely. Partially reversible ischemic neurologic deficits (PRIND) are small strokes longer than 72 hours, with resultant minor neurologic impairment. (*c*) Stroke in evolution (SIE), in which a person experiences gradual weakness on one side of the body. (*d*) Completed stroke (CS), in which a person exhibits symptoms associated with severe cerebral ischemia resulting from an interrupted blood supply to the brain.

Circle of Willis: The union of the anterior and posterior circulation at the base of the brain, often providing a back-up supply of blood in case of occlusion of one of the larger arteries.

Collateral circulation: Secondary or accessory circulation that continues to an area of the brain, following obstruction of a primary vessel, and which can prevent major ischemia.

Contralateral: Pertaining to, situated on, or affecting the opposite side.

Decussation: A crossing over; decussation of pyramids: the anterior part of the lower medulla oblongata in which most of the fibers of each pyramid intersect as they cross the midline and descend as the lateral corticospinal tract.

Deep vein thrombosis (DVT): A thrombosis, most often in the legs or pelvis, which results from phlebitis, injury to a vein, or prolonged bed rest.

Diabetes mellitus: A disorder of carbohydrate metabolism characterized by glucose in the urine, high glucose level in the blood, and resulting from inadequate production or use of insulin.

Dysarthria: Imperfect articulation of speech due to disturbances of muscular control of the lips, mouth, tongue, and vocal cords, resulting from central or peripheral nervous system damage.

Dysarticulation: Difficulty in enunciating words and sentences.

Dysmetria: Difficulty judging distances when trying to coordinate limb movements; inability to properly direct or limit motions.

Dysphagia: Difficulty in swallowing. The condition can range from mild discomfort, such as a feeling that there is a lump in the throat, to a severe inability to control the muscles needed for chewing and swallowing. Dysphagia can seriously compromise the nutritional status of a patient. In general, placing the patient in an upright position, providing a pleasant and calm environment, being sure the lips are closed as the patient begins to swallow, and preparing and serving foods of the proper consistency are helpful. Stroke victims who have difficulty swallowing should be turned, or should turn their heads, to the unaffected side to facilitate swallowing.

Embolism: The sudden blocking of an artery by a moving clot of foreign material (embolus) that has been brought to its site of lodgment by the blood current. Obstructing material is often a blood clot but may be a fat globule, air bubble, piece of tissue, or clump of bacteria. Emboli usually lodge at divisions of an artery, where the vessel narrows.

Endarterectomy: Excision of thickened atheromatous areas of the innermost coat of an artery (intima). Carotid endarterectomy: A surgical procedure in which the diseased carotid artery is opened, a clot removed, and an artificial graft is put in its place.

Extravasation: A discharge or escape, as of blood, from a vessel into the tissues.

Flaccidity: Abnormal muscle tone felt as too little resistance to movement; also called hypotonus. Flaccid: Paralysis of muscles in which there is an absence of reflexes (in lower motor neuron disorders such as poliomyelitis).

Focal: Limited to a specific area, focused.

Hematoma: A localized collection of extravasated blood, usually clotted, in an organ, space, or tissue. Contusions (bruises) and black eyes are familiar forms of hematoma that are seldom serious. Hematomas can occur almost anywhere on the body; they are almost always present with a fracture and are especially serious when they occur inside the skull, where they may produce local pressure on the brain. The most common kinds are epidural (above the dura mater, between it and the skull) and subdural (beneath the dura mater, between the tough casing and the more delicate membranes covering the tissue of the brain, the pia-arachnoid) hematomas.

Hemianesthesia: Anesthesia or absence of sensation on one side of the body.

Hemianopsia (hemianopia): Defective vision or blindness in one-half the visual field, usually applied to bilateral defects caused by a single lesion, often as a result of CVA. The individual is unable to perceive objects to the side of the visual midline. The visual loss is contralateral (i.e., on the side opposite the brain lesion). Homonymous hemianopsia: Both visual fields, either the right halves or left halves, are defective on the same side.

Hemiparesis: Paresis or weakness affecting one side of the body.

Hemiplegia: Paralysis of one side of the body; usually caused by a brain lesion, such as a tumor, or by a cerebral vascular accident. The paralysis occurs on the side opposite the brain disorder, as most of the fibers in the motor tracts of the brain cross to the opposite side in the medulla oblongata; therefore damage to the right hemisphere of the brain affects motor control of the left half of the body.

Hemorrhage: The escape of blood from a ruptured vessel.

Hemorrhagic stroke: A type of stroke that occurs when blood escapes the normal vessels and enters the brain tissue or the subarachnoid space. Intracerebral hemorrhage: A type of hemorrhagic stroke that occurs when blood escapes a cerebral vessel and directly enters the brain tissue.

Subarachnoid hemorrhage: A type of hemorrhagic stroke that occurs when blood escapes its normal vessel, usually from an aneurysm, and spreads to the cerebrospinal fluid surrounding the brain.

Horner's syndrome: Sinking in of the eyeball, ptosis of the upper eyelid, slight elevation of the lower lid, constriction of the pupil, narrowing of the palpebral fissure, anhidrosis, and cooling on the affected side of the face caused by paralysis of the cervical sympathetic nerve supply at the T1 spinal level.

Hyperemia: An excess of blood in a part; following a stroke, an area in the brain in which blood vessels are congested and swollen.

Hyperlipidemia: A general term for elevated concentration of any or all of the lipids in the plasma.

Hypertension: Persistently high blood pressure.

Hypertonus: See spasticity.

Hypotonus: See flaccidity.

Hypoxia: A broad term meaning diminished availability of oxygen to the body tissues.

Incontinence: Inability to control excretory functions.

Infarction: A localized area of ischemic necrosis produced by occlusion of the arterial supply or the venous drainage of the part.

Intima: The innermost coat of a blood vessel; also called tunica intima.

Impulsion: A blind obedience to internal drives, without regard for acceptance by others or pressure from the superego; seen in children and in adults with weak defensive organization.

Ipsilateral: Situated on or affecting the same side.

Ischemia: Deficiency of blood in a part, caused by functional constriction or actual obstruction of a blood vessel, often leading to necrosis of surrounding tissue. Ischemic stroke: A deficiency of blood to the brain caused by a occlusion of an artery from a thrombus or embolism.

Lacuna: A small pit or hollow cavity.

Lacunar strokes: Small infarcts usually in the deep noncortical parts of the cerebrum and brainstem resulting from an occlusion of small branches of larger cerebral arteries.

Lipohyalinosis: A condition characterized by fat and hyaline degeneration.

Neologism: A newly coined word; in psychiatry, a word whose meaning may be known only to the patient using it; also seen in aphasics.

Osmotic agent: An agent (e.g., drug) that increases osmosis, which is the passage of pure solvent from a solution of lesser to one of greater solute concentration when the two solutions are separated by a membrane that selectively prevents the passage of solute molecules, but is permeable to the solvent.

Paraphasia: Partial aphasia in which wrong words are used or words are used in wrong and senseless combinations. Paraphasic errors: substitution of words or sounds, which reduces intelligibility or distorts meaning.

Penumbra: During an infarct, this refers to the zone of injury in the brain that is downstream from the infarcted zone that may be served by collateral blood vessels.

Polycythemia: An increase in the total red cell mass of the blood (viscosity), which results in thickening of the blood and an increased tendency toward clotting. This increased viscosity limits proper flow, diminishing the supply of blood to the brain and other vital tissues, which may cause mental sluggishness, irritability, headache, dizziness, fainting, and acute pain.

Proprioception: From the Latin word for "one's own." Interpretation of stimuli originating in muscles, joints, and other internal tissues that give information about the position and movement of one body part in relation to another. Perception is mediated by sensory nerve endings chiefly in muscles, tendons, and the labyrinth. Proprioceptive input tells the brain when and how muscles are contracting or stretching, and when and how joints are bending, extending, or being pulled or compressed.

Ptosis: Paralytic drooping of the upper eyelid.

Sequela: A morbid condition following or occurring as a consequence of another condition or event.

Reflex sympathetic dystrophy (shoulder-hand syndrome): A neurovascular disorder characterized by severe shoulder pain, along with stiffness, swelling, and pain in the hand, trophic changes, vasomotor instability, and resulting limitation in range of motion of the involved side. Prevention is by early frequent mobilization. Prompt treatment with an aggressive exercise program that includes active muscle contraction, joint movement, and light weight-bearing activities is required to prevent permanent disability.

Spasticity: Abnormal muscle tone felt as too much resistance to movement as a result of hyperactive reflexes and loss of inhibiting influences from higher brain centers. See hypertonus. Spastic: Clonus or rapid series of rhythmic contractions during quick stretch of a muscle due to abnormally increased tension.

Stroke: A sudden and severe attack. Stroke syndrome: A condition with sudden onset caused by acute vascular lesions of the brain (hemorrhage, embolism, thrombosis, rupturing aneurysm), which may be marked by hemiplegia or hemiparesis, vertigo, numbness, aphasia, and dysar-

thria, and often followed by permanent neurologic damage. See CVA.

Subarachnoid: Between the arachnoid and pia mater, which are membrane layers of the brain.

Subclavian steal syndrome: A rare condition in which there is a narrowing of the subclavian artery. When the arm is exercised, blood is "stolen" from the brain and delivered to the exercised arm, often resulting in lightheadness, weakness, and numbness.

Subluxation: Incomplete or partial dislocation. Shoulder subluxation at the glenohumeral joint is commonly seen following a stroke.

Sudeck's atrophy: Potential complication in fracture healing characterized by pain, swelling (over-laying skin is stretched and glossy), and marked joint stiffness; Colles' fracture is one of the most common causes, although overall incidence is small.

Synergy: A grouping of stereotypic movements; correlated action or cooperation by two or more structures. Limb synergies may be elicited as associated reactions or as voluntary movements in early stages of recovery from stroke. When movement of a joint is initiated, all muscles that are linked in a synergy with that movement automatically contract, causing a stereotypic movement pattern.

Thrombus: An aggregation of blood factors, primarily platelets and fibrin with entrapment of cellular elements, frequently causing vascular obstruction at the point of its formation. Thrombosis: The process by which a blood clot forms.

Transient ischemic attack (TIA): A sudden episode of temporary or passing symptoms, typically due to diminished blood flow through the carotid blood vessels, but sometimes related to impaired blood flow through the vertebrobasilar vessels. The symptoms warn of impending stroke; approximately one in three persons experiencing a TIA will have a cerebral vascular accident (stroke) within 5 years. Symptoms can range from obvious loss of sensation or motor function to more subtle changes in speech or mental activity. The person may feel numbness or weakness on both or one side of the body, slurring of speech or inability to talk, staggering or uncoordinated walking, or difficulty in thinking. Double vision or disturbance of vision in one eye is also common. (See CVA).

Unilateral body inattention (neglect): Failure to report, respond, or orient to a unilateral stimulus presented to the body side contralateral to a cerebral lesion. It can result from either defective sensory processing or an attention deficit, resulting in ignoring or impaired use of the extremities.

Unilateral spatial neglect: Inattention to or neglect of visual stimuli presented in the extrapersonal space on the side contralateral to a cerebral lesion, as a result of visual perceptual deficits or impaired attention. It may occur independently of visual deficits or with heminanopsia.

Vertigo: A sensation of rotation or movement of one's self (subjective) or of one's surroundings (objective) in any plane. The term is sometimes used erroneously as a synonym for dizziness. Vertigo may result from diseases of the inner ear or may be due to disturbances of the vestibular centers or pathways in the central nervous system.

Wallenburg's syndrome: The result of lateral damage at the brainstem level (e.g., lateral medullary syndrome). Damaged structures may include the spinothalamic tract, spinal trigeminal tract, nucleus ambiguus, and descending sympathetic fibers. Symptoms of such damage are loss of pain and temperature sensations over the contralateral body (with relative sparing of tactile sensation), loss of pain and temperature sensations over the ipsilateral face, hoarseness and difficulty in swallowing, and ipsilateral Horner's syndrome. If the inferior cerebellar peduncles in the midbrain and vestibular nuclei are damaged, vertigo and ipsilateral cerebellar deficits such as ataxia may result.

Medications

Generic Name	Brand Name	CEREBRAL INFARCTION		Potential Side Effects	Usual Adult Dose	Comments
		Action	Indication			
ANTICOAGULANT: Heparin	Heparin	Inhibition of clotting by interfering with the activity of chemicals in liquid portion of blood that are essential for coagulation	Stroke in evolution, cardiac source of emboli, reduction of DVT formation; does *not* appear as useful in completed cerebral infarct	Thrombocytopenia, increased risk of hemorrhage		
ANTIPLATELETS: Aspirin	Anacin Bayer	Blockage of platelet aggregation	Secondary prevention of stroke and TIAs; works best with men; not as effective with moderate to severe strokes	Gastrointestinal disorders, GI bleeding, ulcers, tinnitus, dizziness		
ANTIPLATELETS:		Inhibits fibrinogen binding and modifies platelet aggregation	Secondary prevention of stroke and TIAs; works equally in men and women	Neutropenia, GI disorders		

THROMBOLYTICS: Streptokinase, urokinase		Converts plasminogen to active plasmin which then lyses thrombin	To be used within hours of an infarction; can result in a high rate of reperfusion of affected area with substantial tissue recovery	Intracerebral hemorrhage
THROMBOLYTICS: Tissue plasminogen activator (TPA)		Involved in the normal formation of thrombus binding to fibrin and the active site of plasminogen	Very early (within 90 min) therapy for cerebral infarction	Intracerebral hemorrhage
HEMORRHAGE				
CALCIUM ANTAGONISTS: Nimodipine	Nimotop	Dilates blood vessels, allowing more blood to flow to the brain; limits flow of calcium into cells	Prevention or reduction of poor neurologic outcome due to vasospasm secondary to aneurysmal subarachnoid hemorrhage	Edema, hypotension; angina, dizziness, depression, abdominal cramping, constipation

3

Developmental Disabilities

MARY STEICHEN YAMAMOTO

The following two cases are representative of the experience parents have had when their child has Down syndrome, a developmental disability.

In the mid-1950s Mr. and Mrs. D. had their first child. Mrs. D., a homemaker in her late 30s, and Mr. D., a bank officer, had tried for many years to have a child. They had both given up when Mrs. D. became pregnant. Shortly after his birth they were told by their doctor that their son was born a "mongoloid" who would be severely retarded and not capable of learning anything. The doctors suggested that they put E.D. in an institution immediately and felt it would be better if they had no further contact with him. Mr. and Mrs. D. were not willing to put him in an institution and wanted him home with them. They took E.D. home with no support from their doctors, family, or the community.

In the late 1980s, Mr. and Mrs. T., both in their 20s, were eagerly awaiting the birth of their second child. Mr. T., a construction worker, and his wife, a bookkeeper, had a 3-year-old son. Mrs. T. had what she described as an easy pregnancy and delivery, resulting in the birth of another son, T.T. Shortly after his birth the doctors told them that they suspected their son had Down syndrome. Mr. and Mrs. T. were devastated. They had heard of Down syndrome but knew little about it. They were frightened and did not know what to expect or how this would affect their family.

They were told that T.T. would have mental retardation that could range from mild to severe. They wanted answers and predictions but were told that they would have to wait, as it was not possible to predict what T.T. would be capable of. Some children with Down syndrome were learning academics in regular classrooms while others remained dependent for many of their basic needs. They were also told that with early intervention, children with Down syndrome were achieving much more independence and higher levels of functioning than had previously been thought possible.

Before T.T. and his parents left the hospital, a referral was made to the local school district for early intervention services to begin within a few months. They were given pamphlets written for parents, describing Down syndrome, which helped to answer many of their questions. Their doctor asked if they would like to be contacted by a parent volunteer from a local group for parents of children with Down syndrome. Although it would take some time for them to come to terms with their son's diagnosis, they knew that there were programs and support available in their community to help their family.

Today E.D. lives in a group home about 30 miles from his parents, who are now quite elderly and can no longer care for him. He takes a bus by himself to visit them twice a week. While he is quite independent, the group home provides the structure and supervision he needs. E.D.'s mother recalls that there were no school programs for him when he was growing up. However, she proudly says that all who know E.D. are very fond of him and he has many special friends. She describes him as a sweet and loving son.

T.T. is now in a special preschool class. His parents feel that he is doing well and are proud of each new accomplishment. Mrs. T. recently gave birth to a baby girl, who was not born with Down syndrome. They are enjoying T.T. but still feel some anxiety about his future.

From these two cases, it is apparent how much attitudes toward and treatment of Down syndrome has changed in this country. This phenomenon applies not just to Down syndrome but to other developmental disabilities as well.

INTRODUCTION

"Developmental disabilities" (DD) encompass a wide variety of chronic conditions that are evident in childhood and interfere significantly with growth and development. The term originated in 1970 with the passage of the Developmental Disabilities Services and Facilities Construction Act (PL91–517) (1). According to this act a *developmental disability* was defined as a disability which:

1. Is attributable to mental retardation, cerebral palsy, epilepsy, or another neurologic condition related to mental retardation or requiring treatment similar to that for mentally retarded individuals;
2. Originates before age 18;
3. Has continued or can be expected to continue indefinitely; and
4. Constitutes a substantial handicap to such individuals (1).

Prior to this time, legislation in the United States provided planning and the provision of services only to those with mental retardation. Those with other developmental conditions who had a need for similiar services were excluded. This

prompted many professionals and consumer parent groups to lobby for legislation and a broader term that would provide services to all. However this original definition does not include autism, specific learning disabilities, or conditions that could not be definitely defined as neurologic in origin. These conditions (with the exception of specific learning disabilities not related to dyslexia) were added in 1975 (PL94–103) as a result of continuing lobbying by concerned individuals and public hearings (1).

The Developmental Disabilities Amendments of 1978 (PL95–602) contained a definition of developmental disabilities for legislative and public policy issues which is widely used today. These amendments to the Developmentally Disabled Assistance and Bill of Rights Act of 1975 defined developmental disability as a severe, chronic disability of a person which:

1. Is attributable to a mental or physical impairment or combination of a mental or physical impairment;
2. Is manifested before the person reaches age 22;
3. Is likely to continue indefinitely;
4. Results in substantial functional limitations in three or more of the following areas of major life activity: (a) self-care, (b) receptive and expressive language, (c) learning, (d) mobility, (e) self-direction, (f) capacity for independent living, and (g) economic self-sufficiency; and
5. Reflects the person's need for a combination and sequence of special interdisciplinary or generic care, treatment, or other services that are of lifelong or extended duration and are individually planned and coordinated (2).

The above definition differs significantly from previous ones by describing DD from a *functional* perspective rather than as a categorical listing of conditions that are considered to be developmental disabilities. For instance, not all persons with mental retardation would be considered developmentally disabled. Those with mental retardation in the mild range, who do not have substantial functional limitations in three or more of the areas listed under point 4 above would not be included in this definition (2). Similarly, no one whose functioning met the criteria would be excluded from services because the condition was not covered by the legislation.

Part 5 of the definition of developmental disability refers to the need for specialized services and treatment. Historically, many general service agencies and agencies providing specialized services to people with disabilities have overlooked or excluded people with developmental disabilities (2). Individuals with disabilities occuring during childhood tend to have more difficulty becoming independent than those who had a normal early developmental period and were independent before becoming disabled.

The services that the person needs change over the lifespan and differ widely from individual to individual. For example, the primary provider of occupational, physical, or speech therapy services for a child with cerebral palsy is usually the school system. As with many developmental disabilities that require extensive medical care, the child's medical needs would be met by a local pediatrician and a variety of specialists. Sometimes these specialists are affiliated with a regional medical center that holds special clinics several times a year. Here the child can be seen at one appointment by various medical team members, including a physiatrist, neurologist, orthopaedist, orthotist, occupational therapist, physical therapist, speech pathologist, and social worker.

As an adult, the person with a developmental disability may need special vocational programs or training and would be eligible for disability or Social Security income. There may be a need for a group home or a supervised living situation if the person is not capable of independent living. The need for medical care would most likely decrease, and the services of fewer team members would be required. A case manager may be needed to coordinate services provided by many separate agencies.

The Developmental Disabilities Assistance and Bill of Rights Act, in addition to the Education For All Handicapped Children Act (PL94–142), has provided a tremendous increase in services to people with developmental disabilities in the past 15 years. PL94–142, which was enacted in 1975, mandated that all school districts provide free, appropriate, public education for all children, regardless of the severity of their disability. This act, most recently amended in 1991 by Public Law 101-476, is now titled, "The Individuals with Disabilities Education Act" (IDEA).

In more recent years, the need for programs to maximize independence for the adult has been recognized, and community-based programs have been increasing. There also has been a shift from institutionalization of the more severely affected individuals to integration in a community.

ETIOLOGY

The causes of DD are usually classified in one of two ways. First, they are classified according to the period in the developmental process during which they occurred, i.e., prenatally, perinatally, or postnatally. The second means of classification is by the nature of the cause, i.e., genetic and/or environmental. There are hundreds of causes of developmental disability (3). Table 3.1 lists some of the more common ones.

With many persons the cause of the developmental disability can not be determined. There is nothing remarkable in the history of the child, parents, or family that could be a contributing factor. In most cases of mental retardation, the cause remains unknown, particularly for those with mild mental retardation, which is over 85%

Table 3.1.
Causes of Developmental Disabilities

	Infections	Trauma	Environmental	Hypoxia	Genetic
PRENATAL	Rubella Cytomegalovirus (CMV) Syphilis AIDS Toxoplasmosis	Accidents	Sperm damage Exposure to chemicals, radiation Use of medications, illegal drugs Fetal alcohol syndrome Toxemia Malnutrition Lack of prenatal care	Specific genetic diseases	Specific gene defects Chromosomal abnormalities
PERINATAL	Herpes simplex II	Misapplication of forceps Birth trauma	Very low birth weight Prematurity Intracranial hemorrhage	Meconium aspiration Prolonged labor Cord wrapped around neck Impaired respiration	
POSTNATAL	Encephalitis Meningitis	Child abuse Accidents	Lead or mercury poisoning Failure to thrive Environmental deprivation Malnutrition	Near drowning Near strangulation	

of the population of persons with mental retardation (4).

One hospital referral clinic for the care of children with mental retardation reports the following distribution of causative factors (5):

1. Genetic disorders and acquired childhood diseases: 4–5%
2. Perinatal difficulties: 10–12%
3. Early alterations of embryonic development: 30+%
4. Unknown causes: 30+%

Prenatal Factors

Prenatal factors include genetic aberrations, environmental influences, or a combination of the two. With genetic aberrations, the problem is either with the genes, which are the basic unit of heredity, or the chromosomes, which carry the genes. Each non–germ cell (cells other than the ovum and spermatozoa) contains 23 pairs of chromosomes, including one pair of sex chromosomes that determine the sex of the person. Males have an X and a Y chromosome, and females have two X chromosomes.

With many developmental disabilities, the gene or chromosome that has caused the condition can be identified specifically. For instance, with Down syndrome, 95% of the cases can be traced to an extra 21st chromosome (6). With others, the specific genetic aberration has not been identified. Factors such as higher incidences of a condition in specific families or increased recurrence rates among siblings suggest that the defect is genetic. For instance, if a woman has given birth to one child with myelodysplasia, a neural tube defect commonly called spina bifida, there is a 5% higher risk that the next child will also be affected and a 10% higher risk if she has two children who are affected (7).

Environmental factors may also be involved. For example, with spina bifida, no specific environmental influence has been proven to be responsible, but water supply, diet, or minor infections in the early weeks of pregnancy have all been proposed as possible contributing factors (8, 9).

GENETIC CAUSES

Genetic causes can be divided into two types: single gene disorders and chromosomal abnormalities (10). In single gene disorders there is a problem with the quality of the genetic material; a specific gene is defective. In chromosomal abnormalities, the problem is with the quantity of material. There is either too much or two little genetic material in a specific chromosome (10).

Single Gene Disorders

Single gene disorders follow specific patterns of transmission: autosomal dominant, autosomal recessive, or sex linked. Table 3.2 describes the transmission patterns and risk factors associated with each type.

The autosomal dominant type is caused by a single altered gene. Either parent may be a carrier or there may have been a spontaneous mutation of the gene. If a parent has the gene, there is a 50% risk of the child being affected in each pregnancy (11). Examples of this are tuberous sclerosis, neurofibromatosis, and myotonic dystrophy.

In the autosomal recessive type, both parents are carriers and disorders are caused by a pair of altered genes on one of the autosomes. Each pregnancy has a 25% risk of the child being affected (11). Examples of this type are phenylketonuria (PKU) and Tay-Sachs disease.

With X-linked disorders, the affected gene is on the sex chromosomes, specifically the X chromosome, and can occur in either parent. Since males have only one X chromosome, if the father has an affected gene he will always have the disorder and cannot be a carrier. Since the female has two X chromosomes, she can either be a carrier of the disorder (if only one X chromosome is affected) or have the disease herself (if both X chromosomes are

Table 3.2.
Single Gene Disorders

Type	Autosomal Dominant	Autosomal Recessive	Sex-Linked
TRANSMISSION PATTERN	Either parent carries gene or spontaneous mutation	Both parents are carriers	Either parent can transmit gene: mother usually a carrier, father cannot be a carrier but can have the disorder
RISK FACTORS	50% risk of child being affected with each pregnancy	25% risk of child being affected with each pregnancy	If mother has affected gene, 25% risk of having affected son or carrier daughter; if father has affected gene, all his daughters will be carriers and his sons will be normal
SEX DISTRIBUTION	Male and female children equally at risk	Male and female children equally at risk	Primarily male children at risk for having disorder, female children at risk for becoming carriers

affected). A carrier mother has a 25% risk of having an affected son. If the father has the affected gene, all his daughters will be carriers, but his sons will not be affected (11).

Examples of X-linked disorders are Duchenne's muscular dystrophy and Hurler syndrome.

Chromosomal Aberrations

Chromosomal aberrations include missing or extra chromosomes, either in part, such as a short arm, or the total chromosome, as is found in the trisomal types. Either the autosomes or sex chromosomes can be affected, with the autosomal type resulting in more serious neuromotor impairments (12). The most common are trisomy 21, 18, and 13. The patterns of transmission are not as readily identified as those of specific gene defects. For instance, with Down syndrome, recent research has shown that even though the age of the mother is a factor, in many cases it is the sperm that contributes the extra chromosome (3).

ENVIRONMENTAL INFLUENCES

There are numerous environmental causes of developmental disabilities, including maternal infections such as rubella, cytomegalovirus, toxoplasmosis, and syphilis. An increasing number of babies are being born to mothers with acquired immune deficiency syndrome (AIDS), which often results in a developmental disability.

Low birth weight due to prematurity or intrauterine growth retardation can also be a contributing factor. Maternal factors associated with low birth weight include smoking, lack of prenatal care, infections, poor nutrition, toxemia, and placental insufficiency. Exposure to industrial chemicals or drugs, including certain over-the-counter prescriptions and illegal substances, can also affect birth weight, particularly during the first trimester of pregnancy.

Perinatal Factors

Two major causative factors of DD in the perinatal period are mechanical injuries at birth and perinatal hypoxia. Mechanical injuries are caused by difficulties of labor because of malposition, malpresentation, disproportion, or other labor complications that result in tears of the meninges, blood vessels, or other substances of the brain.

Factors that cause perinatal hypoxia or anoxia include premature placental separation, massive hemorrage from placenta previa, umbilical cord wrapped around the baby's neck, and meconium aspiration. Very premature infants may also have impaired respiration or an intracranial hemorrhage that can result in brain damage.

If a mother has an active case of herpes simplex II and is shedding the virus at the time of delivery, the baby can acquire the infection in the birth canal, which can cause severe developmental disability. This can be avoided by testing to determine whether the mother has an active case and delivering by cesarean section if she does.

Postnatal Factors

Traumas or infections that result in injury or a lack of oxygen to the brain are a major cause of DD during the postnatal period. Traumas include near-drowning or strangulation, child abuse, and closed head injuries. Infections include encephalitis and meningitis.

Another major postnatal factor is environmental influences. The interplay of an impoverished psychological, social, and economic environment is usually involved. In this type of environment, the child may not receive adequate stimulation and nurturing to support intellectual growth. Depending on the severity of the environmental conditions, this can result in mild-to-severe mental retardation. However, many children from impoverished environments develop normally, which lends some support to a genetic component being at least in part responsible. The tendency of developmental disabilities, particularly milder forms of mental retardation and learning difficul-

ties, to run in families also points toward a genetic component (12).

INCIDENCE

Congress supported the passage of the Developmental Disabilities Amendments (PL95–602) in 1978 because, at that time, there were more than two million persons with developmental disabilities residing in the United States (2). Since the criteria for classification of a DD are currently based on an individual's level of function, rather than upon a medical condition, it is difficult to estimate the number of people affected accurately. Sociocultural factors and inherent variables in methodologic procedures have also hindered efforts at obtaining reliable data.

The most frequent condition among those with developmental disabilities is mental retardation (MR). Estimates of the prevalence of MR in this country range from 1 to 3%, with 1% probably the more accurate figure when different age groups are considered (1, 5, 13).

Cerebral palsy (CP) (discussed in the next section) occurs in 2 to 3 of every 1000 live births in the United States (14). The United Cerebral Palsy Association estimates that 500,000 to 700,000 people in the United States show one or more symptom of CP. They estimate that each year 3000 newborns and 500 preschool children sustain brain damage that results in CP (14).

SIGNS AND SYMPTOMS

Since so many different diagnostic categories result in developmental disabilities, each with its own signs and symptoms, it is not possible to describe them all in this chapter. For information on the signs and symptoms of specific developmental disabilities, the reader is advised to consult *Nelson's Textbook of Pediatrics* (15) or the *Merck Manual* (16). Both these books are available in the reference section of most libraries.

This section discusses two developmental disabilities seen by occupational therapists: mental retardation and cerebral palsy. According to the Member Data Survey conducted by the American Occupational Therapy Association in 1990, 4.9% of registered occupational therapists (OTRs) responding and 11.4% of certified occupational therapy assistants (COTAs) responding indicated that MR was a primary performance deficit of the clients they treated. Cerebral palsy was identified by 9.7% of OTRs and 6% of COTAs as the primary diagnosis (17).

Mental Retardation

It is important to keep in mind that while MR is the major medical diagnosis for many individuals with developmental disabilities, it often occurs in tandem with, or as a secondary manifestation of, another diagnosis. For instance, about 40% of individuals with a diagnosis of pervasive developmental disorder (autism) are mentally retarded (18). In these cases it can be considered a separate diagnosis. With certain genetic conditions such as Down syndrome, it is one of the clinical signs of the condition.

MR is defined by the American Association of Mental Deficiency (AAMD) as "significantly subaverage general intellectual functioning resulting in or associated with impairments in adaptive behavior and manifested during the developmental period" (13). Significantly, subaverage is defined as an IQ of 70 or below on a standardized intelligence test. Impairments in adaptive behavior are limitations in the ability to achieve personal and social self-sufficiency as expected for the individual's age and cultural group. The developmental period is from conception to the 18th birthday (13).

MR is classified according to the severity of the impairment in intellectual functioning. This is determined through standardized intelligence testing (IQ). To be considered mentally retarded, the person's performance on these tests must be two standard deviation units or more below the mean.

The levels of MR as identified by IQ tests are mild, moderate, severe, and profound. A survey conducted from 1983 to 1985 found that almost 90% (89.4) of people with mental retardation were in the mild classification. Six percent were moderate, 3.5% severe, and 1.5% profound (19). Table 3.3 describes the classifications, IQ levels, and general level of functioning as an adult (13, 15, 18). It is important to remember that not all persons in a particular classification will function at exactly that level.

There are two basic groups of people with MR (13). One group, which comprises about 25%, generally demonstrates some central nervous system pathology and includes those whose mental retardation is due to genetic syndromes. IQs tend to be in the moderate range or below, and these individuals have associated handicaps such as a visual or hearing impairment or seizure disorder. Diagnosis is usually made at birth or during early childhood (13).

The second group, which includes most people with MR, demonstrates no obvious signs of MR and no apparent neurologic abnormalities. There are no definite physical signs nor evidence of irregularities on laboratory tests. The level of retardation is usually mild and not diagnosed until after the child has entered school. There are more children from lower socioeconomic backgrounds in this group (13).

Some individuals with MR do not fit the previous categories (13). Some with mild mental retardation may also have a number of neurologic signs. Conversely, some children with a genetic basis for their retardation may come from a lower socioeconomic background and live in significantly disadvantaged environments.

Cerebral Palsy

Cerebral palsy is not a distinct disease but rather a grouping of similar syndromes. It is defined as a disorder of movement and posture due to a defect or lesion of the

Table 3.3.
Levels of Retardation

Classification	IQ Range	When Identified		Adaptive Behavior as Adult
PROFOUND	Below 20	Infancy	Independent functioning: Communication: Occupation:	Requires total supervision Dependent upon others for personal care Very minimal language Minimal participation
SEVERE	20–35	Early childhood	Independent functioning: Communication:	Can contribute partially to self-care with total supervision Can engage in simple conversation Recognizes signs and selected words
			Occupation:	May prepare simple foods, can help with simple household tasks, e.g., bed making, vacuuming, setting and clearing table Requires much supervision
MODERATE	36–50	Early childhood	Independent functioning:	Feeds, bathes, and dresses self; prepares simple foods for self & others; able to care for own hair (wash & comb) May function semiindependently in supervised living situation
			Communication:	Carries on simple conversation, uses complex sentences; recognizes words, reads sentences, ads, & signs with comprehension
			Occupation:	May do simple routine household chores (dusting, garbage, dishwashing); prepares food requiring mixing May function in supported employment or sheltered workshop setting Can learn some functional living skills: shopping, using post office, laundry
MILD	51–70	Elementary school	Independent functioning:	Exercises care for personal grooming, feeding, bathing and toileting; may need health or personal care reminders; may need guidance and assistance when under unusual social or economic stress
			Occupation:	Prepares meals, performs everyday household tasks Can hold semiskilled or simple skilled job

immature brain (14). A child is considered to have cerebral palsy if all of the following characteristics apply:

1. The injury or insult occurs when the brain is still developing. It can occur anytime during the prenatal, perinatal, or postnatal periods, with prenatal factors being responsible in most cases when the cause is known (20). Prenatal factors include maternal infections, metabolic disturbances due to endocrine imbalance, vitamin deficiencies, untreated Rh incompatibilities, cerebral hemorrhage, and fetal malformation. Prematurity and mental retardation in the mother can also be causative factors (7, 20, 21). Previously, cerebral palsy has been associated with a lack of oxygen during labor and delivery, but recent research has cast doubt upon this theory. Many researchers now believe that prenatal problems may actually cause the obstetric difficulties during the birth of some babies with cerebral palsy (20). A recent study published by the National Institutes of Health reported that in 75% of reported cases of cerebral palsy, there were no symptoms of asphyxia during labor and delivery and that in most cases of cerebral palsy the cause is unknown (22). In the postnatal period, infections such as meningitis or encephalitis, accidents that cause anoxia, such as near-drownings or strangulation, injuries due to child abuse, and lead poisoning are common causes (11, 16, 21). There is some disagreement about the upper age limit for a diagnosis of cerebral palsy during the postnatal period, but generally it ranges from 3 to 9 years of age (7, 12).

2. It is nonprogressive; once the damage has occurred, there is no further worsening of the child's condition or further damage to the central nervous system.

3. It always involves a disorder in sensorimotor development that is manifested by abnormal postural tone and characteristic patterns of movement. The severity of the impairment ranges from mild to severe.

4. The sensorimotor disorder originates specifically in the central nervous system. Although some cardiac or orthopaedic problems can result in similar postural and movement abnormalities, they are not classified as such.

5. It is a lifelong disability. Unlike some premature babies who demonstrate temporary posture and movement abnormalities during the first year of life, children with cerebral palsy have permanent abnormalities.

EARLY SIGNS AND SYMPTOMS

The early signs and symptoms common to all types of cerebral palsy are muscle tone, reflex, and postural abnormalities; delayed motor development, and abnormal motor development (7).

Tone Abnormalities. Tone abnormalities may include hypertonicity, hypotonicity, and fluctuating tone, which can shift from hypotonic to hypertonic.

Reflex Abnormalities. With hypertonicity, reflex abnormalities such as hyperreflexia, clonus, overflow, enhanced stretch reflex, and other signs of upper motor neuron lesions are present (7). Retained primitive infantile reflexes and a delay in the acquisition of righting and equilibrium reactions occur in conjunction with all types of abnormal tone. In some cases where hypotonia is present, there may be areflexia, or an absence of primitive reflexes, during the first several months of life, when they should be observable.

Postural Abnormalities. Due to the influence of primitive reflexes and abnormal tone, the child with cerebral palsy assumes abnormal positions at rest and demonstrates predictable postural changes during movement. For instance, a child with hypertonicity in the lower extremities often lies supine with the hips internally rotated and adducted and ankles plantar-flexed. This posture is caused by a combination of high tone in the affected muscles and the crossed extension reflex. A child with hypotonicity typically lies with hips abducted, flexed, and externally rotated because of low muscle tone, weakness in the affected muscles, and the influence of gravity.

Delayed Motor Development. Cerebral palsy is always accompanied by a delay in the attainment of motor milestones. One of the signs that often alerts the pediatrician to the problem is a delay in the ability to sit independently.

Abnormal Motor Behavior. The way in which a child moves when performing skilled motor acts is also affected. Depending upon the type of cerebral palsy, the child may demonstrate a variety of motor abnormalities such as asymmetric hand use, unusual crawling method or gait, uncoordinated reach, or difficulty sucking, chewing, and swallowing.

TYPES OF CEREBRAL PALSY

Types of cerebral palsy are classified neurophysiologically or anatomically (23). Spastic and rigid types, which are characterized by hypertonicity are caused by damage to the pyramidal tract. Dyskinetic types are characterized by deficient voluntary movement and are caused by extrapyramidal damage or in some cases both pyramidal and extrapyramidal (23). Table 3.4 shows the classifications and frequency of the different types. Only the more commonly occurring types are discussed here.

Spastic CP is the most frequent. It is characterized by hypertonicity, retained primitive reflexes in affected parts, and slow, restricted movement. Contractures and deformities are common. It is categorized according to which parts of the body are affected.

Spastic hemiparesis involves one side of the body, with usually the upper extremity more affected (7). Early signs include asymmetrical hand use during the first year or dragging one side of the body when crawling or walking. It begins as flaccid disuse of the involved extremity,

with spasticity developing gradually (7, 23). Most children begin walking after 18 months of age. Ninety percent of those who eventually walk, do so by their third birthday (23). When walking, the child typically hyperextends the knee and the ankle in equinovarus or equinovalgus position on the involved side. The child often lacks righting and equilibrium reactions on the involved side and will avoid weight bearing on this side. The shoulder is held in adduction, internal rotation; the elbow is flexed; forearm is pronated; wrist is flexed and ulnar deviated; and the hand is often fisted. Arm and hand use is limited on the involved side, depending upon the severity. The child may use more primitive patterns of grasping and lacks precise and coordinated movements. In more severe cases, the child may totally neglect the involved side or may use it only as an assist during bilateral activities.

Spastic diplegia involves both lower extremities, with mild incoordination, tremors, or less severe spasticity in the upper extremities. It is most often attributed to premature birth and low birth weight and is, therefore, on the rise as more infants born early survive due to medical advances (7). The ability to sit independently can be delayed up to 3 years of age or older because of inadequate hip flexion and extensor and adductor hypertonicity in the legs (25). Frequently, the child must rely upon the arms for support. The young child will move forward on the floor by pulling along with flexed arms while the legs are stiffly extended. Getting up to a creeping position is difficult due to spasticity in the lower extremities. Similarly, standing posture and gait are affected to varying degrees, depending upon severity. Due to a lack of lower extremity equilibrium reactions, excessive trunk and upper extremity compensatory movements are used when walking. Lumbar lordosis, hip flexion and internal rotation (scissoring), plantar flexion of the ankles, and difficulty shifting weight when walking are common. Many

Table 3.4.
Types of Cerebral Palsy[a]

Classification	Frequency (%)	Characteristics
Spastic	70–80	Hypertonicity, retained primitive reflexes, slow, restricted movement
Hemiparesis	20–25	One side of body affected
Diplegia	25–35	Lower extremities affected, less involvement of upper extremities
Quadriparesis	25–30	All four extremities affected
Dyskinetic	10–12	Includes variety of types of movement disorders
Athetosis	3–5	Slow, writhing movements, face and extremities, distal muscles more affected than proximal
Dystonia	Rare	Rhythmic twisting distortions and tone changes in trunk and proximal part of limbs; slow uncontrolled movements with fixed postures
Chorea	Rare	Rapid irregular jerky movements in face and extremities
Ballismus	Rare	Coarse wide-amplitude flailing or flinging movements, mostly extremities
Ataxia	Rare	Weakness, incoordination, intention tremor, difficulty with rapid or fine movements, nystagmus, wide-based gait, lack of balance
Rigid	4–5	Severe spasticity
Atonia	Rare	Persistent hypotonicity throughout body
Mixed	10–20	Two types of cerebral palsy evident
Spastic-athetoid	10–15	Combination of spastic quadriparesis and athetoid characteristics
Spastic-ataxic	Rare	Combination of spastic quadriparesis and ataxia characteristics
Spastic-rigid	3–5	Combination of spastic quadriparesis and rigid characteristics

[a]Adapted from Molnar G; ed. Pediatric rehabilitation. Baltimore: Williams & Wilkins, 1985.

of these problems result in contractures and deformities, including dorsal spine kyphosis, lumbar spine lordosis, hip subluxation or dislocation, flexor deformities of hips and knees, and equinovarus or equinovalgus deformity of the feet (24).

With spastic quadriparesis the entire body is involved. The disability is more pervasive because the damage or lesions are in the cerebral cortex (7). The arms typically show flexor spasticity, with extensor spasticity in the lower extremities. Due to the influence of the tonic labyrinthine reflex (TLR), shoulder retraction and neck hyperextension are common, partic-ularly in supine position. This results in difficulty with transitional movements such as rolling or coming up to sitting. In prone position, there is increased flexor tone also due to TLR influence, resulting in difficulty with head raising and weight bearing on arms. Independent sitting and standing are difficult for the child because of hypertonicity, primitive reflex involvement, and a lack of righting and equilibrium reactions. Approximately 25% of children with quadriplegia are never able to walk and are dependent upon others for their care because of severe upper extremity impairment (7). Oral musculature is usually affected, with resulting speech and eating difficulties. Mental retardation and seizures are common (23).

Athetosis, another type of cerebral palsy, is characterized by slow, writhing movements of the face and extremities. Head and trunk control is often affected as is the oral musculature. While the spastic types are characterized by hypertonicity in the affected muscle groups and restricted movement, athetoid type is characterized by fluctuating tone and excessive movement. Contractures are rare, but hypermobility may be present. Over two-thirds of those with this type of cerebral palsy have IQs above 90, although their movements and speech disorders often erroneously give the impression of retardation (23).

In mixed type CP, two different types of cerebral palsy occur together, and the damage to the brain is diffuse. The most frequent mixed type is spastic-athetoid, which has the signs of athetosis, while postural tone fluctuates from hypertonicity to hypotonia.

Hypotonia is a common early manifestation of many types of CP. In a small number of cases hypotonia continues throughout life.

ASSOCIATED DISORDERS

Mental Retardation. Estimates of incidence of MR with cerebral palsy range from 40% to 70% (7, 11). It occurs most often and most severely in spastic quadriplegia, rigid, and mixed types. It is seen less often in spastic diplegia, paraplegia, and hemiplegia (7, 11, 22).

Seizure Disorder. Reports of the incidence of seizures in people with CP range from 25% to 60% (7, 11, 22). The incidence varies among the different types. It is most common in spastic hemiplegia and quadriplegia, and lowest in spastic diplegia and dyskinetic types (7, 11, 22). All clinical types of seizures are reported, with grand mal type being the most common (11).

Visual and Hearing Impairments. Visual and hearing impairments occur at a higher rate with CP than in the general population. Strabismus is the most common visual defect, occurring in 20% to 60% of children with CP (22, 25). Other visual and ocular abnormalities include nystagmus, no vertical eye movement, homonymous hemianopsia, and difficulties with visual fixation and tracking (7, 21).

Hearing impairments include sensorineural hearing loss, which occurs in approximately 12% of children under 15 with CP (7). Conductive hearing losses caused by persistent fluid in the ears and middle ear infections in children with severe CP who spend a lot of time lying down have been reported (11).

PROGRESSION/PROGNOSIS

All developmental disabilities are lifelong, but the course and prognosis vary with each of the specific conditions. (For information about specific conditions consult reference 15 or 16). Even within one condition such as cerebral palsy, there is great variation because of the range of severity of involvement. The course of CP varies depending upon type, severity, and the presence of associated problems. With milder involvement, the child will continue to make motor gains and compensate for motor difficulties. With more severe forms, there may be little progress made in attaining developmental milestones and performing functional tasks. As the child grows older, secondary problems such as contractures and deformities will become more common with spastic types. The life span for most persons with cerebral palsy is within the average range (11).

Most developmental disabilities are nonprogressive, that is, once the initial insult to the brain occurs, there is no further damage. The emphasis is on managing the medical aspects of the condition and assisting persons to achieve their highest potential.

However, certain genetic conditions (e.g., muscular dystrophy and Tay-Sachs disease) are progressive, with incremental loss of function and, in some cases, associated early death. The goal for these individuals is to help them achieve the highest level of independence and maintain it as long as possible.

DIAGNOSTICS AND MEDICATIONS

Diagnostics

To determine whether a person meets the criteria for being developmentally disabled, an evaluation must be performed. There are three aspects to this process.

The first involves *a physical examination* to determine what, if any, medical condition the person has and its probable cause. This phase includes a detailed medical and developmental history which is helpful in determining a specific risk or a family history of any specific conditions. The physician looks for certain physical signs or stigmata associated with genetic syndromes. These are listed in Table 3.5.

A thorough neurologic examination should be performed to evaluate the status of the entire central and peripheral nervous systems. This includes assessment of cranial nerves, muscular strength, muscle tone and coordination, deep tendon and primitive reflexes, and cortical sensory function (15).

"Soft" neurologic signs should also be evaluated. These include poor fine and/ or gross motor coordination; strabismus; verbal and motor dyspraxia; immature overflow patterns (mirror movements); immature motor, auditory, or visual sequencing; graphomotor difficulties; constructional dyspraxia; and dysdiadochokinesia (15).

Diagnostic procedures are also performed to determine whether there is an organic basis. These vary, depending upon the findings on the physical examination, and may include various laboratory tests of urine and blood; radiologic examinations such as skull x-rays, computerized tomography (CT scan), and/or chromosomal karotyping (15). Muscle biopsy and an EMG (electromyogram) can aid in diagnosing certain syndromes, and an EEG (electroencephalogram) is indicated if there is evidence of possible seizure activity. Appendix 3.2 describes specific tests.

The second aspect is *the administration of standardized intelligence (IQ) tests*. While many individuals with developmental disabilities have average or above-average intelligence, intelligence testing should still be a part of all diagnostic evaluations, to determine the extent of mental impairment. However, the administration of IQ tests has its limitations and controversies. Many feel that they are culturally biased, that they measure academic functioning rather than adequate social functioning, and that they are not reliable in measuring intelligence in children with IQs below 50 (18).

The third aspect of the evaluation process is the *evaluation of adaptive behavior* as it relates to the major life activity areas described in part 4 of the definition of developmental disability. Adaptive behavior is defined as the performance of the daily activities required for personal and social sufficiency (25). The skills needed for adaptive behavior become more complex and varied as the person ages. For instance, the ability to eat and dress independently is a major skill for the young child, but the child does not need to be able to use a telephone or manage money. Appendix 3.2 lists specific tests used to assess adaptive behavior.

Medications

Drug therapy is not necessarily a part of treatment for many persons with developmental disabilities. However, psychotropic drugs are sometimes used as an adjunct to programming, to promote learning and social interaction and control undesirable or harmful behaviors. The vast majority of medications used are stimulants, neuroleptics (antipsychotics), or antiepileptics (27). Stimulants, which in-

Table 3.5.
Stigmata Associated with Genetic Syndromes

Head
  Maximal occipitofrontal circumference
    below 3rd percentile or above 97th
    percentile

Hair
  Double whorl; sparse or absent hair
  Fine, friable, prematurely gray or
    white locks

Eyes
  Microphthalmia
  Hypertelorism
  Hypotelorism
  Upward-and-outward or downward-
    and-outward slant
  Inner or outer epicanthal folds
  Coloboma of iris or retina
  Brushfield spots
  Eccentrically placed pupil
  Nystagmus
  Telangiectasia

Ears
  Low-set ears
  Simple or abnormal helix formation

Nose
  Flattened bridge
  Small size
  Upturned nares

Face
  Increased length of philtrum
  Hypoplasia of maxilla and/or mandible

Mouth
  Inverted "V" shape of upper lip
    Wide or high-arched palate

Teeth
  Evidence of abnormal enamelog-
    enesis
  Abnormal odontogenesis

Neck
  Short neck
  Lack of full mobility
  Webbing

Extremities
  Unusually short or long limbs
  Increased carrying angle at elbows

Hands
  Short 4th or 5th metacarpals
  Short stubby fingers
  Long, thin tapered fingers
  Broad thumbs
  Clinodactyly
  Abnormal dermatoglyphics
    (e.g., distal triradius)
  Simian line
  Abnormal nails

Feet
  Overlap of toes
  Short stubby toes
  Broad, large big toes
  Deep crease leading from angle of
    1st and 2nd toes
  Abnormal dermatoglyphics

Abdomen
  Protuberant abdomen
  Umbilical hernia

Genitalia
  Ambiguous genitalia
  Micropenis
  Abnormal placement of urethral
    meatus
  Undescended testicles

Chest
  Pectus excavatum or carinatum
  Supernumerary nipples

Skin
  Café au lait spots
  Depigmented nevi
  Adenoma sebaceum
  Malar flush
  Eczema

[a]From Behrman RC, Vaughn U, eds. In Nelson's textbook of pediatrics. 5th ed. Philadelphia: WB Saunders, 1983. With permission.

crease activity in adults, have a reverse action in some children and adolescents who have hyperactivity and conduct problems. They decrease hyperactivity, improve attention, and decrease disruptive, inappropriate, and impulsive behavior. The neuroleptics are used to reduce maladaptive behaviors such as aggression and hyperactivity and to reduce schizophrenic symptoms such as delusions and hallucinations. Antiepileptics are used to control seizures if a seizure disorder is present.

Other medications are also sometimes used in treatment of developmental disabilities. Antianxiety drugs are used to control seizures or to decrease spasticity in medical conditions such as cerebral palsy. Antidepressants are used to treat enuresis, school phobia, depression, and hyperactivity. Lithium is used to treat affective disorders and aggression.

Other drugs used include propranolol (Inderal) for aggression, self-injurious behavior (SIB), and agitation; naloxone (Narcan) to reduce SIB and self-stimulation; and fenfluramine (Pondimin) for the treatment of self-stimulation and decreased activity level. All three of these drugs are sometimes used in the treatment of pervasive developmental disorder (autism) in addition to other disorders. See Appendix 3.3 for a list of specific drugs.

IMPACT ON OCCUPATIONAL PERFORMANCE

Virtually all areas of occupational performance and each of the performance components can be affected by a developmental disability. As stated previously, the Developmental Disabilities Amendments of 1978 identified seven major life activities areas that are affected in persons with developmental disabilities and states that at least three of these must be substantially limited to meet the criteria for being developmentally disabled (2). If these areas are compared with the occupational performance areas and components that are addressed in occupational therapy practice, we see that four of the areas (self-care, mobility, capacity for independent living, and economic self-sufficiency) correspond with the occupational performance areas of activities of daily living and work activities. Two of the areas, learning and self-direction correspond with cognitive and psychosocial performance components.

While all of the occupational performance areas and components can be influenced by a developmental disability, those that are affected will depend upon factors such as medical diagnosis and severity of the disability. Those who have a physical impairment will have more involvement in the sensory integration, neuromuscular, and motor components.

With a mental impairment, the cognitive, psychological, social, and self-management performance components will be most affected. When both physical and mental impairment is present, dysfunction will be more pervasive. The extent to which the occupational performance areas are influenced will depend in part upon the severity of the disability. The following case studies illustrate how a particular developmental disability affects an individual's occupational performance.

CASE STUDIES

Autism

M.L. is a 4-year-old boy with a medical diagnosis of autistic disorder, a subtype of pervasive developmental disorder as identified in the DSM-III-R. Autistic disorder is a developmental disability characterized by impairments in reciprocal social interaction, communication, and imagination, with a markedly restricted repertoire of activities and interests (17). M.L. lives at home with his parents and attends a preschool special education class in an early childhood center. Educationally related services include consultation and monitoring by an occupational therapist. He also receives speech and language therapy.

The occupational performance components affected by M.L.'s disability are sensory integration, cognitive, psychological, social, and self-management skills (Table 3.6). In the sensory integration component, M.L. has difficulty with both sensory awareness and processing. He often seems unaware of his environment and does not attend to environmental stimuli. He has difficulty with processing of all the senses. At times he seeks out tactile experiences excessively, but often he withdraws from touch if it is initiated by others. He is hypersensitive in the oral area. He does not respond to pain unless it is severe. He is hyporeactive to proprioceptive and vestibular stimulation. He often seeks out repetitive proprioceptive and vestibular input. He spins himself in a net swing for extended periods with no signs of dizziness. M.L.'s parents report that he was sensitive to light as a baby and now becomes overwhelmed or excited if he has too much visual stimulation. M.L. is hypersensitive to some environmental sounds such as a microwave oven cooking or the sound test on television, and covers his ears when he hears them. He ignores noxious odors.

In the cognitive integration and cognitive components, M.L.'s attention span, problem solving, and learning are all affected. He attends only briefly, if at all, to most activities. However, he will spend extended periods of time on an activity he enjoys, such as spinning or computer play. If forced to stop an activity before he is ready, he resists and becomes up-

Table 3.6.
Occupational Performance Profile[a]: M.L.

		Work			
		Vocation	Education	Home Management	Care of Others
SENSORIMOTOR	**SENSORY INTEGRATION** Decreased sensory awareness; unable to effectively process sensory input: hyper/hyporeactive		Won't sit at table & eat with peers; excessive self-stimulatory behaviors in classroom		
	NEURO-MUSCULAR Intact				
	MOTOR Intact				
COGNITIVE	**COGNITIVE** Very brief attention span to most activities; limited problem solving; difficulty learning new skills and concepts		Does not attend to structured classroom learning activities; wanders around classroom		
	PSYCHOLOGICAL Rarely initiates activities; lacks self-concept				
PSYCHOSOCIAL	**SOCIAL** Avoids contact with others; difficulty understanding verbal language; does not sustain eye contact; does not communicate with speech; unaware of other's feelings		Will not join small-group activities with peers		
	SELF-MANAGEMENT Becomes agitated and combative if changes in environment and/or needs are not met		Upset if unfamiliar people in classroom; occasionally violent, combative behavior		

(Left margin label spanning the performance component rows: **PERFORMANCE COMPONENTS**)

[a]Grid adapted from Uniform Terminology (2nd ed.). Developed by the occupational therapy faculty at Eastern Michigan University.

| Play/Leisure | | Activities of Daily Living | | | | |
Explora-tion	Perfor-mance	Self-Care	Social-ization	Functional Communi-cation	Functional Mobility	Sexual Expression
Reluctant to try new play activities	Limited rep-ertoire of play activities	Will eat only a few foods with only crunchy tex-ture; becomes agitated & combative when teeth are brushed				
	Does not en-gage in imagi-native play	Not toilet trained; needs assistance with most dressing, grooming, bathing; does not use eating utensils		Has not found alternative means of communicat-ing		
	Spends lim-ited time in play					
		Mother feels uncomfortable taking him out in public due to unpre-dictable and inappropriate behaviors				

Table 3.7.
Occupational Performance Profile[a]: L.N.

			Performance			
			Work Activities			
			Vocation	Education	Home Management	Care of Others
PERFORMANCE COMPONENTS	SENSORIMOTOR	**SENSORY INTEGRATION** Intact				
		NEURO-MUSCULAR Some primitive reflexes influencing movement; limited range of motion in left UE and both LEs; fluctuating muscle tone and spasticity present; limited endurance; decreased head & trunk control		Enrolled in courses at local community college; uses tape recorder for note taking; takes tests verbally; can turn pages of books independently	Dependent in clothing care, cleaning, & meal preparation & clean-up; can use Dustbuster; cares for cat; when shopping needs assistance with wallet; manages own money; dependent in household maintenance	
	COGNITIVE	**MOTOR** Nonambulatory; gross grasp in left UE; right UE used as an assist for bilateral activities; no grasp; dysarthria; difficulty chewing				
		COGNITIVE Intact				
	PSYCHOSOCIAL	**PSYCHOLOGICAL** Intact				
		SOCIAL Intact				
		SELF-MANAGEMENT Depressive episodes; emotional outbursts; frustrated when unable to get needs met				

EXTERNAL FACTORS WHICH INFLUENCE PERFORMANCE: CULTURE; ECONOMY; ENVIRONMENT

[a]Grid adapted from Uniform Terminology (2nd ed.). Developed by the occupational therapy faculty at Eastern Michigan University.

Client initials: L.N.
Diagnosis:
Age:

Areas						
Play or Leisure Activities		Activities of Daily Living				
Exploration	Performance	Self-Care	Socialization	Functional Communication	Functional Mobility	Sexual Expression
Varied interests	Avid reader, enjoys computer games and socializing with friends; participates in church retreats and field trips through local independent living center	Dependent in grooming, bathing, toilet hygiene, dressing; brushes own teeth; transfers self on/ off toilet; self-feeding or finger foods slow and messy; can't grasp eating utensils, usually fed by others; drinks from straw; takes own medications if set up for her		Uses computer for written communication; "Life Alert" emergency system in place; speaker telephone used for telephone communication; can use tape machine if set up; speech is difficult to understand; refuses to use Canon communicator	Can get self in and out of bed; difficulty using public restroom results in some incontinent episodes; needs assistance transferring to shower seat; uses public transportation	

set. M.L. is limited in his problem-solving ability. He has difficulty learning new skills and concepts, even with much repetition.

In psychosocial skills and psychological components, M.L. has deficits in all three areas. He has difficulty initiating activities. He spends much time aimlessly wandering around the room. M.L. avoids interacting with others, particularly unfamiliar persons. He makes only occasional, fleeting eye contact. He does not use speech to communicate but communicates nonverbally through gesturing, guiding the person to what he wants or becoming agitated to express displeasure. He cannot express his thoughts, feelings, and needs in appropriate ways but rather becomes frustrated and upset when trying to communicate. He becomes agitated and at times physically combative if what he wants is in conflict with environmental demands or constraints. He needs consistency in his environment, and he frequently becomes upset with changes in activity, physical space, or people. He is unaware of other people's feelings and has difficulty understanding or relating to what is said to him.

Each of the occupational performance areas are affected, as described in Table 3.6. In the area of work activities, he is too young to be involved in vocation, home maintenance, or care of others. For him, work consists of educational activities. At school, he is unaware of activities going on around him. He doesn't attend to structured learning activities. He generally wanders around the room and resists attempts to engage him in meaningful activities. M.L. does not participate in small-group activities. He is just beginning to be able to tolerate some direct physical and social contact with his classmates. He has recently begun to sit at the table during snack time, but he continues to refuse any food or drink while at school. He has difficulty with changes in his classroom (e.g., teacher leaving the room, stopping an activity he particularly enjoys, going to a different room), and at times he becomes combative.

In the play-leisure area, M.L. is reluctant to try new activities and has a limited repertoire of play activities. He spends proportionally little time engaged in play. He does not engage in imaginative or imitative play and does not play with other children.

In activities of daily living, M.L. has difficulty in self-care, socialization, and functional communication. He needs assistance with self-care activities such as grooming, dressing, and bathing. He is not toilet trained. He becomes agitated and combative when his parents attempt to brush his teeth, because of his sensitivity in the oral area. He will only eat foods with a crunchy texture, and of those only a few different types. He doesn't chew his food. He finger-feeds and can drink from a cup, but he does not use eating utensils.

In the area of socialization, he spends nearly all of his time away from school at home. His mother feels uncomfortable and embarrassed with him in public because of his unpredictable and inappropriate behavior. M.L. has not yet found any alternative means of communicating. He has begun to say ma-ma specifically, but that is his only meaningful language.

Cerebral Palsy

L.N. is a 64-year-old woman with cerebral palsy, spastic quadriplegia type. She has lived alone in an apartment complex for the elderly or disabled for the past 15 years. Before then she was in a nursing home. She supports herself on Supplemental Security Income and Disability payments from the state. A personal-care attendant, who the Department of Social Services provides, comes in each morning and evening to help with activities of daily living such as meal preparation, bathing, and dressing. L.N. has never been employed, but has done volunteer work. She writes articles for a local newsletter on her computer and has worked in her church's Sunday school. She has no family support but has many friends. She enjoys learning and taking classes and is currently enrolled in classes at a local community college. L.N. uses a motorized wheelchair with specialized seating for mobility and uses public transportation.

Table 3.7 lists the occupational performance components and areas that are affected by L.N.'s disability. Affected occupational performance components include neuromuscular, motor, and self-management. Spasticity, fluctuating tone, and primitive reflexes severely restrict L.N.'s functional movement. She has limited range of motion in her left upper extremity and both lower extremities. When reaching with the left arm, she cannot bring it to shoulder height or behind her back. She has a gross grasp in her right upper extremity and can grasp a joystick to operate her electric wheelchair. She cannot write or perform other activities requiring fine motor dexterity. Her left upper extremity is used as an assist for bilateral activities, with no grasping ability present. She can maintain an upright position in sitting, but her weight is shifted to the left (with resulting scoliosis). She can bring her head to an upright position, but neck flexion increases with activities requiring effort. Oral-motor muscles are affected, resulting in severe dysarthria, drooling, and difficulty eating. Endurance is a problem, and L.N. becomes easily fatigued.

In self-management, coping skills and self-control have been affected. L.N. went through depressive episodes when her father and mother died several years ago. She was treated for depression by a psychiatrist who prescribed Haldol. These episodes continue but are not as severe. L.N. becomes frustrated when unable to communicate her needs to others. At times, this leads to an emotional outburst.

All areas of occupational performance are affected. In the work category, L.N. is a student at a local community college. She uses a tape recorder for taking notes and takes examinations verbally.

In home management, L.N. is dependent in clothing care, cleaning her apartment, household maintenance, and meal preparation. She can use a hand-held portable vacuum cleaner for small cleanups. She has a cat that she cares for. She shops independently, but needs assistance getting money out of her wallet at the cash register.

In the leisure area, L.N. has varied interests. She is an avid reader and enjoys computer games. She socializes with friends frequently and enjoys going out into the community. She participates in church retreats and field trips through an independent living center.

All areas of activities of daily living are affected except socialization. In self-care, L.N. is dependent in grooming, bathing, toilet hygiene, and dressing. She brushes her teeth and can transfer on and off the toilet in her apartment with grab bars and the toilet seat at the proper height and position. She can feed herself with her fingers if the food is set up for her, but the process is slow and messy. She drinks from a straw. She takes her own medications if they are set out for her.

In functional communication, L.N. uses a computer for written communication. She uses a speaker phone for telephone communication and can use a tape machine if it is set up for her. If she falls or is in danger at home, she has an emergency alert system that she can activate. Her speech is difficult to understand. She has a Canon communicator but prefers not to use it.

In functional mobility, L.N. can get in and out of bed. Although at home she can transfer herself to and from the toilet, she has difficulty using public restrooms. This sometimes results in incontinent episodes. She needs assistance transferring to the shower seat she uses for bathing. She uses public transportation with no difficulty.

SUGGESTED READINGS

Behrman R, Vaughan V, eds. Nelson's textbook of pediatrics. 12th ed. Philadelphia: WB Saunders, 1992. Good medical reference for common and rare conditions found in childhood. Expensive, but available in reference section of most libraries.

Fraser B, Hensinger R, Phelps J. Physical management of multiple handicaps. A professional's guide. 2nd ed. Baltimore: Brookes Publishing, 1990. Valuable reference for those working with children and adults with severe physical or multiple impairments. Contains chapters on physical management and treatment; seating systems; therapeutic positioning and adaptive equipment; and activities of daily living.

Morris S, Klein M. Pre-feeding skills. Tuscon: Therapy Skill Builders, 1987. Excellent reference for oral motor and feeding therapy for children. Very thorough and good overall approach to feeding issues.

Pratt P, Allen A. Occupational therapy for children. 2nd ed. St. Louis: Mosby, 1989. Good overall reference for occupational therapy practice with children. Has separate chapters on treatment of children with cerebral palsy, mental retardation, and learning disabilities.

REFERENCES

1. Ehlers WH, Prothero JC, Langone J. Mental retardation and other developmental disabilities: a programmed introduction. 3rd ed. Columbus: Charles E. Merrill, 1982.
2. United States statutes at large containing the laws and current resolutions enacted during the second session of the 95th Congress of United States of America 1978. V.92. Part 3. Washington: U.S. Government Printing Office, 1980.
3. Edgerton R. Mental retardation. Cambridge, Massachusetts: Harvard University Press, 1979.
4. Shapiro B, Batshaw M. Mental and emotional disturbances: mental retardation. In: Gellis S, Kagan B, eds. Current pediatric therapy. Philadelphia: WB Saunders, 1986.
5. Rubin L, Crocker A. Developmental disabilities: delivery of medical care for children and adults. In: Developmental disabilities. Philadelphia: Lea & Febiger, 1989.
6. An evaluation and assessment of the state of the science: report of the Study Group on Mental Retardation and Developmental Disabilities. U.S. Department of Health and Human Services. Public Health Service. National Institutes of Health, Sep 1986.
7. Molnar G, ed. Pediatric rehabilitation. Baltimore: Williams & Wilkins, 1985.
8. Leck I. Causation of neural-tube defects: clues from epidemiology. Br Med Bull 1974;30:158.
9. Allum N. Spina bifida: the treatment and care of spina bifida children. London: George Allen & Unwin, 1975.
10. Smith D. Clinical diagnosis and nature of chromosomal abnormalities. In: Yunis J, ed. New chromosomal syndromes. New York: Academic Press, 1977.
11. Blackman J. Medical aspects of developmental disabilities in children birth to three. Iowa City: The University of Iowa, 1983.
12. Harris S, Tada W. Genetic disorders. In: Umphred D, ed. Neurological rehabilitation. St. Louis: CV Mosby, 1990.
13. Grossman H. Classifications in mental retardation. Washington D.C.: American Association on Mental Deficiency, 1983.
14. Bax M. Terminology and classification of cerebral palsy. Dev Med Child Neurol 1964;6:295–297.

15. Taft L. Mental retardation. In: Behrman R, Vaughan V, eds. Nelson's textbook of pediatrics, 12th ed. Philadelphia: WB Saunders, 1992.

16. Berkow R, Fletcher A, eds. The Merck manual of diagnosis and therapy. 15th ed. Rahway: Merck Sharp & Dohme Research Laboratories, 1987:2110.

17. American Occupational Therapy Association. "1990 Member Data Survey Summary Report." OT Week, vol 5, no 22.

18. Kaplan H, Sadock B. Clinical psychiatry. Baltimore: Williams & Wilkins, 1988:393.

19. La Plante M. Data on disability from the national health interview survey, 1983–1985. In: Chartbook on disability in the United States. National Institute on Disability and Rehabilitation Research. Washington D.C.: U.S. Department of Education, 1989.

20. Brody J. Research sheds new light on causes of cerebral palsy. In: the Ann Arbor News. Dec 28, 1989:D3.

21. Lefkofsky S. Introduction to cerebral palsy. Detroit: Wayne State University School of Medicine. 1973.

22. Researchers find asphyxia not responsible for most CP. In O.T. Week, Sep 22, 1988:2.

23. Avery ME, First LR, eds. Pediatric medicine. Baltimore: Williams & Wilkins 1989:1298.

24. Bobath K. A neurological basis for the treatment of cerebral palsy. Philadelphia: JB Lippincott, 1980.

25. Hiles D, Wallar P, McFarlane F. Current concepts in the management of strabismus in children with cerebral palsy. Ann Opthalmol 1975;7:789.

26. Sparrow S, et al. Vineland adaptive behavior scales, interview edition, survey form manual. Circle Pines, MN: American Guidance Service, 1984.

27. Gadow K, Poling A. Pharmacotherapy and mental retardation. Boston: Little, Brown & Co, 1988.

Glossary

Areflexia: Absence of the reflexes.

Ataxia: Incoordination occurring in the absence of apraxia, paresis, rigidity, spasticity, or involuntary movement manifested when voluntary muscular movements are attempted. In posterior column damage of the spinal cord, there is a loss of proprioception and incoordination due to misjudgment of limb position with balance problems. Cerebellar ataxia produces a reeling, wide-based gait in an individual.

Athetoid: Resembling athetosis or repetitive involuntary, slow, sinuous, writhing movements. Classification of cerebral palsy in which involuntary purposeless movement occurs when an individual attempts purposeful motion. The abnormal movements may occur not only in the limb being moved but may also involve an "overflow" of activity to all the other limbs with an exaggeration of reflexes.

Atonia: Absence or lack of normal muscle tone.

Acquired immune deficiency syndrome (AIDS): A disease caused by immunologic action of one's own cells or antibodies on components of the body.

Autosomal: Pertaining to any of the 22 pairs of chromosomes in man not concerned with determination of sex.

Recessive gene: One that produces an effect in the organism when it is transmitted by both parents. Dominant gene: One that produces an effect in an organism regardless of the state of the corresponding allele (e.g., brown eye color)

Ballismus: Violent flinging movements of the limbs, sometimes affecting only one side of the body (hemiballismus).

Chorea: The ceaseless occurrence of rapid, jerky involuntary movements such as seen in Huntington's or Sydenham's disease.

Chromosome: In animal cells, a structure in the nucleus, containing a linear thread of DNA, which transmits genetic information and is associated with RNA and histones.

Clonus: Alternate involuntary muscular contraction and relaxation in rapid succession.

Conduction: Conveyance of energy, as of sound.

Contracture: Abnormal shortening of muscle tissue, rendering the muscle highly resistant to stretching that can lead to permanent disability. In many cases contractures can be prevented by range-of-motion exercises (active or passive) and by adequate support of the joints to eliminate constant shortening or stretching of the muscles and surrounding tissue.

Constructional dyspraxia (apraxia): A failure to produce or replicate a specific design or object from parts in two or three dimensions, either drawings or block designs. The failure may manifest spontaneously, upon command, or by copying.

Deep tendon reflexes: A reflected action or movement (reflex) elicited by a sharp tap on the appropriate tendon to induce brief stretch of the muscle.

Diplegia: Paralysis of like parts on either side of the body. In cerebral palsy, diplegia describes involvement of the lower extremities predominantly, with only mildly affected upper extremities.

Duchenne's muscular dystrophy: One of a group of genetically determined, painless, degenerative myopathies that are progressive, as the muscles gradually weaken and eventually atrophy. Duchenne's type affects children and is not detected until age 2 or 3. It is also called pseudohypertrophic muscular dystrophy because at the beginning, the muscles (especially those in the calves) appear healthy and bulging when actually they are already weakened and their size is due to excess fat.

Dysdiadochokinesia: An impaired ability to accomplish repeated alternating movements rapidly and smoothly, e.g., sequential alternating movements like pronation and supination of the forearm.

Dyskinesia: Impairment of the power of voluntary movement.

Dyspraxia: A partial loss of ability to perform coordinated movements.

Embryo: A new organism in the earliest stage of development; the human young from the time of fertilization of the ovum until the beginning of the third month. After the second month the unborn baby is usually referred to as the fetus.

Encephalitis: Inflammation of the brain.

Enuresis: Involuntary discharge of urine, usually referring to involuntary discharge of urine during sleep at night; bed-wetting beyond the age when bladder control should have been achieved.

Equilibrium reactions: Balance in developmental positions is achieved by these reactions in which the postural muscles contract to maintain or regain an upright position during walking, standing, or sitting.

Equinovalgus (talipes equinovalgus): A foot deformity in which the heel is abducted (turned outward) and everted and the foot is plantar flexed.

Equinovarus (talipes equinovarus): A foot deformity in which the heel is adducted (turned inward) and inverted and the foot is plantar flexed.

Flaccid: Paralysis of muscles in which there is an absence of reflexes (in lower motor neuron disorders such as poliomyelitis). Flaccidity (hypotonus): Abnormal muscle tone felt as too little resistance to movement. Also called hypotonus.

Gene: The basic unit of heredity. Each gene occupies a certain location on a chromosome. Hereditary traits are controlled by pairs of genes in the same position on a pair of chromosomes.

Genetic aberrations: Deviations within the information system in living cells, the genetic code that determines the amino acid sequence of polypeptides, causing hereditary abnormalities.

Grand mal seizures: A type of epilepsy (recurrent paroxysmal disorder of cerebral function characterized by sudden, brief attack of altered consciousness, motor activity, or sensory phenomena) that is generalized and affects the entire brain. The seizure proceeds with loss of consciousness; falling; and tonic then clonic contractions of the muscles. The attack usually lasts 2 to 5 minutes.

Graphomotor: Pertaining to movements involved in writing.

Hearing loss: Conductive: Defects in the auditory system which interfere with sound waves reaching the cochlea. Locus of lesion is usually in the outer or middle ear (e.g., external auditory meatus, tympanic membrane, auditory (eustachian) tube, auditory ossicles). Sensorineural: Defects to the auditory pathways within the central nervous system, beginning with the cochlea and auditory nerve and including the brain stem and cerebral cortex. Mixed: Both conductive and sensorineural defects.

Hemiparesis: Paresis or weakness affecting one side of the body.

Hemianopsia (hemianopia): Defective vision or blindness in one-half the visual field, usually applied to bilateral defects caused by a single lesion, often as a result of CVA. The individual is unable to perceive objects to the side of the visual midline. The visual loss is contralateral (i.e., it is on the side opposite of the brain lesion). Homonymous hemianopsia: Both visual fields, either the right halves or left halves, are defective on the same side.

Hurler syndrome: The prototypic form of mucopolysaccharidosis, with gargoyle-like facies, dwarfism, severe somatic and skeletal changes, severe mental retardation, cloudy corneas, deafness, cardiovascular defects, hepatosplenomegaly, and joint contractures. It is due to an enzyme deficiency and is transmitted as an autosomal recessive trait

Hyperreflexia: Exaggeration of reflexes during standard stretch of a muscle

Hypertonicity (spasticity): Abnormal muscle tone felt as too much resistance to movement as a result of hyperactive reflexes and loss of inhibiting influences from higher brain centers. Spastic: Clonus or rapid series of rhythmic contractions during quick stretch of a muscle caused by abnormally increased tension

Hypotonicity: See flaccid

Hypoxia: A broad term meaning diminished availability of oxygen to the body tissues with many and varied causes

Intrauterine: Within the uterus

Kyphosis: Abnormally increased convexity in the curvature of the thoracic spine viewed from the side, resulting from an acquired disease, an injury, or a congenital disorder or disease

Lordosis: Forward curvature of the lumbar spine

Meconium: Dark green mucilaginous material in the intestine of the full-term fetus; it constitutes the first stools passed by the newborn infant

Meningitis: Inflammation of the meninges

Myelodysplasia: Neural tube defect of the spinal cord, referred to as spina bifida

Nystagmus (nystaxis): Involuntary, rapid, rhythmic movement (horizontal, vertical, rotatory, or mixed, i.e. two types) of the eyeball

Orthotic: Pertaining to the use or application of an orthosis. Orthosis: An orthopaedic appliance or apparatus used to support, align, prevent, or correct deformities or to improve function of movable parts of the body

Orthotist: A person skilled in orthotics and practicing its application

Overflow: See athetosis

Phenylketonuria (PKU): A congenital disease due to a defect in the metabolism of the amino acid phenylalanine. The condition is hereditary and transmitted recessively through apparently healthy parents who, if tested, will show signs of the disease. It results from lack of an enzyme, phenylalanine hydroxylase, necessary for the conversion of the amino acid phenylalanine into tyrosine. If untreated, the condition results in mental retardation and other abnormalities

Physiatrist: A physician who specializes in physiatrics, that branch of medicine using physical therapy, physical agents such as light, heat, water, and electricity, and mechanical apparatus, in the diagnosis, prevention, and treatment of bodily disorders

Placental insufficiency: The major function of the placenta is to allow diffusion of nutrients from the mother's blood into the fetus's blood and diffusion of waste products from the fetus back to the mother. This two-way process takes place across the placental membrane, which is semipermeable; that is, it acts as a selective filter, allowing some materials to pass through and holding back others. A problem with the placenta can create a deficiency such as low birth weight due to inadequate nutrition

Placenta previa: Low implantation of the placenta so that it partially or completely covers the cervical os (orifice). The condition is more frequent in women who have had multiple pregnancies or are over 35. When the cervix begins to dilate at the onset of labor and the upper and lower uterine segments differentiate, the placenta is stretched and pulled from the uterine wall, producing bleeding. The life of the fetus is in jeopardy because of anoxia resulting from separation of the placenta from its blood supply. If the bleeding continues, the life of the mother is also at risk

Reflex: The total of any particular stereotyped, automatic response mediated by the nervous system. A reflex is built into the nervous system and does not need conscious thought to take effect. Reflex responses to stimuli begin to develop in fetal life and continue to be clearly apparent in motor behavior in early infancy. In adults, they become apparent in motor behavior as a result of stress and/or fatigue. Reflex motor patterns continue to underlie the organized voluntary movements used in daily activities and sports. Primitive reflexes: Innate primary reactions found in newborns and indicative of severe brain damage if present beyond their usual time of disappearance. Adult patients with closed head injury or stroke may manifest these signs; absence on reevaluation is a sign of progress in recovery. Examples include placing reactions, Moro reflex, grasp reflex, rooting reflex, and sucking reflex

Psychotropic: Exerting an effect on the mind; capable of modifying mental activity; a drug that affects the mental state. There are several classes of psychotropic drugs such as antidepressants, lithium, neuroleptics (major tranquilizers), and antianxiety agents (minor tranquilizers)

Quadriparesis: Partial or incomplete paralysis of all four extremities

Rh factor: Genetically determined antigens present on the surface of erythrocytes (red blood cells). Presence or absence of Rh factor is especially important in pregnancies. If the mother is Rh negative and the fetus is Rh positive, the Rh antigens in the fetal tissues diffuse through the placental membrane and enter the mother's blood. Her body reacts by forming anti-Rh agglutinins, which diffuse back through the placental membrane into the fetal circulation and cause clumping of the fetal erythrocytes. This is known as Rh incompatibility

Righting reactions: Response to stimuli in which an active righting movement brings the head and body into a normal relationship with each other in space; ability to assume an optimal position when there has been a departure from it

Rigidity: Difficulties initiating movement and slow performance of active movements as well as increased resistance to passive movements due to increased muscle tone. There are different types of rigidity, including cogwheel seen in Parkinson's disease and clasp-knife rigidity seen in upper motor neuron diseases

Strabismus: Deviation of the eye in which the visual axes assume a position relative to each other different from that required by the physiological conditions; also called squint

Stretch reflex: Reflex contraction of a muscle in response to passive longitudinal stretching

Subluxation: Incomplete or partial dislocation. Shoulder subluxation at the glenohumeral joint is commonly seen following a stroke or can be caused by a contracture

Tay-Sach's disease: The hereditary infantile form of a progressive disorder marked by degeneration of brain tissue and the maculas (with the formation of a cherry-red spot on both retinas) and by dementia, blindness, and death. This disease is a sphingolipidosis in which the inborn error of metabolism is an enzyme deficiency that results in accumulation of gangliosides in the brain.

Diagnostic Tests

Medical tests
Laboratory tests
   Chromosomal karyotype
   Aminoaciduria
   Urinary mucopolysaccharides
   Urinary reducing substances
   Urinary ketoacids
   Blood lead level
   Serum uric acid
   Serum ammonia
   Serum neuroenzymes
   Skin histamine test
CT scan
Muscle biopsy
EEG
EMG
Intelligence tests
Stanford-Binet
Wechsler intelligence scales
Peabody vocabulary test
Kullman-Binet

Adaptive behavior scales
Note: there are over 100 of these but these are most often used

Adaptive behavior inventory for children
Adaptive behavior scale—public school version
Vineland adaptive behavior scales
American Association of Mental Deficiency adaptive behavior scales

Medications

Brand Name	Generic
Stimulants	
Ritalin	Methylphenidate
Dexedrine	Dextroamphetamine
Antidepressants	
Elavil	Amitriptyline
Tofranil	Imipramine
	Desipramine
Antianxiety	
Valium	Diazepam
Antipsychotics	
Thorazine	Chlorpromazine
Haldol	Haloperidol
Navane	Thiothixene
Stelazine	Trifluoperazine
	Lithium bicarbonate
Antiepileptics	
Depakene	Clonazepam
Dilantin	Valproic acid
Tegretol	Phenytoin
Zarontin	Phenobarbital
	Primidone
	Carbamazepine
	Ethosuximide
Others	
Inderal	Propranolol
Pondimin	Fenfluramine
Narcan	Naloxone
	hydrochloride

4

Hand Injuries

JOANNE PHILLIPS ESTES

The hand is one of the most important organs of the human body. It is vital to human function. The hand implements desires of the human brain (1). It is responsible for carrying out many functional activities. It is used for prehension and manipulation of objects. Most importantly, though, our hands allow us to explore and control our environment.

The hand's tactile sensibility (ability to feel) is very important to function. It ranks with the human eye as a prime mechanism for sensory perception (2). The hand is also used for communication. We express ourselves nonverbally and give comfort to others with our hands. Finally, the hand has aesthetic value. It is critical to our self-image. "In some respects, disfigurement of the hand has more emotional impact than disfigurement of the face, since one sees his own face only in the mirror but constantly views his own hands" (2). To summarize, the hand is vitally essential to the performance of all areas of occupational performance.

Function of the hand depends on the smooth performance of several anatomical systems, including the integumentary (skin), vasculature, muscular (including tendons), skeletal, and nervous systems. Depending on the system(s) involved, a patient can have different problems. It is not unusual for trauma to the hand to involve most or all of the above systems simultaneously. One must understand normal function and interactions of each

system as well as principles and stages of healing. The three categories of injuries discussed here are upper extremity wrist fracture (Colles' fracture), hand flexor tendon repair, and upper extremity peripheral nerve repair.

ETIOLOGY

The hand is vulnerable to direct injury and trauma. It is exposed to more injuries because it is used for most functional activities and because it is at the end of an appendage. Dysfunction can also be due to disease or congenital anomalies. Both cause disruption of one or more of the above systems. However, injury is the greatest cause of functional impairment in the hand (2). Hand injuries are often caused by industrial, household, or leisure accidents.

Bone fractures occur as the result of direct trauma (1). Colles' fracture is a fracture of the distal radius bone, most commonly caused by falling on an outstretched hand (3) (Fig. 4.1).

Severed tendons result from a laceration. The sharp object can be a knife blade, broken glass, or tin can. Tendon lacerations can occur in conjunction with other injuries. Crush injuries and fractures may also sever a tendon.

Nerve injuries can be caused by severe blunt trauma or stretch injuries (see Neuropraxia and Axonotmesis in Appendix 4.1). Complete nerve severance can result from

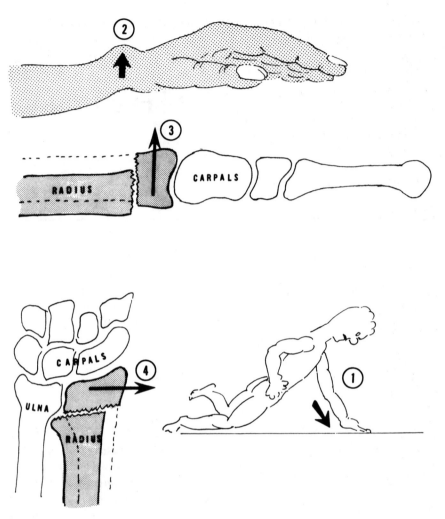

Figure 4.1. Colles' fracture. (1) Fracture usually occurs from a fall upon the outstretched hand. (2) The typical "dinner fork" or "silver-fork" deformity is noted. (3) The distal fragment is displaced backward (dorsally) and (4) outward (radially). (Reprinted with permission from Caillet R. Hand pain and impairment. 3rd ed. Philadelphia: FA Davis, 1982:138.)

an accident, crush injury, or violent incident. Nerve injuries can also occur in conjunction with fractures and tendon injuries.

INCIDENCE/PREVALENCE

Upper extremity injuries account for one-third of all injuries (4). Again, injuries result from home, leisure, or vocational activity accidents or trauma. Approximately the same number of injuries occur in the home as in industry or on the farm. The injuries sustained at home, however, are generally less severe (2).

Those most prone to upper extremity injury are young, productive individuals (2). In the United States in 1979, upper extremity injuries "collectively accounted for about 95 million days of restricted activity and 16 million days of absence from work" (2). Hand injuries are responsible for more lost days from work than any other kind of occupational injury (5). These injuries have a significant impact on the national economy. In 1987, hand injuries cost our economy 42.4 billion dollars in wages, medical expenses, and insurance administration (5).

The Colles' fracture is the most common wrist fracture (6), and it occurs most often in people over the age of 50. Females are more likely to sustain this injury than males, due to weakened, osteoporotic bones (6).

SIGNS/SYMPTOMS

Colles' Fracture

The clinical signs of a Colles' fracture are structural breaks in the continuity of the radius as shown in radiographic (x-ray) studies. There is also swelling in the affected limb. The examiner will observe gross angular or rotational deformities of the fractured bone. These deformities of the radius are "displacement backwards, tilt backwards, and tilt in a radial direction" (8). The ulnar styloid is also usually (but not always) avulsed.

These deformities give the appearance of an upside down dinner fork. Thus, it is called a "dinner fork" deformity (Fig. 4.1) (5). The examiner can move the fracture fragments upon palpation. If there is a break in the skin at the fracture site, it is termed an open fracture. If not, it is a closed fracture.

A fracture has two symptoms. The patient will complain of localized tenderness at the fracture site and experience a sharp, piercing pain in the area of the fractured bone.

Flexor Tendon Repair

The primary sign of a severed flexor tendon is lack of active flexion. The actions of each tendon are tested individually by having the patient perform isolated finger flexion movements.

Flexor tendon injuries can be observed in the resting hand. The normal posture of a resting hand is forearm supination, wrist extension, and digits flexed at all joints. The degree of flexion increases from index finger to little finger. When a flexor tendon is cut, the involved digits distal to the cut are extended when the upper extremity is placed in the above-described resting position (7).

Peripheral Nerve Injury

A severed nerve results in loss of motor and sensory function to areas innervated by that nerve. The losses occur distal to the site of nerve lacerations. See Table 4.1 for motor and sensory distribution of the median, radial, and ulnar nerves in the hand. Loss of nerve function also results in dry skin in the area of nerve distribution. This is due to loss of the sudomotor response of sweating, since sympathetic nerves travel in the arm with sensory nerves.

PROGNOSIS/PROGRESSION

Because of advanced microsurgical techniques, the prognosis/progression of return of function is changing. Surgeons are creating new techniques and thus saving limbs that previously might have been amputated. The prognosis or progression of an upper extremity or hand injury depends on many factors. The ultimate goal of medical and therapeutic management is to restore maximum functional use of the involved extremity. Factors that can influence the healing process (and ultimately the prognosis) include type, severity, and location of injury or complications in the healing process. The prognosis of Colles' fracture, flexor tendon repair, and peripheral nerve repair are discussed individually below.

Colles' Fracture

The prognosis for a Colles' fracture is determined by the quality of the healing process. Healing begins immediately after the fracture occurs. In adults, union of a fracture takes approximately 3 to 4 months (3). Plentiful blood supply and immobilization with a plaster cast can facilitate union. The cast typically extends from the forearm to (but not including) the metacarpal heads (5).

Table 4.1.
Nerve Distribution in the Hand

	Sensory Loss	Motor Loss
MEDIAN NERVE	Thenar eminence	Weakness of wrist flexors
	Palmar thumb Palmar surface of radial two and one-half digits	Lack of thumb flexion and opposition Lack of index and middle digit flexion Poor pinch
RADIAL NERVE	Radial border dorsum of hand (thumb, proximal two-thirds of first two and one-half digits	Wrist drop Lack of finger and thumb extension

ULNAR NERVE	Palmar ulnar one and one-half digits
	Dorsal ulnar one and one-half digits
		Loss of ulnar wrist flexion
		"Claw hand" deformity:
		    Hyperextension of MCP ring and little fingers
		    PIP flexion of ring and little fingers
		Inability to hold paper between thumb and index finger
		Weakness in finger spreading

Most Colles' fractures are stable enough for cast removal after 6 to 8 weeks (2). At this time, clinical union has occurred. Clinical union occurs when, upon examination, there is no pain or movement of the fracture pieces. The cast is replaced with a protective removable wrist brace or splint, and the splint is worn for an additional 6 to 8 weeks.

Abnormal healing can occur. There are three types of abnormal healing: malunion, delayed union, and nonunion. In a malunion, fracture healing has occurred at the normal time but in an unsatisfactory position. A delayed union fracture eventually heals but takes a considerably longer time to do so. A nonunion occurs when a fracture fails to completely heal by bony union. Causes of abnormal healing include open fractures, fractures separated by soft tissue interposition, or poor blood supply (6).

The goal of Colles' fracture management is to restore functional use of the involved extremity. Complications such as infection from open fractures or following surgery can impede the healing process and prognosis. It can also cause osteo-

myelitis and may lead to loss of limb function or loss of limb (6). Vascular damage from the injury or fracture fragments can lead to hemorrhaging and place the patient's life and limb in danger (6). Neurological complications can occur from a compressed median nerve during healing. This produces a carpal tunnel syndrome (see Appendix 4.1).

Sudeck's atrophy or osteodystrophy is a late-occurring complication found particularly following a Colles' fracture. The cause and nature of this condition are ill-understood, and incidence is low (3). Reflex sympathetic dystrophy (RSD), another potentially disabling complication, causes eventual atrophy of tissues with joint contractures, chronic edema, and fibrosis (6).

In general, during healing of a Colles' fracture, a patient experiences decreased functional use of the involved extremity. Specifically, edema and decreased range of motion (ROM) (especially in the wrist), strength, and grip are noted. Disuse of the hand because of any of the above complications can result in pain, stiffness, and decreased strength or ROM of the fingers, wrist, forearm, elbow, and shoulder. Twenty percent of Colles' fracture patients have residual symptoms, and 10% have significant functional impairment (9).

Flexor Tendon Repair

Flexor tendons must be able to glide within their sheaths to function efficiently. The flexor tendon sheath is a fibrous tunnel. It is synovium-lined and produces synovial fluid, which helps the tendon glide smoothly and assists with tendon nutrition and healing.

The goal following tendon repair is normal hand function. If this is to occur, there must be no adhesion formation within the tendon sheath (8). Adhesion formation prevents free, gliding movement. "Fixed adhesions preventing gliding are the major problem with tendon repairs" (2).

The actual prognosis for functional return depends on the location of tendon laceration. Tendons repaired in the forearm or dorsal hand usually function well (2). Laceration of a hand flexor tendon is a serious injury. Some type of permanent disability usually follows this injury (7).

For classification purposes, the hand is divided into five zones (Fig. 4.2). Zone II

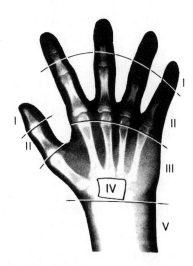

Figure 4.2. Hand flexor tendon zones. (Reprinted with permission from Ariyan S. The hand book. 1st ed. New York: McGraw-Hill, 1989:146.

is called "no man's land." Tendon lacerations here have the poorest prognosis for functional return because of the anatomical structures in this area. Here the tendons lie in their sheaths beneath a tendon fibrous pulley system, and any scarring will cause adhesions (4). Also, following suturing, a tendon usually swells. This area has no room for expansion, and ischemic necrosis occurs (5). Postoperative management aimed at minimizing adhesion formation is critical for optimal functional return.

In general, flexor tendon lacerations in the other zones have a more favorable prognosis for functional recovery, because structures around these tendons are less complex and the areas are not as prone to scarring.

Peripheral Nerve Repair

Peripheral nerve injury prognosis depends on the type of injury. In order to understand the three types of injury, one must understand the structural anatomy of a nerve (Fig. 4.3). A neurapraxia is a nerve injury with no physical disruption of axons (2). This type of injury usually results from a contusion. The nerve is intact, but conduction is impaired. This injury has the best prognosis. Full recovery is expected. It can occur within several days and is usually complete in 3 months.

An axonotmesis is a moderate injury. Here the axon and myelin sheath are damaged. The endoneurial tubes remain intact. These provide the axons with tubes where they can regrow. Patients experience loss of motor and sensory function. Recovery is expected to be complete, but it will take longer than a neurapraxia.

The third, and most serious, type of nerve injury is a neurotmesis. Here there is a complete laceration of the nerve, which is divided and must be surgically repaired. Recovery from this injury depends on "precise surgical approximation of proximal-to-distal segments, providing the regenerating axons with appropriate neural tubes leading to their end organs" (2).

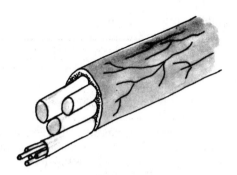

Figure 4.3. Parts of a peripheral nerve. "Individual axons are enclosed by an endoneurium. These units bunched together form fasciculi (or funiculi) and are covered by perineurium. These fasciculi bunched together form the nerve, which is covered by an epineurium" (11). (Reprinted with permission from Ariyan, S. The hand book. 1st ed. New York: McGraw-Hill, 1989:172.

Recovery from a severed nerve is never complete (2). A major influencing factor is the precision with which the axons were realigned. "Never can alignment be so perfect that all axons enter their own awaiting Schwann tubes, and remyelination is also imperfect" (2). The more distal (farther away from its brachial plexus origin) the lesion, however, the better the prognosis.

It is difficult to predict the degree of recovery following a nerve repair. In general, a patient can expect to have functional power in muscles innervated by repaired nerves. However, their strength will be less than normal.

Sensory recovery can be expected to be greater than the protective level (2). If there is not much evidence of sensory return in the first few months, the ultimate prognosis for return is poor (2). A good prognosis, however, is indicated when progressive recovery of sensibility occurs in the first few months. In this case, sensory recovery will not reach a plateau for 4 to 5 years (2).

If the nerve takes a long time to heal (i.e., the injury is very proximal or close to its brachial plexus origin), other problems may arise. Muscles will atrophy and scarring will take place in the interval (10). This muscle wasting spreads rapidly after

2 months and is maximal after 3 months (5). In this case, a poor prognosis is due not to failure of the nerve repair but rather to disuse of noninjured structures during the recovery period. Nevertheless, impaired functional use of the involved extremity is the result.

DIAGNOSTICS

A physician performs a systematic evaluation of the upper extremity to diagnose structural injury. Radiographic studies (x-rays) show fractured bones. Electromyographic (EMG) studies show motor nerve function. Manual muscle tests (MMT) and ROM evaluations also test extent of motor nerve function. A Froment's sign test indicates nerve function for thumb adduction. Weber's two-point discrimination test, Phalen's test, and Tinel's sign can be used to determine sensory function. Finally, one is able to diagnose lacerated flexor tendons with observation of the position of a resting hand (i.e., when a flexor tendon is completely lacerated the digit rests in extension (1)). See Appendix 4.2 for further explanation of the above diagnostic tools.

MEDICATION

Following an upper extremity injury, the primary medication is for pain relief. This can consists of nonprescriptive analgesics such as aspirin or Tylenol. Prescriptive narcotic pain relievers may also be given for relief of more severe pain. Common narcotic pain relievers are Tylenol-3 or Percocet. See Appendix 4.3 for a listing of pain-relief medication.

IMPACT ON OCCUPATIONAL PERFORMANCE

The function of several performance components may be compromised by a hand injury. A patient with a hand injury has impairment that varies from minimal to absent. Degree of impairment depends on severity of the injury as well as the anatomical structures involved (Table 4.2).

Table 4.2.
Occupational Performance Components—Hand Injury

Sensory Motor Component	Cognitive Integration & Cognitive Components	Psychosocial Skills & Psychologic Components

1. **Sensory integration**
  a. Sensory awareness
  b. **Sensory processing**
    1. **Tactile**
    2. Proprioceptive
    3. Vestibular
    4. Visual
    5. Auditory
    6. Gustatory
    7. Olfactory
  c. **Perceptual skills**
    1. Stereognosis
    2. **Kinesthesia**
    3. Body scheme
    4. Right-left discrimination
    5. Form constancy
    6. Position in space
    7. Visual-closure
    8. Figure ground
    9. Depth perception
    10. Topographic orientation
	1. Level of arousal
	2. Orientation
	3. Recognition
	4. **Attention span**
	5. Memory
	  a. Short-term
	  b. Long-term
	  c. Remote
	  d. Recent
	6. Sequencing
	7. Categorization
	8. Concept formation
	9. Intellectual operations in space
	10. Problem solving
	11. Generalization of learning
	12. Integration of learning
	13. Synthesis of learning
		1. **Psychologic**
		  a. **Roles**
		  b. **Values**
		  c. **Interests**
		  d. **Initiation of activity**
		  e. Termination of activity
		  f. **Self-concept**
		2. **Social**
		  a. **Social conduct**
		  b. **Conversation**
		  c. **Self-expression**
		3. **Self-management**
		  a. **Coping skills**
		  b. **Time management**
		  c. **Self-control**

2. **Neuromuscular**
  a. Reflex
  b. **Range of motion**
  c. **Muscle tone**
  d. **Strength**
  e. **Endurance**
  f. Postural control
  g. **Soft tissue integrity**		

3. **Motor**
  a. **Activity tolerance**
  b. Gross motor coordination
  c. Crossing the midline
  d. Laterality
  e. Bilateral integration
  f. Praxis
  g. **Fine motor coordination**
  h. Visual-motor integration
  i. Oral-motor control
	Note: All occupational performance areas can potentially be affected.	

Table 4.2. (Continued)

Occupational Performance Areas

Activities of Daily Living	Work Activities	Play/Leisure Activities

1. Grooming
2. Oral hygiene
3. Bathing
4. Toilet hygiene
5. Dressing
6. Feeding and eating
7. Medication routine
8. Socialization
9. Functional communication
10. Functional mobility
11. Sexual expression
	1. Home management
	  a. Clothing care
	  b. Cleaning
	  c. Meal preparation and cleanup
	  d. Shopping
	  e. Money management
	  f. Household maintenance
	  g. Safety procedures
	2. Care of others
	3. Educational activities
	4. Vocational activities
	  a. Vocational exploration
	  b. Job acquisition
	  c. Work or job performance
	  d. Retirement planning
		1. Play or leisure exploration
		2. Play or leisure performance

The major performance component compromised in a hand injury is sensory motor. If a peripheral nerve is involved, tactile function (light touch, pressure, temperature, pain, or two-point stimuli) will be impaired. In all hand injuries, neuromuscular and motor components are primary areas affected. Diminished function in these areas could be the result of direct injury to a structure (e.g., muscle). Diminished neuromuscular and motor function of noninvolved structures on an injured extremity also could result from disuse of that extremity.

One's psychosocial skill and psychologic components may also be affected by a UE injury. Severe injuries may result in mangled appearances and diminished function, which can impair one's self-concept. Self-expression may be compromised if one cannot use the hand in conversation. Finally, a patient may be unable to implement previous coping skills or develop new ones, especially if physical activity is used as a coping technique.

The degree to which occupational performance is affected after a hand injury depends on many variables including age, sex, and home situation. Hand dominance is also a variable. The injury will certainly have a more detrimental influence on function if the dominant extremity is involved. Finally, the severity and type of injury also determines the extent to which occupational performance is affected. A hand injury causes potential dysfunction in all three occupational performance areas (work, play, and ADL).

Two case studies describe the impact of an upper extremity injury upon two very different individuals.

CASE STUDIES

Colles' Fracture

B.T. is a 65-year-old female who sustained a right upper extremity Colles' fracture after falling on ice. Her fracture was reduced (i.e., fracture fragments manipulated and realigned) and forearm and wrist casted. One week after casting, she complained of stiffness, swelling, pain, and decreased movement in her right hand.

B.T. is a widow who lives alone. She has a son and daughter who live in the area but work outside the home and are very busy with their own young children. Prior to her accident, she was independent. She

Table 4.3.
Occupational Performance Components—Colles' Fracture Case Study[a]

Sensory Motor Component	Cognitive Integration & Cognitive Components	Psychosocial Skills & Psychologic Components
1. Sensory integration	1. Level of arousal	1. Psychologic
a. Sensory awareness	2. Orientation	***a. Roles**
b. Sensory processing	3. Recognition	b. Values
*1. Tactile	4. Attention span	c. Interests
2- Proprioceptive	5. Memory	d. Initiation of activity
3. Vestibular	a. Short-term	e. Termination of activity
*4. Visual	b. Long-term	***f. Self-concept**
5. Auditory	c. Remote	2. Social
6. Gustatory	d. Recent	a. Social conduct
7. Olfactory	6. Sequencing	b. Conversation
c. Perceptual skills	7. Categorization	c. Self-expression
1. Stereognosis	8. Concept formation	3. Self-management
2. Kinesthesia	9. Intellectual operations in space	***a. Coping skills**
3. Body scheme	10. Problem solving	b. Time management
4. Right-left discrimination	11. Generalization of learning	c. Self-control
5. Form constancy	12. Integration of learning	
6. Position in space	13. Synthesis of learning	
7. Visual-closure		
8. Figure ground		
9. Depth perception		
10. Topographic orientation		
2. Neuromuscular		
a. Reflex		
b. Range of motion		
*c. Muscle tone		
*d. Strength		
*e. Endurance		
*f. Postural control		
*g. Soft tissue integrity		
3. Motor		
*a. Activity tolerance		
*b. Gross motor coordination		
*c. Crossing the midline		
d. Laterality		
e. Bilateral integration		
f. Praxis		
*g. Fine motor coordination		
h. Visual-motor integration		
*i. Oral-motor control		

Table 4.3.   (Continued)

Occupational Performance Areas

Activities of Daily Living	Work Activities	Play/Leisure Activities

1. Grooming
2. Oral hygiene
*3. **Bathing**
*4. **Toilet hygiene**
*5. **Dressing**
6. Feeding and eating
7. Medication routine
8. Socialization
9. Functional communication
*10. **Functional mobility**
11. Sexual expression
	1. Home management
	*a. **Clothing care**
	*b. **Cleaning**
	*c. **Meal preparation and cleanup**
	*d. **Shopping**
	e. Money management
	*f. **Household maintenance**
	g. Safety procedures
	*2. **Care of others**
	3. Educational activities
	4. Vocational activities
	   a. Vocational exploration
	   b. Job acquisition
	  *c. **Work or job performance**
	   d. Retirement planning
		*1. **Play or leisure exploration**
		*2. **Play or leisure performance**

performed her ADL and home-management activities independently. B.T.'s leisure activities consisted of going to church and associated church activities, playing bridge, doing volunteer work at the local hospital, needlecraft activities, and gardening. Often she baby-sat her young school-age grandchildren, as she enjoyed their company. She drove herself to her activities.

Several occupational performance components are affected by B.T.'s injury. (See Table 4.3 for a chart of B.T.'s occupational performance deficit profile.) She displays deficits in neuromuscular control as well as motor function. Her activity tolerance is approximately 3 minutes for those activities that involve right upper extremity only. She further reports that pain, tenderness, and stiffness in her wrist and hand prevent her from using that arm functionally. B.T. uses her right upper extremity for light stability only.

B.T. has difficulties in psychosocial/psychologic adjustment. Before the accident, she prided herself in her ability to take care of herself and her home independently. Now she has a negative self-concept. B.T. also has difficulty coping with her situation. Before her accident, she relied heavily on leisure activities for life enjoyment, and now she is unable to do this.

B.T. injured her dominant extremity. This has a significant impact on her functional capabilities. Virtually all areas of occupational performance are affected. She can perform most ADLs using her left upper extremity functionally and right upper extremity for light support. It takes her much longer to complete tasks than before.

In work activities, B.T. manages most tasks independently, but not to the extent she previously did.

Simple tasks tire her out. B.T. prepares simple meals. She relies on an electric can opener and microwave oven. B.T. continues to maintain her home with outside assistance (yard work, repair people).

Leisure activity performance has been the most affected. B.T. has essentially stayed home since the injury. She is afraid to take the bus. Furthermore, she is afraid of falling and reinjuring herself.

Severed Nerve

J.L. is a 32-year-old construction worker who sustained a laceration to his left wrist at work. He was using a saw, became momentarily distracted, and was cut. He severed all finger flexor tendons and his median nerve. The tendons and nerve were surgically repaired.

J.L. has been married for 10 years. He and his wife have three children, ages eight, six, and two. His wife hasn't worked outside the home since the birth of their first child. Prior to that, she was a secretary. They've always managed to make ends meet financially but have never been able to save much money. They recently purchased and moved into a new home. Both he and his wife have parents and siblings in the area. The families are close, and they often socialize together.

In his leisure time, J.L. enjoyed playing sports and games with his children. He also enjoyed attending sports events and watching them on television. In the summertime he played softball, and he bowled in the winter. He enjoyed going to bars after work with co-workers, and he and his wife occasionally went to movies or dined out with friends or family.

Table 4.4.
Occupational Performance Components—Severed Nerve Case Study[a]

Sensory Motor Component	Cognitive Integration & Cognitive Components	Psychosocial Skills & Psychologic Components

1. Sensory integration
  a. Sensory awareness
  b. Sensory processing
    *1. Tactile
    2. Proprioceptive
    3. Vestibular
    *4. Visual
    5. Auditory
    6. Gustatory
    7. Olfactory
  c. Perceptual skills
    1. Stereognosis
    2. Kinesthesia
    3. Body scheme
    4. Right-left discrimination
    5. Form constancy
    6. Position in space
    7. Visual-closure
    8. Figure ground
    9. Depth perception
    10. Topographic orientation
 	
2. Neuromuscular
  a. Reflex
  b. Range of motion
  *c. Muscle tone
  *d. Strength
  *e. Endurance
  f. Postural control
  g. Soft tissue integrity
 	
3. Motor
  *a. Activity tolerance
  *b. Gross motor coordination
  c. Crossing the midline
  d. Laterality
  e. Bilateral integration
  f. Praxis
  *g. Fine motor coordination
  h. Visual-motor integration
  i. Oral-motor control
	1. Level of arousal
	2. Orientation
	3. Recognition
	4. Attention span
	5. Memory
	  a. Short-term
	  b. Long-term
	  c. Remote
	  d. Recent
	6. Sequencing
	7. Categorization
	8. Concept formation
	9. Intellectual operations in space
	10. Problem solving
	11. Generalization of learning
	12. Integration of learning
	13. Synthesis of learning
		1. Psychologic
		  *a. Roles
		  b. Values
		  c. Interests
		  d. Initiation of activity
		  e. Termination of activity
		  *f. Self-concept
		2. Social
		  a. Social conduct
		  b. Conversation
		  c. Self-expression
		3. Self-management
		  *a. Coping skills
		  b. Time management
		  c. Self-control

Table 4.4. (Continued)

Occupational Therapy Performance Areas

Activities of Daily Living	Work Activities	Play/Leisure Activities
1. rooming	1. Home management	*1. **Play or leisure exploration**
2. Oral hygiene	a. Clothing care	*2. **Play or leisure performance**
3. Bathing	b. Cleaning	
4. Toilet hygiene	c. Meal preparation and cleanup	
*5. **Dressing**	d. Shopping	
*6. **Feeding and eating**	e. Money management	
7. Medication routine	*f. **Household maintenance**	
8. Socialization	g. Safety procedures	
*9. **Functional communication**	*2. **Care of others**	
*10. **Functional mobility**	3. Educational activities	
*11. **Sexual expression**	4. Vocational activities	
	a. Vocational exploration	
	b. Job acquisition	
	*c. **Work or job performance**	
	d. Retirement planning	

Asterisks indicate components affected by condition.

J.L. has a high school education. He's worked in construction for 14 years and likes his job. He is right-hand dominant. It has been 3 weeks since his injury and repairs.

This injury caused deficits in J.L.'s occupational performance. (See Table 4.4 for a chart of J.L.'s occupational performance deficit profile.) The severed nerve results in decreased sensory processing function. Neuromuscular abilities are limited by the lacerated nerve and tendons, as well as a splint designed to protect the sutures. Active flexion of digits cannot be determined at this time because this motion might rupture the repaired structures. Likewise, we cannot evaluate muscle strength, grip, or pinch. J.L.'s musculoskeletal endurance is normal for activities in which he can participate.

J.L. is experiencing major difficulties in psychosocial/psychologic functioning. He has difficulty adjusting to lack of a "worker" role. Furthermore, he's afraid he won't be able to return to his previous job, qualify for other work, or provide for his family. For these reasons, J.L. has a negative self-concept.

Socially, J.L. is loud, argumentative, and disruptive. He also has difficulty with self-management. J.L. can't identify his stress or coping mechanisms. He has begun to drink at bars with friends more and more. At home, he primarily lies on the couch, watches TV, and criticizes his wife. Finally, J.L. has little self-control and loses his temper often.

His injury has affected J.L.'s function in several occupational performance areas. He performs all one-handed self-care tasks independently and is able to drive a car. He has difficulty with socialization and sexual expression. J.L. feels "deformed" in appearance and therefore feels unable to perform sexual activity.

J.L. essentially performs no work or play activities. He shows no initiative to assist his wife with housework or child care. J.L. continues to watch sports on TV but does not participate anymore. Furthermore, he has not explored new leisure activities.

REFERENCES

1. American Society for Surgery of the Hand. The hand examination and diagnosis, 1978.
2. Beasley R. Hand injuries. Philadelphia: WB Saunders, 1981.
3. Adams JC. Outline of fractures. New York: Churchill-Livingstone, 1983.
4. Padretti L. Occupational therapy practice skills for physical dysfunction, 2nd ed. St. Louis: CV Mosby, 1985.
5. Kasdan M. Occupational hand and upper extremity injuries and disease. Philadelphia: Hanley & Belfus, 1991.
6. Smigielski M. Lecture: Upper extremity orthopedics. Ypsilanti, MI, Feb 4, 1986.
7. Caillet R. Hand pain and impairment. Philadelphia: FA Davis, 1983.
8. Lamb DW, Hooper, G. Hand conditions. New York: Churchill-Livingstone, 1984.

9. Hughes S. A new short textbook of orthopedics and traumatology. London, England: Hodder & Stroughton, 1989.

10. Lidstrom A. Fractures of the distal end of the radius: a clinical and statistical study of end results. Acta Orthop Scand 1959;(suppl) 41:X.

11. Dorland's illustrated medical dictionary. 25th ed. Philadelphia: WB Saunders, 1974.

12. Aryian S. The hand book. New York: McGraw-Hill, 1989.

13. Physicians' desk reference. 44th ed. Oradell, NJ: Medical Economics Company, 1990.

14. Trombly, C. Occupational therapy for physical dysfunction. 3rd ed. Baltimore: Williams & Wilkins, 1989.

Glossary

Adhesion: Union or joining of two body structures that are usually separate; also, any fibrous band that connects them. Adhesions are usually painless and cause no difficulties, although occasionally they produce obstruction or malfunction by distorting an organ and preventing normal smooth function of the parts.

Analgesic: Pain-relieving agent.

Anomalies: Marked deviation from normal.

Antiinflammatory: An agent that suppresses the inflammatory process; inflammation is characterized by classic signs of pain, heat, redness, swelling, and loss of function (10).

Antiplatelet: Interferes with platelet function (10). Blood platelets (thrombocytes) are disc-shaped, nonnucleated blood elements with very fragile membranes, responsible for coagulation and clotting of the blood.

Antipyretic: An agent that reduces fever.

Atrophy: Wasting away in the size of a muscle, which may result from decreased activity.

Avulsion: The tearing away of a structure.

Axonotmesis: Type of nerve injury usually due to blunt trauma or stretch injuries; axons and the myelin sheath are physically disrupted, but tubes and endoneural tissues (connective tissue) remain intact, resulting in degeneration of the axon distal to the injury site; axon can regrow in original neural tube and regeneration is spontaneous and of good quality (2). See Neurotmesis.

Carpal tunnel syndrome: Condition in which the median nerve becomes compressed in the carpal tunnel; can cause numbness, tingling, and weakness in median nerve distribution area of the hand.

Colles' fracture: The transverse fracture of the distal end of the radius (just above wrist) with displacement of hand backward and outward.

Contracture: "Condition of fixed high resistance to passive stretch of a muscle, resulting from fibrosis of the tissues supporting the muscles of the joints, or from disorders of the muscle fibers" (10). Resistance to stretching can lead to permanent disability. In many cases contractures can be prevented by range-of-motion exercises (active or passive) and by adequate support of the joints to eliminate constant shortening or stretching of the muscles and surrounding tissue.

Contusion: A bruise, usually an injury where the skin is not broken. In a contusion, blood from the broken vessels accumulates in surrounding tissue, producing pain, swelling, and tenderness. A discoloration results from blood seepage under the surface of the skin.

Endoneurium: The interstitial connective tissue in a peripheral nerve, separating individual nerve fibers.

Delayed union: Complication in fracture healing where the fracture takes considerably longer than normally expected to heal.

Diaphoresis: Profuse perspiration or sweating.

Edema: Presence of abnormally large amounts of fluid in intercellular tissue spaces (10); swelling.

Fibrosis: Formation of tissue composed of fibers.

Hepatic: Pertaining to the liver.

Hyperesthesia: "Abnormally increased hypersensitivity of the skin" (10) or a state of abnormally increased sensitivity to stimuli.

Inflammatory phase: First phase of bone fracture healing; blood clots form in the fracture ends with no blood supply to those areas; there is vasodilation and edema with inflammatory cells.

Ischemic necrosis: Deficiency of blood supply to a body part, causing death of a tissue.

Laceration: A wound produced by tearing, as distinguished from a cut or incision.

Malaise: "A vague feeling of bodily discomfort" (10) or a feeling of uneasiness or indisposition.

Malunion: Complication in fracture healing in which the fracture heals in the normal amount of time but with incorrect position and deformity of the healed bone.

Nonunion: Complication in fracture healing in which there is fibrous union rather than bony union so that the ends of the fractured bone fail to unite.

Neurapraxia: Nerve injury in which there is damage to the myelin sheath around axons, but axons remain intact (no physical disruption) (2); failure of nerve conduction in the absence of structural changes, caused by blunt injury, compression, or ischemia.

Neuroma: A new growth or tumor made up largely of nerve cells and nerve fibers (10).

Neurotmesis: A type of nerve injury in which there is complete or partial severance of all structures of a nerve, with disruption of the axon and its myelin sheath and the connective tissue elements. (See Axonotmesis)

Osteodystrophy: Abnormal development of bone.

Osteomyelitis: Inflammation of bone, localized or generalized, due to pyogenic infection. It may result in bone destruction, in stiffening of joints if the infection spreads to the joint, and in extreme cases occurring before the end of the growth period, in the shortening of a limb if the growth center is destroyed.

Osteoporosis: Demineralization of bone; abnormal diminution of density and weight of the bone. A decreased mass per unit volume of normally mineralized bone compared with age- and sex-matched controls. It is the most prevalent bone disease in the world.

Paresthesia: Abnormal sensation; burning or prickling (10).

Protective level of sensation: One of the two subsystems of the somatosensory system, currently called the primary level. (The other subsystem is the discriminative level). The protective level receives and interprets simple sensations such as touch, pain, and extremes of temperatures and allows persons to defend or protect themselves (13).

Range of motion: "Arc of motion through which a joint passes" (4). For example, the elbow normally moves from 0° (extended straight) to 135–150° (fully flexed).

Reflex sympathetic dystrophy (shoulder-hand syndrome): A neurovascular disorder characterized by severe shoulder pain, with stiffness, swelling, and pain in the hand, trophic changes, vasomotor instability, and resulting limitation in range of motion of the involved side. Prevention is by early frequent mobilization. Prompt treatment with an aggressive exercise program that includes active muscle contraction, joint movement, and light weight-bearing activities is required to prevent permanent disability.

Remodeling phase: Third phase in fracture healing; after the union is complete "the bone often forms a bulbous collar which surrounds the bone" (3); the mass varies in size.

Reparative phase: Second phase in fracture healing; repair cells begin to work; new bone and cartilage forms about the fracture site.

Sudeck's atrophy: Potential complication in fracture healing; characterized by pain, swelling (overlaying skin is stretched and glossy), and marked joint stiffness (3); Colles' fracture is one of the commonest causes of Sudeck's atrophy; overall incidence is low (3).

Sudomotor: Stimulating the sweat glands (10).

Vasculature: The vascular (blood vessel) system.

APPENDIX **4.2**

Diagnostic Tests

Electromyography (EMG): Insertion of fine needles into skeletal muscle to stimulate and record neuromuscular function.

Froment's sign: Test for thumb adduction (adductor pollicis muscle, ulnar nerve). When this muscle is weak or nonfunctional, a patient's thumb interphalangeal (IP) joint will flex when forcibly holding a piece of paper between the thumb and radial side of the index finger proximal phalanx (1).

Manual muscle test (MMT): Tests extent of nerve function by assessing strength of muscles against manual resistance provided by an examiner.

Phalen's test: Tests nerve function. A patient rests both elbows on a table top. The examiner passively fully flexes both wrists. If there is paresthesia or hyperesthesia along the median or ulnar nerve sensory distribution within 60 seconds, these nerves are compromised.

Radiographic studies (x-ray): Diagnostic films of internal body structures produced by the action of x-rays or gamma rays on sensitized film. For a possible fracture, the films should include good lengths of bone above and below the suspected fracture site. Two views should be taken, usually anteroposterior and lateral, perpendicular to one another.

Tinel's sign: A subjective evaluation in which tapping along an injured nerve will cause paresthesias (numbness) over the area of regeneration.

Weber's two-point discrimination test: Touching the skin with two blunt points simultaneously placed along a longitudinal line of the finger while the patient's vision is occluded. The patient indicates whether one or two points were felt. Normal range for volar fingertips is up to 5 mm distance between the two points and 6 to 12 mm on the dorsum of the hand. A failure of more than 10 mm on the volar fingertips will impair functional grip (5).

Medications

Generic Name	Brand Name	Action	Indication	Potential Side Effects	Usual Adult Dose
Aspirin	Anacin Bayer Bufferin	Analgesic, antipyretic, antiinflammatory, antiplatelet	Relief of minor aches and pains	Tinnitus, dizziness, gastrointestinal distress	One to two tablets/caplets; may be repeated every 4 hours; maximum 12 tablets/caplets per day
Acetaminophen	Tylenol Extra-Strength Tylenol	Clinically proven analgesic and antipyretic	Provides safe and quick temporary relief from minor aches and pains; if aspirin allergy is present, this is an excellent alternative	Massive overdose may cause hepatic toxicity; early symptoms of hepatic toxicity may include nausea, vomiting, diaphoresis, general malaise	One to two tablets/capsules three to four times daily
Ibuprofen	Motrin	Nonsteroidal antiinflammatory agent, analgesic, and antipyretic	Controls pain & inflammation; statistically significant reduction in mild gastrointestinal side effects; mild-to-moderate pain relief	Serious gastrointestinal toxicity; bleeding, ulceration, perforation can occur with or without warning symptoms with chronic use	1200–3200 mg; do not exceed 3200 mg daily
Propoxyphene	Darvon Darvocet	Centrally acting narcotic agent	Relief of mild-to-moderate pain	Dizziness, sedation, nausea, vomiting; limit alcohol intake; do not prescribe for suicidal or addiction-prone patients; prescribe with caution for persons taking tranquilizers or antidepressant drugs or persons who use alcohol in excess	65 mg every 4 hours
Oxycodone	Percocet Percodan	Narcotic, analgesic & sedative	Relief of moderate-to-severe pain	Lightheadedness; dizziness; sedation; nausea; vomiting; potentially habit-forming; psychologic dependence and tolerance can develop	One tablet every 6 hours; may be adjusted for more severe pain or for those who have become tolerant of analgesic agents

5

Schizophrenia

YVONNE R. TESKE

Opinions vary about what schizophrenia is. We know that it affects the central nervous system, and biologic, psychologic, and social function. Schizophrenia interrupts life. Schizophrenia affects people who have it differently than some other illnesses do because it changes who they are. Sylvia Frumkin, the subject of the book *Is There No Place On Earth for Me?*, relates her feelings about herself during a therapy session with her mother and a social worker. Sylvia is imagining that she lives on a make-believe planet called Verna where life was less demanding. Her social worker, exasperated with Sylvia's tendency to escape from reality in the therapy session, challenges her:

> Cut out the nonsense about Verna— you're right here in this office . . . . This is the real world. Come back from the make-believe."
>
> Sylvia responded, "You live in the real world, and my parents live in the real world. I'd prefer to live in an imaginary place like Verna. In my world, I can be anyone I want to be. But what does your world have to offer me . . .? In your world I'm nothing." (1, p. 239)

Besides having to contend with the subjective sense of losing yourself, which accompanies schizophrenia, people who have schizophrenia face the stigma placed on them by members of the community. Editors of a daily newspaper in a mid-sized community call the responses of city council members to a local housing problem "schizoid" (2). A front-page article in the same newspaper labels the winter weather "schizophrenic," having "multiple personalities." Writers use these words to dramatize the unpredictability of the winter climate. The words have a negative connotation, which places a stigma on people who have schizophrenia and their families, ignoring the many people with schizophrenia in our communities who lead meaningful lives.

Regularly, newspapers, magazines, and journals have reports about studies of schizophrenia, many about its etiology. The study of schizophrenia is a good example of how scientific inquiry works. Investigators conduct many studies of key questions until a clear picture emerges. Most studies involve small numbers of patients and families when compared with the 900,000 people who have schizophrenia. No one study alone can solve the problem of schizophrenia. The Schizophrenia Research Branch of the National Institute of Mental Health funds and coordinates many studies, and in turn publishes research results in the *Schizophrenia Bulletin*.

Scientists and clinicians do not all share the same view of schizophrenia; two different perspectives guide study and treatment (3). Because schizophrenia is complex and the exact cause is unknown, both perspectives are based on assumptions.

One perspective is that schizophrenia is a single disease or illness. People who believe this assume that schizophrenia, like other diseases, has one known cause, pattern of onset, incidence, clinical picture, and treatment. This perspective guides psychiatric diagnosis and treatment in the United States. Psychiatric diagnostic guidelines in the United States define schizophrenia narrowly as an illness or disease that can be specifically diagnosed and medically treated. Within this perspective, people can be admitted to treatment programs that include medication and other interventions.

The second perspective about schizophrenia is that it is a clinical syndrome, not one disease. Instead, schizophrenia is several different disorders with similar symptoms, grouped together and called schizophrenia. In this perspective, no single, typical, clinical picture of schizophrenia exists. The cause and clinical picture are heterogeneous. This perspective guides much of the scientific research into the etiology of schizophrenia. Attempts to narrowly define schizophrenia for research purposes can miss important factors in etiology. Scientists now prefer to cast their nets over a broad area to include many possible causes.

ETIOLOGY

We know that schizophrenia affects all components of occupational performance, but we do not know what causes schizophrenia. The varied symptoms and problems suggest a complex etiology.

Schizophrenia may be genetic, nongenetic, or result from the interaction of both genetic and nongenetic factors (4, 5). Perhaps several possible causes must be present for a person to be diagnosed with schizophrenia. We can think of the possible causes as risk factors. Beyond generally knowing that the cause of schizophrenia is genetic and/or nongenetic, scientists want to discover how the risk factors lead to the genetic or nongenetic causes.

Genetic Causes

Through studies of twins, adopted offspring, and families, scientists believe now that schizophrenia is not caused by a single gene, genetic factor, or genetic location. Studies show strong support for many factors and many genes being involved in the inheritance of schizophrenia (6). Several different fields of genetics contribute to understanding the cause of schizophrenia—genetic epidemiology, pathophysiologic genetics, and molecular genetics.

Genetic epidemiology is the study of patterns of incidence, prevalence, and covariance of schizophrenia in families. Schizophrenia runs in families, and the best established risk factor for schizophrenia is genetic. Scientists develop theories or models to describe how genes can possibly transmit schizophrenia and test them by studying twins, adopted offspring, and families. If a genetic factor causes schizophrenia, then twins who share all of their genes (monozygotic) should have a greater chance of both twins having schizophrenia than twins who share only half their genes (dizygotic). Data from 11 studies, which included 1300 pairs of same-sex twins, show a 50% concordance rate for monozygotic twins, and a 12–14% concordance rate in dizygotic twins. This means that if one of a pair of monozygotic twins has schizophrenia, the chance of the other having the disorder is 50%. On the other hand, if one dizygotic twin has schizophrenia, the chance of the other having it is 12–14% (7).

For a nontwin, the risk of having schizophrenia if an immediate family member has the clinical syndrome is 10 times the risk in the general population (8). Though schizophrenia runs in families, 85–90% of cases of schizophrenia show no family history of the disease (9).

Pathophysiologic genetics is the study of inherited biological weaknesses. Scientists look for measurable psychophysiologic irregularities that appear to be genetically associated or linked with schizophrenia. More specifically, linkage is the tendency of two alleles (one of several forms of a gene) at different positions on the same chromosome to be inherited together. Linkage between unique psychophysiologic irregularities and schizophrenia is important because linkages do not change over time like behavioral symptoms do. The consistent and stable irregularities are called markers. Because they are stable, markers are studied intensively as a way to understand the cause of disease.

One example of psychophysiologic genetic marker is irregular smooth-pursuit eye movements (SPEM) (10). Most of us can follow moving objects across our visual field with slow, coordinated eye movements. Slow and fast eye movements work together. Once the object starts to move, a short, fast eye movement helps the retina catch up. When the object crosses the retina, the fast movements are inhibited, and slow pursuit of the object takes over. In schizophrenia, rapid eye movements are not inhibited, and they interrupt slow eye pursuits. People without SPEM cannot pursue a moving object smoothly or move their heads across a line of print. The abnormal genetic marker also appears in nonschizophrenia family members of people who have schizophrenia.

Molecular genetics applies recombinant DNA (deoxyribonucleic acid) techniques to the study of linkages. Scientists identify irregularities that suggest chromosomal abnormalities. Then, using highly sophisticated and complex methods, they study the biochemical structures and mechanisms within the genes and chromosomes which might explain how schizophrenia is inherited. Scientists are beginning to identify specific biochemical substances in and map patterns of genes and chromosomes, attempting to correlate the specific schizophrenia trait with DNA sequences in large extended families (11).

Nongenetic Causes

Nongenetic causes, often called environmental stressors, which are considered risk factors in schizophrenia are nonspecific. No single factor has been commonly linked with schizophrenia. Diet, stress, birth injuries and complications, viral infections, general health, stressful life events, and cultural factors are risk factors (8). Others are gender and seasonal birth. Males are more likely to have an early onset of schizophrenia than females. A greater proportion of schizophrenics are born in the winter months than nonschizophrenic psychiatric patients, although the pattern of an increased number of winter births is less strong in the southern United States (12). Several explanations have been given for the seasonal birth phenomenon, but no conclusions have been confirmed. The phenomenon may be related to infectious disease rates in the winter months (13).

Mechanisms

Brain anatomy of people with schizophrenia has been studied through autopsy and with neuroimaging techniques in living patients. Autopsies have shown decreased size of some portions of the brain in schizophrenic patients. Scientists disagree about the degree of shrinkage and the cause of the abnormalities. Brain areas identified are the internal pallidum, limbic portions of the temporal lobe, dentate gyrus, subiculum of the hippocampus, parahippocampal gyrus, and amygdala. Scientists regard the abnormalities in the limbic structures as critical, since the limbic structures contribute to memory, regulation of affect, and emotional responsiveness (6). Memory and emotional expression are problems of people with schizophrenia.

Neuroimaging techniques including computer tomography (CT) scanning and magnetic resonance imaging (MRI) have shown enlarged lateral and third cerebral ventricles. However not all people with schizophrenia have enlarged cerebral ventricles. The characteristic is normally distributed over the population of schizophrenia cases.

In addition to differences in brain anatomy, neurophysiologic abnormalities are also evident in schizophrenia (14). One mechanism that scientists believe causes some of the symptoms of schizophrenia is the abnormal function of the neurotransmitter dopamine in the brain. Detecting and measuring abnormalities in dopamine function is difficult. Currently scientists believe that hyperactivity or hypoactivity of the dopamine system causes some of the symptoms of schizophrenia. Other abnormalities seen in some people with schizophrenia are in the vestibular system and sensory reception.

One problem in studying the mechanisms of schizophrenia is finding patients who have never been on medications for treatment. Most people who have been diagnosed with schizophrenia have taken medication. Those who have never taken medication may differ from most people who have the clinical syndrome. The results of studies using a few unusual subjects may not apply to most people with schizophrenia.

INCIDENCE AND PREVALENCE

Best estimates are that 1% of the general population in the United States has schizophrenia (6). According to statistics from the National Institute for Mental Health, over a 6-month period, approximately 1.5 million persons are counted who have schizophrenia (15). That is 1 of every 100 adult Americans. During 1986, 900,000 persons diagnosed with schizophrenia were treated in inpatient and outpatient programs in the United States. On one day in April 1986, a national count was taken to find out how many people were being treated for mental illness. For schizophrenia, 396,000 people were being cared for in organized inpatient, outpatient, and partial-care settings that day (15). According to the World Health Organization, people around the world are at equal risk.

Schizophrenia usually begins between ages 15 and 45. About a tenth of affected persons are younger than 20, and a tenth are above 45 (16). Most are poor, generally because of the way the disease affects the ability to earn a living.

SIGNS AND SYMPTOMS

Schizophrenia was first described as a health condition in 1809 by John Haslam of Bethlem Hospital in London and by Philippe Pinel in Paris (16). Today physicians note that no clinical signs or symptoms are unique to schizophrenia; all can be seen in people with other psychiatric disorders. To further complicate the clinical picture, symptoms change in a person over time. The confusing array of symptoms lends credence to the idea that schizophrenia is a clinical syndrome encompassing many different disorders.

Remember that schizophrenia is categorized as a psychosis. People who are psychotic cannot distinguish reality from fantasy or evaluate the world beyond the self, a problem called poor reality testing. The person creates a new reality with a unique and very individual view of the world. This unique worldview is apparent in the patient's symptoms.

Symptoms of schizophrenia are sometimes organized into two major groups, positive and negative (5). Positive symptoms are excessive or distorted behaviors, when compared with normal function. The term florid is used to describe these excessive behaviors. Positive symptoms are hallucinations and delusions, disorganized speech, and disorganized behavior.

An hallucination is a false perception. People who have hallucinations have a strong sense that what they perceive is real even without related or adequate stimuli from the environment. One person describes seeing rabbits, cats, bugs, and people from the past appear and disappear during a long drive (17). You may notice grins, laughter, and moving lips as patients listen and sometimes talk to the voices they hear. Hallucinations seen in schizophrenia may be auditory, visual, olfactory, gustatory, and/or tactile.

Delusions are false beliefs that persist in spite of evidence that makes them invalid. The beliefs are not logical conclusions based on reality, yet they are firmly set in the mind. The person cannot be argued out of them. Delusions reflect a system of thinking that is unique to the person holding them. Examples of kinds of delusions are delusions of persecution, grandeur, and reference.

Delusions of persecution are false beliefs that the person is being harassed, cheated with ill-treatment, persistently annoyed, or bothered. One person believed that the FBI was pursuing him because he saw dark-colored cars without license plates taking turns driving behind him (16). The person may feel harassed by politicians, political parties, and the government, and may try to start legal action against the persecutors.

Delusions of grandeur are false beliefs that the person's value, worth, or importance are greater than evidence shows. For example, one patient had a well-organized belief that everyone existed on one of seven levels. He believed that most people were on the first, second, or third level, but that he was on the seventh level, close to God. He said he felt protected, that personal criticism didn't matter.

Persons who have delusions of reference definitely believe that events, objects, or other people have to do with them. The comments of others and daily events take on unusual and personal meaning, often negative. For example, one young woman, discussed later in this chapter, felt that other people were calling her a whore. She believed that she heard the telephone ringing, and when she answered it, she heard a caller label her a whore.

Positive symptoms do not easily relate to dysfunction in one specific anatomic area of the brain. However the abnormal neurochemical mechanism that probably causes positive symptoms is excessive dopamine activity (5).

Whereas positive symptoms are an excess or distortion of normal behavior, negative symptoms are defects, a loss of normal behavior. Persons with negative symptoms show limited amounts and meaning of speech. They speak very little, and what they do say lacks rich, informative meaning. Verbal and nonverbal emotional expression are decreased. Affective blunting is the term used to describe the lack of facial expression. People with negative symptoms show avolition, the lack of will, drive, or energy. They do not experience pleasure normally (ahedonia). The ability to relate to other people decreases.

Negative symptoms correspond to a loss of frontal lobe function. The frontal lobes govern cognitive and psychosocial performance in creative and abstract thinking, volition and affect, communication, and social judgment (6).

While no universal clinical picture of schizophrenia exists, problems in cognitive and psychosocial performance are seen in most persons who have the syndrome. Motor problems are not universally seen. The most common motor problem is SPEM, described earlier. Some uncertainty exists about whether the inability to make direct eye contact, the lack of facial affect, and limited spontaneous speech are motor, cognitive, or psychosocial problems or a combination of problems.

COURSE AND PROGNOSIS

The course and prognosis of schizophrenia are highly individual. No common pattern applies to most people with schizophrenia. Scientists and therapists are interested in understanding the course and outcome of schizophrenia, so they can predict which patients will have a short-term interruption of their lives and which will have chronic disability. Several predictive factors appear to be valid for some subgroups of schizophrenia (5, 6).

Short-term Interruption	Chronic/Disability
Acute onset	Slow onset
Late onset	Early onset
Social support	No social support
Precipitating factors	No precipitating factors
(Reactive)	(Process)
Positive symptoms	Negative symptoms

The course of schizophrenia may occur in three phases: onset, middle, and late (18). Onset is the time when people have acute symptoms of psychosis and personality symptoms that are not psychotic. Psychotic symptoms are hallucinations, delusions, and disordered thinking. An example of a nonpsychotic personality symptom is social withdrawal.

In the middle course of schizophrenia, people have periods of fluctuation when symptoms are active then quiet, or continued psychosis. Usually, personal deterioration occurs in the onset and middle courses. Then, in the late course, the clinical syndrome either improves or worsens. Five to 10 years after onset, the schizophrenic process plateaus (19). People who have had the clinical syndrome for more than 10 years are called chronic schizophrenics. Those for whom schizophrenia has stabilized are still good candidates for rehabilitation programs.

Investigators have used individual case studies to learn about the course of schizophrenia (20). Overall, the cases show that schizophrenia is not a condition with a steady course of improvement or deterioration. Instead, case analyses show shifts in symptoms and function. A person may experience a moratorium, a stable period that seems to provide strength. Or, a person may experience change points, brief periods of increased function or deterioration that are responses to individual or environmental factors. Within a given period, a person may seem to reach a ceiling in functional level, and when attempting to reach beyond the ceiling, may break down. The functional breakdown, when symptoms reappear, is called decompensation.

The outcome of schizophrenia is usually worse than that of other major mental illnesses. Long-term studies have not shown that treatment changes the natural course of schizophrenia, but scientists have drawn several conclusions. One is that schizophrenia is frequently disabling for a lifetime, 3 to 4 decades. Bleuler (21) reports that in persons with schizophrenia,

25% recover completely without further need for treatment, 50% show fluctuating symptoms over decades, and 25% have persistent problems. People with schizophrenia may also have other mental illnesses. About half of those with persistent problems have lifelong invalidism.

People with schizophrenia die sooner than other people. The mortality rate in schizophrenia is two times that of the general population. They have an increased risk of suicide, accidents, and physical illness such as infections and cardiovascular disease. People with schizophrenia have high rates of problematic drinking or alcoholic use disorders. Men's lives may be shortened by 10 years, and women's by 9 years. Men may deteriorate more than women in the course of the condition. One reason may be that schizophrenic women are more likely to be married than schizophrenic men (22, 23). Remember that the outcome of schizophrenia is highly individual; just as the etiology and symptoms vary, so does the outcome.

DIAGNOSIS

A diagnosis of schizophrenia is inferred through the speech and behavior of the person. Clinicians look for five major types of problems: hallucinations and delusions, cognitive impairment, affective disturbances, social withdrawal, and neurologic deficits. Diagnosis is difficult because the clinical syndrome shares most of its signs and symptoms with other psychiatric conditions. To increase the accuracy of the diagnosis, open and structured interviews, the mental status examination, history, psychologic tests, and neurologic examinations are all used.

The need to make reliable diagnoses has led to the development of several published, structured interviews. While the psychiatrist most often conducts the interview with the patient, information (for example about social relationships and task performance in daily life) can also be provided by family members and health professionals like occupational therapists. The entire treatment team can be trained to administer structured interviews or to contribute relevant information. On any intervention team, all members assume the responsibility for understanding diagnostic measures and sharing information from their own discipline.

The lack of agreement about exactly what schizophrenia is means that no one best way is available for diagnosis. Clinicians and scientists are exploring different ways to classify schizophrenia. In the United States, clinicians use criteria determined by the American Psychiatric Association, the *Diagnosis and Statistical Manual of Mental Disorders*, edition 3, revised (DSM III-R) (24). This manual contains diagnostic criteria and guidelines for all psychiatric disorders. The criteria consist of narrowly defined, specific symptoms to increase the accuracy of diagnosis and treatment and to differentiate schizophrenia from other diagnoses such as depression. The criteria limit diagnosis of schizophrenia to people who have had some symptoms continuously for at least 6 months and the major psychotic symptoms for 1 week. The International Classification of Diseases, edition 9 (ICD-9) (25) frequently is used outside the United States. The match between diagnosis and treatment is critical, especially when medications are part of the regimen.

The DSM III-R gives criteria for five subtypes of schizophrenia: paranoid, catatonic, disorganized, undifferentiated, and residual (Table 5.1). To be diagnosed with paranoid schizophrenia, a person must have one or more well-organized delusions or frequent auditory hallucinations, all related to a single theme.

A person who has catatonic schizophrenia may be immobile or agitated. This subtype of schizophrenia, rarely seen in the United States today, is characterized by disorganization and the lack of inhibitions and habits. The subtype undifferentiated schizophrenia is used when the person can not be easily categorized. The subtype residual schizophrenia is used for people who have had at least one past episode of schizophrenia. They currently have no psychotic symptoms, but may have negative symptoms.

TREATMENT

Treatment of schizophrenia includes pharmacotherapy, individual and group psychotherapy, and psychosocial programs. Psychiatrists treat 90% of new admissions for all forms of mental illnesses with medications, 74% with individual therapy, and 52% with group therapy (15). Psychiatrists and other clinicians actively discuss the pros and cons of pharmacotherapy and psychotherapy, but psychiatric literature suggests that both methods of treatment are useful, either alone or in combination. The choice of treatment depends on many factors. The philosophy that guides the use of medications is that schizophrenia is a biologic illness; the patient must adjust to the symptoms. No medical cure exists. The philosophy that guides the use of psychotherapy is that the schizophrenic person has psychologic problems that can be cured or lessened.

Pharmacotherapy

Neuroleptic drugs are used to treat the symptoms of schizophrenia. They are dopamine antagonists because they oppose the excessive activity of the neurotransmitter, dopamine, in the brain. By affecting the action of dopamine, the drugs reduce the positive, psychotic symptoms of hallucinations, delusions, and thought disorders. For this reason they are called antipsychotic drugs. Without severe psychotic symptoms, patients can communicate more effectively, improving social relationships. Patients when first given medications in acute admissions wards, appear sedated. Then, after weeks or months, neuroleptic drugs reduce psychotic processes.

The five families of drugs are shown in Table 5.2. Three possible side effects of the antipsychotic drugs are extrapyrami-

Table 5.1.
Characteristics of Schizophrenia Subtypes[a]

Subtype	Characteristics
Paranoid	Onset after late 20s, delusions of persecution or grandeur, hostile, reserved, intelligent, social skills
Catatonic	Psychomotor dysfunction-rigidity, stupor, agitation, negativism, mutism
Disorganized (hebephrenic)	Onset before age 25, primitive, aimless, disorganized, sloppy, loose thinking, poor reality testing, silly, grimaces, lacks social skills
Undifferentiated	Hallucinations, delusions; disorganized speech, thought, and behavior; meets the criteria for more than one subtype or does not fit into any one subtype
Residual	Has had schizophrenia in past, now no psychotic symptoms, may have negative symptoms, illogical thinking, eccentric behavior

[a] Information taken from DSM III-R, Washington: American Psychiatric Association, 1987; and Kaplan HI, Sadock BJ, Synopsis of psychiatry, behavioral sciences, clinical psychiatry. 5th ed. Baltimore: Williams & Wilkins, 1988.

Table 5.2.
Neuroleptic Drugs Used to Treat Schizophrenia[a]

Drug Type	Side Effects		
	Extrapyramidal	Sedative	Anticholinergic
Phenothiazines			
Chlorpromazine (Thorazine)	Mild	Mild	Strong
Prochlorperazine (Compazine)	Strong	Moderate	Weak
Thioridazine (Mellaril)	Weak	Strong	Strong
Trifluoperazine (Stelazine)	Strong	Weak	Weak
Thioxanthenes			
Thiothixene (Navane)	Strong	Weak	Weak
Butyrophenones			
Haloperidol (Haldol)	Strong	Weak	Weak
Dihydroindolones			
Molindone (Moban)	Strong	Weak	Weak
Dibenzoxapines	Strong	Weak	Weak
Loxapine (Loxitane)			

[a] Information taken from Rothstein JM, Roy SH, Wolf SL. The rehabilitation specialist's handbook. Philadelphia: FA Davis, 1991.

dal, sedative, and anticholinergic. Typical neuroleptic drugs like haloperidol produce extrapyramidal side effects in some, but not all, patients. Patients show changes in muscle tone, coordination, and activity level. Specific side effects are dystonia, parkinsonism, akathisia, tardive dyskinesia, and tardive dystonia.

Dystonia appears in the first few days of treatment for about 10% of patients. Dys-

tonic movements are involuntary. They may be slow muscle contractions or spasms that involve the neck, jaw, tongue, eyes, and the entire body. The involuntary movement can be painful and frightening. As a result, patients may refuse to take neuroleptic drugs if they experience dystonia.

Patients who have akathisia feel physically uncomfortable. They move and adjust their bodies constantly to relieve the feeling of muscle discomfort. Observers note the agitation, restlessness, pacing, and repeated sitting down and standing up.

Tardive dyskinesia and tardive dystonia are delayed effects of neuroleptic drugs. (The word tardive means late.) The symptoms usually occur after 6 months of drug treatment. Tardive dyskinesia is involuntary. Patients have repetitive rapid, jerky, and writhing movements in the limbs, trunk, and head. Mouth, tongue, and jaw movements are most common. Approximately half of chronic, institutionalized patients have tardive dyskinesia. Tardive dystonia is the late appearance of dystonia.

Anticholinergic effects are caused by the drug's action on acetylcholine at several locations in the parasympathetic system. For example, acetylcholine action can be blocked at postganglionic cholinergic nerve endings, on blood vessels, and in the central nervous system. As a result, patients may experience side effects such as dry mouth, tachycardia, decreased gastric secretions with no decrease in acidity, and decreased tone and motility in the gastrointestinal tract and bladder.

The adverse effects of neuroleptic drugs can be treated in two ways. One is to reduce drug doses after the acute phase of schizophrenia. Psychiatrists prescribe minimal doses to maintain patients and control symptoms. Dosage reduction can decrease adverse effects and improve the patients' feelings of well-being (26).

The second way to treat neuroleptic drug adverse effects is to give antiparkinsonian drugs. The use of these drugs is controversial. Advantages are that the adverse side effects and patients' negative reactions to the effects are reduced. Patients are not frightened by the bizarre neurologic reactions and are more compliant with treatment. A disadvantage is that the additional drugs may not be necessary; all patients do not have adverse side effects. The patient's response to a combination of medications is very individual. For some, no satisfactory combination may be found. Occupational ther-

apists can carefully observe patients to note changes in muscle tone and coordination.

Some neuroleptic drugs are atypical, having no extrapyramidal effects, e.g., clozapine. Clozapine was developed to treat the 20% of patients with schizophrenia who do not respond to neuroleptic drugs. Patients, families, and clinicians welcomed the new medication with hope. However, the drug has major side effects and is expensive.

Clozapine, developed by Sandoz Pharmaceuticals under the name Clozaril, caused agranulocytosis in 1–2% of Americans who were involved in drug trials before marketing. Agranulocytosis is the marked decrease of granular leukocytes or white blood cells. Patients die from infections. Lesions appear in the throat and other mucous membranes, gastrointestinal tract, and skin. In addition, 5% of patients have seizures, and 25% have increased heart rates.

To protect themselves from liability suits, Sandoz requires that the drug be administered by Casemark, a home-care company. The company requires weekly blood tests and tracks patients. Drug purchase, administration, and monitoring procedures cost about $9000 a year for each patient. Sandoz threatened to remove the drug from the market unless it was allowed this protection. Recently, Sandoz and clinicians have said they are hopeful that alternative administration and monitoring agencies can be developed that would make the drug affordable to the patients who need it (27).

Psychotherapy

Psychotherapists care for the psychologic problems of a person with schizophrenia. Therapists use exploratory, directive, and supportive approaches to help patients see themselves as individuals separate from other people. Psychotherapy usually occurs when a patient is on medications, but sometimes happens when the patient is not receiving pharmacotherapy. Psychotherapists can help patients value themselves and their accomplishments. Patients can learn to feel less apathetic and more comfortable with independent actions. One problem that arises in psychotherapy is that it depends on a close relationship between therapist and patient. Schizophrenic patients have a reduced ability to form close relationships. They need, but fear, the relationship (28).

Psychosocial Treatment

The goals of psychosocial treatment are to develop, improve, or maintain (a) social skills and adaptation, (b) vocational functioning, (c) subjective well-being, and (d) family information and education. Psychosocial treatment includes such interventions as educational groups for families, social skills training, budgeting, transportation, employment groups, and living arrangements. Occupational therapy, music therapy, art therapy, recreational therapy, psychology, nursing, and social work are disciplines usually involved in psychosocial treatment. Generally, the treatment should be psychoeducational and supportive. No strong evidence shows that individual, group, or milieu therapy has an impact during the acute phase of illness (26). An effective approach to treatment is short-term hospital stay, aftercare planning, and long-term community-based treatment efforts.

The purpose of social skills training is to increase the social adaptation and skills necessary to function in the family and community. Inadequate social skills are a major source of stress for some people with schizophrenia. They often show social skills deficits even when other symptoms are controlled by drugs or are in remission (30). Not all people with schizophrenia have social problems. Those with positive symptoms often can function well between episodes. They may not have a history of interpersonal difficulties. People with negative symptoms are more likely to have ongoing interpersonal problems.

Treatment in social skills training programs usually includes interpersonal and instrumental, daily living skills. Training is usually based on learning theory and behavioral therapy principles such as modeling and reinforcement. Social skills programs use special techniques developed for targeted behaviors. Several studies suggest that social skills training can lead to improvement in targeted behaviors. The results are unclear about whether patients can generalize what they have learned to the many social problems in their lives.

Different models of social skill training are used. One of the most documented and studied is the motor skills model (29). In the motor skills model, social skills consist of a series of specific behaviors that are verbal—forming words, voice tone, volume—and nonverbal—gaze and gestures. Most people respond to cues in social situations automatically. However, people with schizophrenia do not, for many reasons. In social skills training, specific behaviors like eye contact are practiced repeatedly in behavioral rehearsal or role play. The behaviors are practiced until they become automatic. Studies of the results of motor skills training show positive effects on eye contact, response speed in conversation, voice tone, statements of appreciation, and assertiveness. According to Bellack (29), large studies have shown that patients with schizophrenia can acquire and maintain new skills and that social skills training can significantly reduce relapses. The motor skills model of social skills training does not target cognitive skills like attending and information processing.

Recently, therapists have developed a problem-solving approach to social skills training which includes cognitive skills. The problem-solving approach works on the primary problems of processing social input and carrying out problem-solving steps in social interaction. Some clinicians have noted limitations in the problem-solving training model. The social interaction skills taught in problem-solving training may not accurately represent both aspects, the actual skills in normal problem-solving and the skills needed by people with schizophrenia. This is a problem of validity. Investigators and clinicians need to study the complexities of attention, information processing, and problem solving to develop skill-specific, effective, training programs.

The purpose of education as a family intervention is to prevent the relapse of the family member with schizophrenia. Through education, stress on the family from caring for a family member after a short hospitalization can be reduced. Family education usually includes a variety of topics: information about schizophrenia, communication training, instruction in coping skills, and support (9). Generally, these family programs can reduce the negative climate in the family.

PERFORMANCE COMPONENTS AND OCCUPATIONAL PERFORMANCE

The following description of cognitive, psychologic, and social performance involves problems that most people with schizophrenia have to some degree.

Performance Areas

Cognitive Performance

Information processing is a theory that behavioral scientists use to explain how a person perceives, processes, and acts on information. People with schizophrenia show deficits in nearly every aspect of information processing (10).

We perceive information through sensory input. Once received, we process information using the memory to relate the information to past experience and ideas. Affect and language are important in memory. Affect has an organizing role in memory. The kind of emotion we have about an experience (e.g., whether we feel anger, love, or no strong feelings) helps to determine if and how we remember it.

Information processing requires language skills to receive and understand what is said and to communicate the intended meaning to others. Both receptive and productive language are impaired in schizophrenia. Listeners find the speech of people with schizophrenia unpredictable and incoherent because it does not seem to refer to the immediate conversation or events. People with schizophrenia sometimes do not know they are unclear. They leave out important cues that listeners need to understand conversation. On the other hand, when people with schizophrenia listen to others, they find normal speech less predictable than people without schizophrenia do. That is, people with schizophrenia may have difficulty comprehending normal speech.

We use affect, language, and memory in thought processes ranging from simple categorization of similarities and differences to complex problem solving and evaluation. We output information through motor performance in speech and movement. People with schizophrenia show deficits in receiving sensory input in the form of perception and information processing using memory, affect, and language. They also have problems in the output of information processing, expressive and receptive language.

Effective information processing depends on attention. To attend, we must filter out irrelevant information. Our filters consist of our needs, intentions, expectations, and the content of the stimulus itself. All facets of attention— orienting, sustaining attention, selective attention, concentration, preparation, capacity, and controlled processing—are affected by schizophrenia. No one area of the brain governs attention. Instead, several different areas and mechanisms influence the ability to attend. When the ability to attend is interrupted, information processing (including the resulting task performance) is difficult or impossible. This is the situation for many people with schizophrenia.

Psychologic Performance

A major characteristic of schizophrenia is affective dysfunction, especially for people with negative symptoms. People with schizophrenia have a reduced capacity for emotional expression. They cannot respond to feelings, inner sensations, and changes in feelings and actions. Emotional expression is complicated, with several elements involved including information processing. Information from events or situations that could potentially evoke emotion must be processed before a person can experience and show a response. We must be able to retrieve related memories, expectations, and styles of coping for the event we are experiencing. In addition, individual emotions have unique expressive and physiologic responses. Also, we have unique ways of acting on each emotion, so that for example, your response to anger is different from another person's. In schizophrenia, we can see evidence of these problems in a patient's unchanging facial expression and few expressive gestures.

One of the symptoms of schizophrenia is "extreme perplexity about one's own identity" (24; p. 189). People with schizophrenia report feeling a loss of their own identity and alienation from others. We define ourselves through others in an ongoing, changing process. We compare and contrast ourselves with others, and in turn, others give us feedback on how they see us. Identity depends on some agreement between ourselves and others about ourselves. Lack of agreement can lead to the alienation people with schizophrenia report. Lack of agreement also leads to the difficulties others have in understanding the person with schizophrenia.

The concepts of private and public self are helpful when considering schizophrenia. Our private selves are known mostly to us. Within our private selves, we reflect on ourselves as people. We make self-observations, are self-conscious, and relate to ourselves. Private selves are not on public view. However, our public selves are open to view. This is the self known to others.

Usually the two selves overlap, but in schizophrenia, the overlap between private self and public self may be small. The struggle for identity goes on in both parts of the self, the private and the public. In the private self, the person struggles with hallucinations, delusions, and disturbances in emotions. At the same time, family members see the changes in performance, habits, roles, relationships, and ambitions. The person experiences a loss of self and is aware of the loss. The family experiences the changes in the person as a loss of a familiar family member (30).

Social Performance

People with schizophrenia are highly sensitive to emotional cues from others. This is particularly true of negative cues like criticism. They usually have problems in relationships with friends and peers, who eventually find that their schizophrenic friend responds best to emotionally muted communication.

Sensitivity to criticism and reaction to emotional conversation are symptoms that affect the family life of a person with schizophrenia. A family that is high in emotional expression (EE) can exacerbate symptoms of a family member. Families can be high EE or low EE. High EE families have members who are hostile, critical, intrusive, and/or overinvolved in interaction with the person who has schizophrenia. The family member with schizophrenia doesn't seem to get used to the negative climate as some other people might, but instead, seems hypersensitive to criticism and hostility. The family member also lacks the social skills to protect against what is perceived as an attack.

A negative emotional climate in the family of a discharged patient is one of the most reliable predictors of patient relapse in the year after discharge (29). Patients living with high EE families are continually exposed to intense interactions. The patients feel extreme stress, especially if the family shows excessive criticism and hostility.

Overinvolvement by the family is not associated with intense affect, but probably is a response to the long-standing problems of the family member with schizophrenia. Living with a person who has schizophrenia can be stressful, and family members may react to the stress.

The person with schizophrenia may find environments in which communication is vague, unclear, or inaccurate to be personally harmful or destructive, whereas other people may not react negatively. In some families, members may not share a common focus of attention or be able to understand another member's point of view. Vague, diffuse communication and implied messages are confusing for people with schizophrenia.

People with schizophrenia show less social drive and so have less interaction with other people. Reduced interaction may be a secondary effect of problems in emotional expression, information processing, and emotional sensitivity. One of the best predictors of later schizophrenia in children is the shy-withdrawal picture, children who cannot comfortably interact with others.

Occupational Performance

Schizophrenia affects all aspects of occupational performance because of the pervasive central nervous system symptoms (Table 5.3). During onset, positive or negative symptoms will interrupt a person's performance in work activities, play or leisure activities, and activities of daily living. For some people the interruption may be temporary. Periods of stability can mean a return to performance in daily life. However, for others, occupational performance will be continuously altered in some of the following ways.

Work

Many people with schizophrenia are able to work. Some are assisted by medication, psychotherapy, and rehabilitation. Difficulties with eye pursuits, tremors as a result of medications, attention, information processing, and reality testing can affect vocational activities. These senso-rimotor and cognitive abilities provide the foundations for task performance and decision making on the job. Workers usually manage several tasks and decisions at a time, while they simultaneously respond to demands for increased performance from supervisors. Many jobs can be thought of as a series of ongoing problems that must be solved. People with schizophrenia have difficulties with problem solving because successful problem solving requires immediate and spontaneous attention and information processing. The inability to make the kind of judgments necessary for safety can also be a vocational problem.

Living with a condition as profound as schizophrenia can affect a person's identity and esteem. People with schizophrenia may experience little meaning or pleasure at a job because of their symptoms. Evaluation and criticism that are part of most job situations further complicate job satisfaction for the emotionally sensitive person with schizophrenia. Fearful of making mistakes that will bring criticism, the worker may become immobilized, may be dependent, or refuse to work. The usual feedback from supervisors and other authority figures sometimes threatens people with schizophrenia so much they resign, even when the supervisor is satisfied with their work.

Communication is made difficult by expressive and receptive language problems. Remember that a mutual lack of clarity exists when a schizophrenic person communicates with someone else. Few jobs are so isolated that communication is unnecessary.

Some of the same problems that interfere with vocational performance also affect educational performance. However the educational environment has some unique performance requirements. The perceptual-cognitive problems in schizophrenia make learning difficult. Reading can be especially difficult because of the need for slow-pursuit eye movements, attention, and information processing. All academic tasks require the complex interplay of these abilities.

In addition, criticism in the form of evaluation from peers and teachers can make school performance stressful. School is a social environment, requiring ongoing verbal and nonverbal communication,

and as we have said, communication is a problem for people with schizophrenia.

Depending on the individual, a person with schizophrenia can live in the community. The type of setting, supervised or independent, depends on the severity of problems with decision making, prob-

Table 5.3.
Occupational Performance Components

Sensory Motor Component	Cognitive Integration & Cognitive Components	Psychosocial Skills & Psychological Components
1. **Sensory integration**	1. **Level of arousal**	1. **Psychological**
a. **Sensory awareness**	2. **Orientation**	a. **Roles**
b. **Sensory processing**	3. Recognition	b. **Values**
1. Tactile	4. **Attention span**	c. **Interests**
2. Proprioceptive	5. **Memory**	d. **Initiation of activity**
3. Vestibular	a. **Short-term**	e. Termination of activity
4. **Visual**	b. **Long-term**	f. **Self-concept**
5. **Auditory**	c. **Remote**	2. **Social**
6. Gustatory	d. **Recent**	a. **Social conduct**
7. Olfactory	6. **Sequencing**	b. **Conversation**
c. **Perceptual skills**	7. **Categorization**	c. **Self-expression**
1. Stereognosis	8. **Concept formation**	3. **Self-management**
2. Kinesthesic	9. Intellectual operations in	a. **Coping skills**
3. Body scheme	space	b. **Time management**
4. Right-left dis-	10. **Problem solving**	c. **Self-control**
crimination	11. **Generalization of learning**	
5. Form constancy	12. **Integration of learning**	
6. Position in space	13. **Synthesis of learning**	
7. Visual-closure		
8. **Figure ground**		
9. Depth perception		
10. Topographic ori-		
entation		
2. Neuromuscular		
a. Reflex		
b. Range of motion	*Note:* All occupational performance areas can be affected de-	
c. Muscle tone	pending on phase of schizophrenia: onset, middle, late and/or	
d. Strength	prognosis.	
e. Endurance		
f. Postural control		
g. Soft tissue integrity		
3. **Motor**		
a. **Activity tolerance**		
b. Gross motor coordi-		
nation		
c. Crossing the midline		
d. Laterality		
e. Bilateral integration		
f. Praxis		
g. Fine motor coordina-		
tion		
h. **Visual-motor integra-**		
tion		
i. **Oral-motor control**		

Table 5.3 (Continued)

Occupational Performance Areas
(Effects depend on degree of disability)

Activities of Daily Living	Work Activities	Play/Leisure Activities
1. Grooming	1. Home management	1. Play or leisure exploration
2. Oral hygiene	a. Clothing care	2. Play or leisure perfor-
3. Bathing	b. Cleaning	mance
4. Toilet hygiene	c. Meal preparation and	
5. Dressing	cleanup	
6. Feeding and eating	d. Shopping	
7. Medication routine	e. Money management	
8. Socialization	f. Household maintenance	
9. Functional communica-	g. Safety procedures	
tion	2. Care of others	
10. Functional mobility	3. Educational activities	
11. Sexual expression	4. Vocational activities	
	a. Vocational exploration	
	b. Job acquisition	
	c. Work or job perfor-	
	mance	
	d. Retirement planning	

lem solving, judgment, task performance, and communication. An effective home manager must organize an environment to meet basic needs for safety, nutrition, money management, and cleanliness. In addition, unexpected events are part of daily living. In daily life, people with schizophrenia may be preoccupied with managing their own thoughts and behaviors that are interfering with performance. Reality testing may be faulty. These problems can make home management, nurturing children, and caring for the needs and meeting the demands of other people, a difficult challenge for the person with schizophrenia.

Leisure

The ability to select and perform pleasurable activities is required for satisfactory leisure time. The diminished ability to experience pleasure seen in schizophrenia means that participation in leisure activities does not bring the critical satisfaction and reward that make the activities worth doing. Schizophrenic patients may have difficulty thinking of activities they want to do. In addition to ahedonia, their visual tracking and cognitive problems may have prevented them from doing many activities. In the past, when they attempted to participate, they may have failed. The lack of successful activity experience in the past and the presence of current symptoms may make schizophrenic patients unmotivated in leisure activities.

Daily Living

Performance in activities of daily living is difficult if a schizophrenic person has active cognitive symptoms, sensorimotor side effects of medications, or overall deterioration. Most people perform grooming, hygiene, and dressing tasks by following a personal routine. We organize a routine to meet the reality-based demands of our lives. We can also attend to each basic task, figure out the best way to perform it, and perform the sequence of steps necessary for successful accomplishment. Schizophrenia symptoms can make all aspects of task performance a struggle.

Most of us perform daily living activities in a place we have chosen to live. We have the money to buy essential supplies. We may also have family and friends to support our self-care and socialization. The person with schizophrenia may lack many of these supports.

Several environmental factors influence performance across all areas of occupational performance. Emotional and financial support from family and friends help performance. Social and financial support may no longer be in place for the long-term, chronic schizophrenic. The person may not be able to afford housing or may have been asked to leave an apartment or room because of social, financial, and other problems. People with schizophrenia may not be able to get necessary rest and nutrition when they are homeless or living in environments that do not support health. Patients who have tried to sleep in shelters with 100 or more people complain about being constantly tired and hungry. During the day, they hunt for a place to take a shower and wash clothes.

Two different ways to explain and analyze schizophrenia are used. One is through scientific research into the causes, disease processes, and behaviors. Scientists look for relationships between mechanisms and behaviors. Patterns allow scientists and clinicians to make predictions about how schizophrenia affects people.

The second way to understand schizophrenia is through the life stories of people with the condition. Life stories help us to understand the development and meaning of schizophrenia at a personal level. Causes of schizophrenia are not explained in life stories, but the ways in which the condition affects function can be understood. The following two case studies show how schizophrenia has changed the occupational performance and the daily lives of two people who have the condition.

CASE STUDIES

C.S.

C.S. is a 19-year-old woman who is admitted to the inpatient, acute care ward of a psychiatric hospital. She was picked up by state police when she was seen wandering on the shoulder of an expressway. Drivers reported that she seemed dazed and was walking dangerously close to traffic. Her husband and parents had been trying to find her.

C.S. is tall and slim, with pale complexion and wispy blond hair. She wears sunglasses, dramatic eye makeup, and pale lipstick. Contrasting with the dramatic sunglasses and makeup, she pulls a long white T-shirt over her clothes and wears one of her many hats. Her face shows little expression of feeling or warmth. Her placid affect is interrupted occasionally by expressions of alarm in response to voices she hears.

Two years ago, her family moved to Detroit from the Tennessee hills where they had farmed for generations. The family, including seven children, moved because her father was offered a job by a relative. Back in Tennessee, the parents and children were active in a fundamentalist church. She describes them as "very religious." Both parents spent their days farming and caring for their children and grandchildren. When the family moved to Detroit, several of their married children and their families also came North.

As a child, the family left C.S. alone because they felt she was different. They said they didn't know how to manage her. She found school difficult because she couldn't attend to school work or relate to peers. She stayed away from school, sometimes spending her days with her mother. Most of the time she wandered by herself. She could not attend to school tasks, especially when they were presented to the group of students together. She found the presence and activity of peers very distracting. In the classroom, she seemed a shy person, described by family members as a "scared rabbit." She did not complete high school because of poor attendance and learning difficulties.

At puberty, her family reports they began setting limits and imposing stricter control over her wandering. They hoped she would "mature." She responded by becoming confused.

Once in Detroit, C.S. met a new boyfriend who included her in his group of friends. She eventually became sexually involved with him. Both report feeling guilty above having sexual intercourse. They decided to marry, and were married 1 year before the hospitalization.

In the last year C.S. has begun to hear the telephone ring when it does not. When she answers the phone, she hears voices calling her a whore and other accusations. Besides hearing accusatory voices, she believes that people are talking about her, making derogatory remarks about her sexual behavior, and calling her a prostitute. Though her husband is supportive, she is neglecting routine household tasks. He feels uncomfortable leaving her alone for safety reasons.

Physicians have diagnosed her as paranoid schizophrenic because of her well-organized auditory hallucinations and delusion of reference. Generally she shows positive symptoms, but she does not show active hostility.

Table 5.4.
Occupational Performance Profile[a]—C.S.

| | | Performance Areas | | |
| | | Work Activities | | |
	Vocation	Education	Home Management	Care of Others
SENSORIMOTOR — **SENSORY INTEGRATION** Hallucinations, limited visual pursuit	Has never held a job	Limited reading	Can't follow written directions	
NEUROMUSCULAR				
MOTOR				
COGNITIVE — **COGNITIVE** Lacks attention, concentration, limited information processing & problem solving		School dropout	Unsafe at home	
PSYCHOLOGICAL Delusions, fearful, confused about self, placid affect				
PSYCHOSOCIAL — **SOCIAL** Values confused, role crisis, low trust, unclear communication		Inadequate communication with others		
SELF-MANAGEMENT Lacks habits, routine, time sense, & time management			Can't organize day	
EXTERNAL FACTORS WHICH INFLUENCE PERFORMANCE				
CULTURE, ECONOMY, ENVIRONMENT	Move to Detroit Recent marriage			

(Left margin vertical labels: PERFORMANCE COMPONENTS)

[a]Grid adapted from Uniform Terminology (2nd ed.). Developed by the occupational therapy faculty at Eastern Michigan University.

C.S.'s major deficits in sensorimotor function are slow eye-pursuit movements and auditory hallucinations (Table 5.4). Her cognitive function is limited by her lack of attention and concentration and inadequate information processing. When she tries to work, delusions interrupt her task performance.

In the psychologic area, She is distant, fearful, and confused. She imitates the clothing and manner of other people by wearing costumes instead of usual clothes. She expresses confusion about her sexual upbringing and values.

C.S. has a few casual friends. Generally though, communication between herself and others is often unclear. She misinterprets what others say, and others ask, "What does she mean?" In spite of communication difficulties, others seek her out to talk because they find her appealing.

She makes no effort to follow a daily routine or to control her time to make her days satisfying. Overall, she has had little successful experience in work, leisure, or activities of daily living. She has never held a job and shows no interest in working. C.S. has ex-

Client initials: **C.S.**
Diagnosis: **Schizophrenia**
Age: **19**

| Play or Leisure Activities | | Activities of Daily Living | | | | |
Exploration	Performance	Self-Care	Socialization	Functional Communication	Functional Mobility	Sexual Expression
		Dresses, eats independently				
No successful leisure activity						
Lacks interests						
			Isolated, few friends	Unclear communication		
Does not initiate activity		Lacks routine				Confusion about marriage

pressed interest in learning to sew and cook. She is enthusiastic because she wants to make gifts for her nieces and nephews. However, sewing a simple basting stitch with a needle and thread is difficult because of SPEM and distractions from hallucinations.

In leisure activities, she has no specific interests or performance abilities. She goes along on social occasions, but not to participate. In leisure as in other areas of occupation, C.S. cannot perform simple tasks and interact with anyone at the same time. This is a problem because even instruction can be distracting. In activities of daily living, she is able to perform all self-care tasks.

C.S. was treated as an inpatient for 3 months in a milieu treatment unit. She received both neuroleptic drugs and psychotherapy. Her structured daily routine included individual and group occupational therapy, recreational therapy, music therapy, and ward activities. After discharge she returned home to live with her husband. She could perform very simple

Table 5.5.
Occupational Performance Profile[a]—J.R.

| | | Performance Areas | | |
| | | Work Activities | | |
	Vocation	Education	Home Management	Care of Others
SENSORY INTEGRATION Hallucinations, altered body scheme, dreams	Could not work			None
NEUROMUSCULAR Fatigue				
MOTOR				
COGNITIVE Delusions, decline in information processing, concentration		Completed college degrees		
PSYCHOLOGICAL Alienated, frightened, change in self Decline in self-esteem		Complete withdrawal from people and activity		
SOCIAL Altered communication, isolated				
SELF-MANAGEMENT Lost coping skills				

The left margin reads vertically: PERFORMANCE COMPONENTS, with sub-groupings SENSORIMOTOR, COGNITIVE, PSYCHOSOCIAL.

EXTERNAL FACTORS WHICH INFLUENCE PERFORMANCE:
CULTURE,   First time—joined military, left home
ECONOMY,   Second time—broke engagement, mother had cancer, job
ENVIRONMENT   problems

[a]Grid adapted from Uniform Terminology (2nd ed.). Developed by the occupational therapy faculty at Eastern Michigan University.

home-management tasks with some satisfaction. One year later she was rehospitalized with an increase in psychotic symptoms. She was discharged home again once symptoms were controlled.

J.R.

J.R. is a 45-year-old man who has had schizophrenia for about 25 years. When he was 20 years old, after 1 1/2 years at a community college and unable to

decide on a career, he joined the army. At the end of the first month of basic training, he became fearful of others in the barracks. They seemed robot-like, inhuman, and without emotions. He became suspicious. He suspected that the military training was brainwashing the trainees. J.R.'s fears distracted him and made performance increasingly difficult. As his suspicions increased, he became more and more alienated and lonely.

Sleep at night brought no respite from the suspicion and loneliness of each day. He was kept awake

	Client initials:	**J.R.**
	Diagnosis:	**Schizophrenia**
	Age:	**45**

Play or Leisure Activities		Activities of Daily Living				
Exploration	Performance	Self-Care	Socialization	Functional Communication	Functional Mobility	Sexual Expression
Decrease in satisfying leisure activities						
				Lost fiance		
		Poor diet and sleep				

at night by his dreams. In his dreams, fantasy princesses sent messages to him in riddles and popular songs. Feeling that he had been singled out to receive important messages, he tried to decode and write down his dreams. As the dreams and alienation continued, J.R. became fearful of public places.

When he went to the military physicians, he was given pills for his fatigue and anxiety, which he was afraid to take. He then left the military, feeling very ill. After one restful year, he was able to return to college and complete a degree in business.

For 10 years, he worked for a public relations firm. Then several stressful events caused depression and the return of disturbing dreams. His mother died of cancer. He broke his engagement to his live-in companion, and at the same time, he uncovered corrupt, unethical practices at his job.

J.R. tried psychotherapy but stopped going when he continued to feel overwhelmed with his life. He gradually withdrew into a world in which he heard constant conversation, singing, and nonsensical words in the background. He felt physical changes and experienced detachment from his own body. Finally, he became so frightened that he called his former psychotherapist in desperation. During the following 5 years of therapy, which included drugs, J.R. returned to work as a public relations writer at a different firm.

During his periods of illness, constant fatigue and malaise disturbed his ability to cope with sensory input (Table 5.5). He was overly responsive to noise and unable to screen out background sounds and movement. He also experienced hallucinations.

His cognitive performance was marked by poor memory, distractibility, and delusions. He was unable to make simple decisions in daily life and often felt confused.

Fearfulness and anxiety affected J.R.'s psychologic function. Nervousness, impatience, and irritability caused him to feel lonely and alienated, even from himself. In social situations, he was fearful of populated areas and had poor eye contact in the few situations when he did interact with others.

The case study shows that his performance in work, leisure, and activities of daily living was altered during his two acute periods. During periods of stability, he was able to work, live in a close relationship with another person, and lead a satisfying life.

Enhancing Occupational Performance in Schizophrenia

Over the years, J.R. and others like him have discovered specific techniques that help them gain control over their own behavior, their environment, and their schizophrenia. In the physical and sensorimotor area, performance can be enhanced by adequate rest, regular exercise, and a balanced diet. Physical behaviors such as pacing, curling up in a ball, and rocking comfort them when they feel fearful or stressed. These behaviors become socially acceptable if you think of a hammock, rocking chair, sleeping, and walking.

Planning and following a daily schedule are ways to control distractions. Too much free, unstructured time creates anxiety, while overscheduling results in poor decision making and fatigue. Many people plan brief periods in which they can concentrate intensely.

List making enhances both cognitive and psychologic function. Writing down important things helps memory, and accomplishing the listed tasks helps self-esteem. Reality testing can be assisted by having one close person who can give feedback on perceptions of reality.

People with schizophrenia find that social relationships seem to be better with people who have similar interests. In social situations, they have learned to ask for simple, clear communication and to avoid talking to themselves or their voices when around other people. They can force themselves to look at, or a little past, the other person from time to time during conversation. Social support groups provide necessary opportunities to be around people who are understanding.

People with schizophrenia often feel that work is necessary for self-esteem, that too much leisure time creates stress, and that activities of daily living must be compulsively organized. In all areas of occupation, successful task performance may require more time and more persistance than for other people, but the feelings of mastery and competence that result are invaluable.

REFERENCES

1. Sheehan S. Is there no place on earth for me? Boston: Houghton Mifflin, 1982.
2. Ann Arbor News, April 26, 1990.
3. Carpenter WT Jr. Approaches to knowledge and understanding of schizophrenia. Schizophr Bull 1987;13:1–8.
4. Andreason NC. The diagnosis of schizophrenia. Schizophr Bull 1987;13:9–22.
5. Andreason NC. Clinical phenomenon. Schizophr Bull 1988; 14:345–364.
6. Gottesman II, McGuffin P, Farmer AE. Clinical genetics as clues to the "real" genetics of schizophrenia (a decade of modest gains while playing for time). Schizophr Bull 1987;13:23–48.
7. McGue M, Gottesman II. Genetic linkage in schizophrenia: perspectives from genetic epidemiology. Schizophr Bull 1989;15:453–464.
8. Eaves L. Genetics, immunology, and virology. Schizophr Bull 1988; 14:365–382.
9. Goldstein MJ. Psychosocial issues Schizophr Bull 1987;13:157–172.
10. Holzman PS. Basic behavioral sciences. Schizophr Bull 1988;14:413–426.
11. Pato CN, Lander ES, Schulz SC. Prospects for the genetic analysis of schizophrenia. Schizophr Bull 1989;15:365–372.
12. Torrey EF, Bowler AE. The seasonality of schizophrenic births: a reply to Marc S. Lewis. Schizophr Bull 1990;16:1–3.

13. Watson CG. Schizophrenic birth seasonality and the age incidence artifact. Schizophr Bull 1990;16:5–9.

14. Friedhoff AJ. Neurochemistry and neuropharmacology. Schizophr Bull 1988;14:399–412.

15. Rosenstein M, Milazzo SL, Manderschield R. Care of persons with schizophrenia: a statistical profile. Schizophr Bull 1989;15:45–58.

16. Gottesman II, Wolfgram DL. Schizophrenia genesis: the origins of madness. New York: WH Freeman, 1991.

17. Anonymous. First person account: birds of a psychic feather. Schizophr Bull 1990;16:165–168.

18. Carpenter WT Jr, Kirkpatrick B. The heterogeneity of the long term course of schizophrenia. Schizophr Bull 1988;14:645–652.

19. McGlashan TH. A selective review of recent North American long term follow-up studies of schizophrenia. Schizophr Bull 1988;14:645–652.

20. Breier A. Small sample studies: unique contributions for large sample outcome studies. Schizophr Bull 1988;14:589–593.

21. Bleuler M. The schizophrenic disorders: long term patient and family studies. Clemens SM, translator. New Haven: Yale University Press, 1978.

22. Allebeck P. Schizophrenia: a life shortening disease. Schizophr Bull 1989;15:81–89.

23. Tsaung MT, Woolson RF, Fleming JA. Premature deaths in schizophrenia and affective disorders: an analysis of survival curves and variables affecting the shortened survival. Arch Gen Psychiatry 1980b;37:979–983.

24. American Psychiatric Association: Diagnostic and statistical manual of mental disorders, ed. 3-R. Washington D.C.: American Psychiatric Association, 1987.

25. World Health Organization: International classification of diseases, rev 9. Geneva: World Health Organization, 1977.

26. Kane JM. Treatment of schizophrenia. Schizophr Bull 1987;13:133–156.

27. O'Connor J. Psychiatrists patient advocates demand clozapine be made more affordable. Psychiatric news, Washington, D.C.: American Psychiatric Association; June 15, 1990.

28. Katz HM. A new agenda for psychotherapy of schizophrenia: response to Coursey. Schizophr Bull 1989;15:355–358.

29. Bellack AS, Morrison RL, Mueser KT. Social problem solving in schizophrenia. Schizophr Bull 1989;15:101–116.

30. Estroff SE. Self identity and subjective experiences of schizophrenia: in search of the subject. Schizophr Bull 1989;15:189–196.

Glossary

Agranulocytosis: A great majority of cases are caused by sensitization to drugs or chemicals that affect the bone marrow, leading to a marked decrease of granular leukocytes (white blood cells) e.g., leukopenia often leading to an increased susceptibility to bacterial and fungal infections. Manifestations are high fever, chills, prostration, and ulceration of mucous membranes.

Akathisia: A condition marked by motor restlessness and anxiety (considered an extrapyramidal symptom and a common side effect of neuroleptic drugs). Persons with this disorder feel quivering of muscles, an urge to move about constantly, and an inability to sit still.

Anticholinergic: Blocking the passage of impulses through the parasympathetic nerves (parasympatholytic).

Decompensation: In psychiatry, the failure of defense mechanisms such that there is a functional breakdown and symptoms reappear, as occurs in relapses of schizophrenics.

Delusion: A false belief, based on incorrect inference about external reality, not consistent with an individual's intelligence and cultural background, which cannot be corrected by reasoning.

Dizygotic (or dizygous) twins: Twins resulting from the simultaneous fertilization of 2 ova by 2 spermatozoa. Recurrence in families is common. (Synonym: Fraternal twins).

Dystonia: Impairment of muscular tonus manifested as an abnormal persistence of limb and trunk postures; body is bent or twisted in abnormal, relatively fixed positions with possible accompanying muscular facial spasms or torticollis (considered an extrapyramidal symptom).

Extrapyramidal: Any of a group of clinical disorders marked by abnormal involuntary movements, alterations in muscle tone, and postural disturbances (including parkinsonism, chorea, athetosis). Functional unit: Nuclei and fibers (excluding the pyramidal tract) of the brain involved in motor activities that control and coordinate, especially the postural, static, supporting, and locomotor mechanisms. Structures include the corpus striatum, subthalamic nucleus, substantia nigra, and red nucleus, with their interconnections with the reticular formation, cerebellum, and cerebrum; some authorities include the cerebellum and vestibular nuclei.

Florid: Excessive behaviors.

Genetic epidemiology: The study of patterns of incidence, prevalence, and covariance of disorders in families.

Genetic marker: A gene having alleles that are all expressed in the phenotype, that is, they are codominant. Markers are used to determine consistent and stable irregularities in the sequential order of bases in DNA to pinpoint disorders of heredity.

Hallucination: False sensory perceptions not associated with real external stimuli; there may or may not be a delusional interpretation of the hallucinatory experience. Hallucinations indicate a psychotic disturbance only when associated with impairment in reality testing.

Molecular genetics: Application of recombinant DNA techniques to the study of linkages to identify irregularities that suggest chromosomal abnormalities as a factor in various disorders.

Monozygotic (or monozygous) twins: Twins resulting from the division into 2 embryos of a single zygote, following fertilization of a single ovum by a single spermatozoon. Recurrence within families is rare. (Synonym: Identical or one-egg twins.)

Neurophysiology: Scientific study of physiology of the nervous system.

Pathophysiologic genetics: Scientific study of inherited biological weaknesses (physiology of disordered function).

Psychophysiology: Scientific study of interaction and interrelations of psychic and physiologic factors

Psychosis: Inability to distinguish reality from fantasy; impaired reality testing, with creation of new reality.

SPEM (Smooth-pursuit eye movements): The ability to track an item with the eyes without excessive jerking.

Tardive dyskinesia: Disturbed coordination and motor activity in the voluntary motor nervous system characterized by choreiform movements of the buccal-facial muscles and less commonly the extremities. Rarely, focal or generalized dystonia may also be seen. Tardive: applied to a disease in which the characteristic lesion is late-appearing.

6

Mood Disorders

VIRGINIA ALLEN DICKIE

Betsy is at the door waiting for the occupational therapist to arrive on the unit. "I want to go to the O.T. shop right now. I have to make presents for all of my nieces and nephews and for my two sisters. I want to make some pillows like my roommate made, but I want mine to be larger, and I need lots more colors, and . . ." The occupational therapist interrupts Betsy as she pauses to catch her breath, explaining that he will have to check to see if there is a doctor's referral for occupational therapy. He adds that, in any case, the occupational therapy group session will not begin for another 10 minutes.

As he walks down the hall, the therapist thinks to himself that most of that 10 minutes will be spent in Elizabeth's room, encouraging her to leave her bed and "try out" occupational therapy. As he predicted, Elizabeth is curled up on her bed and refuses the therapist's request that she get up and join the group. At first she doesn't say anything. Then she responds to the therapist's gentle encouragement with short statements: "I don't feel good," "I didn't sleep last night," "I'm not good at making things," "Nothing I do ever turns out," "I just don't feel like doing anything." Only after considerable persuading, does Elizabeth consent to come to the clinic and "only to watch." She joins the therapist as he approaches the door. Betsy is waiting there impatiently, telling everyone who is near of her plans to make a set of pillows for each of her relatives.

Betsy and Elizabeth have both been admitted to a psychiatric ward because a mood disorder has caused each of them to be unable to function in her normal environment. As different as their problems seem in this brief description, they could in fact be the same person at different times in the course of a bipolar disorder; Betsy in a manic episode and Elizabeth in a depressed episode. Or Elizabeth might be suffering with a major depression. In either case, each of these women is severely incapacitated in all occupational performance areas.

This chapter discusses mood disorders; how they are classified and diagnosed, how they differ from the "moods" we all feel normally, and research and theories regarding their etiology. Standard treatment approaches are reviewed. The impact of mood disorders on occupational performance is described and then examined in more detail in two case studies.

WHAT IS A MOOD DISORDER?

Mood disorders always involve a disturbed mood, which may be either depressed or manic (1). Each of us has had a disturbed mood many times. How then do mood disorders differ from the normal experience of being "down," "having the blues," or feeling elated? Stated simply, mood disorders differ in apparent cause, in severity, in duration, and in impact on functioning. Our personal experiences of emotional "ups and downs" can help us to understand a little bit about how a person with a mood disorder might be feeling, but to even begin to comprehend clinical depression or bipolar disorder, we must multiply the feelings we have experienced—imagine feeling so bad that there is no reason to get out of bed day after day, or always feeling as if there is a heavy weight on your shoulders, or feeling "high" for several weeks. The novelist William Styron described his own depression as a "smothering" illness (2).

There is danger of misunderstanding mood disorders, though, if we only use our own experiences with changes in mood to try to comprehend these problems. We have developed methods to handle our ups and downs; for example, we get together with a friend, take a walk, help someone else, or exercise. Because we can manage unpleasant moods, we may feel that everyone else should be able to do the same thing. It is not that easy for people who have a mood disorder. Their disturbed moods do not respond to such "do-it-yourself" approaches.

We must also avoid thinking that these disorders are unimportant because they are somewhat like our normal feelings. Mood disorders disrupt occupational functioning, destroy family and social supports, and can result in serious consequences including death if they are not treated. The good news is that treatment for mood disorders is usually very successful (3). The bad news is that only a fraction of the people with depression (by far the more common of the two broad types of mood disorders) receive treatment (4).

CLASSIFICATION OF MOOD DISORDERS

The *Diagnostic and Statistical Manual of Mental Disorders* (DSM-III-R) sets forth criteria that must be met for the mood disturbance to be considered pathologic (1). These criteria include both symptoms and minimum duration, as well as the necessity of ruling out other physical or mental disorders as the cause.

Mood disorders are classified into *bipolar disorders* and *depressive disorders*. A person diagnosed with a mood disorder must have a pattern of *mood episodes*. Mood episodes are *mood syndromes* that have no known cause other than the mood disorder. A mood *syndrome* can occur separately or as part of another disorder.

A person must have had one or more manic or hypomanic episodes to be diagnosed with a bipolar disorder. Characteristics of manic and hypomanic episodes are discussed later in this chapter. A person with a bipolar disorder usually has experienced a major depressive episode, but this is not essential to the bipolar diagnosis.

Bipolar disorders are separated into two types, *bipolar disorder*, which requires that the person has had one or more manic episodes, and *cyclothymia*, which is characterized by recurrent hypomanic episodes and periods of depression. It may be helpful to think of a bipolar disorder as more extreme, more episodic, and more serious, and to think of cyclothymia as less extreme and more an enduring part of the individual's character. Generally a person with cyclothymia is not admitted to an inpatient psychiatric unit solely for treatment related to this diagnosis.

There are also two types of depressive disorders, *major depression* and *dysthymia*. In either case, the person must have had one or more periods of depression, without ever having either a manic or hypomanic episode. A person with major depression has had one or more major depressive episodes. A person who has experienced a depressed mood for the majority of days during the past 2 years without ever (during the first 2 years) meeting the criteria for a major depressive episode, is said to have dysthymia. Dysthymia is less severe, more long-standing, and lacks the episodic quality of major depression. In the past it was sometimes called a neurotic depression. After the initial 2 years, a person may have a major depression in addition to dysthymia if diagnostic criteria for both are met.

Scientists and clinicians continue to argue about whether or not bipolar disorders and depressive disorders are part of a single continuum, whether or not there are distinct subtypes of both, and what these might be (4). Both syndromes are expressed in a wide variety of ways in different individuals and at different times by the same person. This chapter will adhere to the DSM-III-R classification system, generally ignoring questions of subtypes, but adding information from other sources as pertinent. The DSM-III-R system will continue to be modified in further revisions and editions based on research and clinical experience that supports or refutes existing classification criteria. As these changes occur in the future, you should compare new editions with previous systems for clarification.

A wide variety of terms are used to describe mood disorders within clinical settings. Many of these terms are derived from past classification systems or from particular theoretical perspectives. If you find yourself in this situation it is best to seek clarification within the setting. DSM-III-R is currently used nationwide to code psychiatric disorders for reimbursement and reporting purposes and to ensure consistency in research. Thus, when other terminology is used, it is usually in addition to this system.

It is easiest to discuss depressive disorders and bipolar disorders separately because their etiology and treatment are different and because they are very different in clinical manifestations when the person with a bipolar disorder is in the manic phase. Keep in mind that this distinction may not be nearly so clear in reality. Neither dysthymia nor cyclothymia will be discussed.

You may see patients with any of these conditions in any setting. If a mood disorder coexists with other conditions, treatment of problems relating to those conditions may be seriously affected by the mood disorder.

DEPRESSIVE DISORDERS

Incidence and Prevalence

Depression is the most common psychiatric disorder. In a study of over 20,000 adults, the National Institute for Mental Health (NIMH) found an incidence of major depression of 3.0% in a 6-month period and a lifetime incidence of 5.8% (5). When people with bipolar disorders and dysthymia are included, 5.85% of the population can be expected to suffer from mood disorders in a 6-month period and 8.3% during their lifetime (5). Major depression cost the United States more than $16 billion a year in 1986; $14.2 billion of that was indirect: lost productivity, family care costs, and costs of morbidity and mortality (5).

Depression cuts across all social, racial, and economic groups. Studies differ on whether or not rates differ between socioeconomic groups, but rates between racial groups are similar. Physicians may underdiagnose mood disorders in people of a different race from their own (6). (Psychiatric diagnosis requires relating behaviors and symptoms to the individual's own life and situation. This increases the risk of misdiagnosis when there is significant difference between physician and patient.) Women have twice the risk of men in developing depression during their lifetime according to Kaplan (6). Depression is more common in people who are single than in those who are married (6). Epidemiologic studies may give different rates, which may reflect use of different reporting systems or different protocols for identification and diagnosis. Depression affects people of all ages, from infancy to old age, with the highest rate of occurrence in the 25- to 44-year age range (5). Recently there has been concern about the growing rate of depression in children and adolescents. It is not clear if this is due to a true change in rate or to improved diagnostic procedures and/or increased awareness that depression is common in younger persons.

Depression often goes unrecognized and untreated, and thus mental health statistics may underrepresent actual occurrences.

Etiology of Depression

People suffering from depression, their friends and families, and many professionals working with them tend to look for external causes or environmental events to explain the terrible suffering that this disease creates. When a person commits suicide, it is rare to see the act attributed to depression without some additional cause given for the mood disorder. Explanations over centuries have included mysterious changes in body "humors," unusual amounts of stress, real or perceived losses of important people at an early age, recent losses or bad luck, anger turned inward, and on and on. A "melancholic" mood was once thought desirable in artistic individuals as a sign of sensitivity (7); thus people who are depressed must be extra sensitive.

Today we are much closer to understanding what causes depression, although the exact mechanisms of the disease are unclear. What is very clear is that there is no simple or single answer! Depression appears to be a biopsychosocial phenomenon in both cause and expression. It may be a clinical picture that can be caused by a variety of different factors, or it may be a number of different disorders.

Problems in Research

When you read research reports about the cause of depression, you must look carefully at the way investigators have conducted their studies. What condition(s) are they studying? What questions are they asking? What are their methods?

It is often difficult to sort out cause from effect for an existing problem. Much depression research has been conducted with people after they have been diagnosed as depressed, thus the psychosocial antecedents are seen through the lens of

the illness and may be distorted. This illness alters the individuals' functioning in life roles and relationships. Even the biologic differences that are supported in many studies could be a result rather than a cause of the depression. Longitudinal studies of a population from birth to death would help us to understand who becomes depressed and why. Medical records in countries (such as Denmark) that have socialized medicine are helpful in this regard. Research studies may study people with true depressive disorders or study subjects who are more inclined than the controls to express a depressed mood on some test or scale. For example, studies are often done with groups of medical students or college students enrolled in psychology courses. The results may say more about different personality types than about depression as a psychiatric disorder. (They also focus on a very limited population.) These studies do not look at clinical depression, but many of them are very interesting, and they may help us understand how people with depressed moods think and function. Use caution, however, in applying the findings in such studies to people with major depression.

Research on depression is further complicated by the possibility that depression is not a single entity. The clinical syndrome may be the outward manifestation of a variety of processes. Investigators also disagree as to whether or not there are subtypes of depression, what they might be, and if they represent different syndromes. Look carefully at studies to see what criteria have been used to group the subjects. Different subtypes of depression are not yet clearly linked to different causes, but failure to distinguish subtypes or patterns of variation may flaw research results.

Biologic Theories of Etiology

Medications are very effective in alleviating symptoms of major depression in most people. This is one of the most obvious indicators that depression has biologic components. Antidepressant medications affect the neurotransmitters serotonin and/or norepinephrine. Simplistically, antidepressants cause an increased availability of these neurotransmitters for transmission of nerve impulses. Because of this, we can assume that there is some decreased level or blockage of serotonin and/or norepinephrine in the brains of depressed persons (or at least in those who respond well to drug treatment).

Neuroendocrine studies of patients with depression show irregularities related to the limbic-hypothalamic-pituitary-adrenal axis (6). One commonly used test, the dexamethasone suppression test (DST), shows abnormal cortisol secretions in at least 50% of the patients with depression. For these patients, the cortisol levels return to normal as clinical improvements occur. A great deal of research is being done using the DST, and it is sometimes used clinically to attempt to distinguish types of depression, but the changes it shows are not specific to depression and are not consistent among those who are depressed. Nonetheless, it and other endocrine studies lend support to a biologic component in depression.

Other research areas that support a biologic factor in depression include sleep studies that show depressed persons having disrupted sleep and decreased REM latency (6, 8) and studies of immune function that show changes of cellular response in persons who are depressed. Additional evidence for a biologic cause or component of depression comes from the similarity of symptoms in people with known brain lesions and our knowledge of the functions of specific areas of the brain. Some physiologic symptoms of depression (e.g., lack of sexual interest, sleep difficulties, and decreased appetite) occur with dysfunction of the hypothalamus (6). Problems such as slowness, lack of energy, and difficulty thinking are similar to problems seen in people with basal ganglia lesions.

Genetics

A number of studies show increased rates of depression in biologic family members of depressed persons and in monozygotic (identical) twins. These associations are significant but not nearly as strong as they are for bipolar disorder.

Seasonal Disorders

Ancient writing about depression ascribed a depression-like state to seasonal patterns that modern research has confirmed exist for some individuals. DSM-III-R provides criteria for diagnosing a seasonal pattern, most notably that the onset of each episode occurs within the same 60-day period for at least 3 separate years and that remission occurs within a certain period for each episode (1). Winter depression has distinct symptoms in addition to the time that it occurs. These include overeating, oversleeping, and craving for carbohydrates (9). Light deficiency is implicated as the cause of winter depression, and people with this diagnosis respond well to phototherapy (prescribed exposure to light). (Records of the use of light to treat depression date back 2000 years!) The cause of summer depression is less clear, but it may be related to heat (9). In addition to clear seasonal disorders, data on suicides and on onset of depressive episodes (nonseasonal) also reveal seasonal patterns. Suicide rates peak in late spring and early summer with a smaller peak in late fall and early winter, and the onset of mood disorders peaks in both spring (March through May) and fall (September through November) (9).

Seasonal mood disorders may provide clues to the cause of mood disorders in general. For this reason, research interest is developing in this area. The hypothalamus, already implicated in many biologically focused studies of depression, monitors and regulates the body's exposure and response to such things as light and heat. Appetite and weight, physical activity, sleep, and body temperature are all regulated by the hypothalamus, the autonomic nervous system, the hypothalamic-pituitary-adrenal axis, and the hypothalamic-pituitary-thyroid axis. Thus mood disorders that involve change in appetite, activity, sleep, and/or energy level may result from changes in these areas of the central nervous system.

Psychosocial Theories of Etiology

The psychosocial theories and explanations of the etiology of depression have varying degrees of support from research, but have major impact on the methods of psychotherapy that clinicians use for depressed persons. Many theories exist. Four approaches are discussed here to illustrate the variety of these perspectives.

Psychodynamic theories characterize depression as evolving from an internal state often involving extreme emotional dependence on others. Many different psychodynamic theories have been proposed over many years, most rooted in Freud's theories of psychosexual development and intrapsychic conflict. Depression is seen as the "consequence of underlying conflict" (10). The following description is my somewhat simplistic version of a psychodynamic approach to explaining how depression occurs.

Depressed individuals never developed the ability to find meaning in life except through other persons and probably experienced some early childhood loss or deprivation from mother or another significant person. They depend upon others to make choices and only know that a job is well done if told so by an important person. Their lives are defined totally by significant others. (In psychodynamic terms this person is referred to as an object.)

Now, imagine yourself as a significant other—could you possibly be all things to another person, someone who depended upon you exclusively? Even if you tried, inevitably you would fail as you acted to meet your own needs and those of the social system. Unless you were acting from your own psychopathology, you would

probably grow to feel burdened by the other person's extreme dependency and would try to encourage him or her to rely upon you less. The person who has this dependency sees these attitudes and actions of the significant other as loses, failures, rejections, or betrayals. These perceived "loses" may range from outright rejection (e.g., a spouse leaving) to more symbolic losses (birth of a sibling and consequent need to share mother's time and attention). The loss "event" may be a sharing of affection with an additional person (best friend gets a boyfriend) or a lack of availability of the other caused by a life event (hospitalization, move to another part of the country). It may simply be perceived indifference to the person's concerns, a sharp word, a lack of response.

The spiral into depression starts with the loss. The individual is faced with a terrible problem—he or she relies totally upon a special person, who has let them down. Becoming angry with that person only increases the chance that that person will not come back or will continue to be less available. Thus it is not safe to show this anger, and angry feelings generate both fear and guilt. At this point the anger is turned inward. The individual feels responsible for the loss or letdown. Anger with oneself seems safer, but it results in depression, which is destructive to self.

This description of a psychodynamic theory of depression does not begin to cover the multiple and complex approaches that have been put forth over the years. There are many theories in the literature. In his review of psychotherapies for depression, Karasu summarizes modern dynamic theory as combining "such psychoanalytic formulations as early childhood disappointment and loss . . . damaged self-esteem . . . persistence of narcissistic rage beneath an unloved and punished self . . . a sense of helplessness and hopelessness, and difficulties in autonomy and intimacy." (10).

Psychodynamic theories are not well supported by research, but are often cited in postulating possible causes for a person's depression. These theories form the basis for psychodynamic therapies for depression. Today such therapy takes many forms other than traditional Freudian psychoanalysis—most notably it is shorter-term, and the therapist takes a more active role in treatment.

Existential explanations of depression look at the correlation of depression with the person's life and see the relationship of depression to prolonged periods when it is difficult to find meaning in life or to major changes, often the attainment of long-sought goals.

Many of us find meaning in life by striving toward achieving something (e.g., job promotion, graduation from college, marriage, retirement). We expect that when we reach this goal we will be very happy (or at least content), will be able to do what we want to do, or will be recognized by others. But two things happen when you reach your goals. The first is that you no longer have the goal! You have lost something that has been important in guiding your life over a long period of time. The second effect is that the result of reaching the goal may not be what you expected. Happiness is not a guaranteed result. Other things may be going wrong; The promotion may mean more work, longer hours, and loss of friends from the old office. Graduation may decrease exciting intellectual stimulation. Marriage entails a great deal of adjustment. Retirement may exchange a hated job for boredom. The loss of goals and/or the failure of achievements to meet expectations may result in depression.

Again we have a theoretical perspective that lacks significant research support, but the existential view may be helpful in understanding some of the reactions we have to our successes—there may be a reason for feeling letdown or blue when we and the world around us expect a happy response!

Cognitive Theory

A number of theorists have contributed to the cognitive view of depression, but

Aaron Beck and his associates are the people most associated with this approach today. Beck developed a paradigm to explain the relationship of cognitive patterns to the characteristic symptoms of depression (11). Depression is caused by problems in thinking. He described three cognitive patterns that differentiate depressed people from others in the way that they think.

First, depressed individuals have a negative view of the world. They consistently interpret their experiences in the worst light or distort events in a negative direction. Less than total success may be seen as failure (e.g., getting an A− instead of an A may be seen as a defeat). Depressed persons may consider themselves deprived over minor things (e.g., having less money to spend on clothes than a friend has). They tend to overreact to feedback from others, interpreting neutral signs in a negative way (e.g., when her husband doesn't say anything about her new dress, the woman interprets this to mean that he thinks it is ugly).

The second area of cognitive distortion is in the individuals' view of themselves. A negative view of self is displayed in a tendency to blame oneself for anything that goes wrong and to view this as a major shortcoming in one's character. The student is convinced that he is stupid because he didn't get a good grade on a test. The woman "knows" she is a terrible mother because her son misbehaves in nursery school. When a girl turns him down for a date, the boy knows it is because he is totally unattractive to the opposite sex. Depressed persons simply do not like, nor see any reason to like, themselves.

The third cognitive distortion is a negative view of the future. Not only is the world a terrible place and the self a terrible person, but there is no reason to expect things to get better in the short run or in the long run. The future is seen as a continuation of the current unpleasantness, and this continuity with the present differentiates the depressed person's view of the future from normal anxiety about the future.

In addition to these three cognitive distortions, depressed people have deeply felt silent assumptions that distort the conclusions they draw from events, and they exhibit illogical thinking (10). For example, an isolated event such as a critical comment will be used to make broad generalizations about one's own worth, or others' attitudes toward oneself. Depressed persons may hold themselves responsible for events, when this could not possibly be the case.

In Beck's view, the symptoms of depression are a result of distorted thinking. Beck further elaborated his theories and developed a treatment approach that helps patients to identify the way in which they develop negative cognitions. Errors in thinking are identified, and alternate patterns are developed and practiced in short-term and time-limited therapy. This treatment approach has been effective for many people, but it must be used in conjunction with medications when a person has a major depressive episode.

Some of Beck's statements about distorted cognitions may be questioned in light of research that shows that depressed persons may *accurately* assess their own role in success and failure in laboratory test situations, while "normals" tend to distort their responsibility for negative results, to place themselves in the best light (12, 13). This research does show that depressed persons place more emphasis on their failures than on their successes. Beck's theory is reasonably supported by research in its ability to describe the differences between depressed and nondepressed persons. It is not clear, however, that negative or distorted cognitions cause the clinical entity called depression. Again it is the question of which came first.

There are a number of other cognitive theories of depression, as well as elaboration of Beck's work by others. Two theories that are frequently cited are Ellis' theory of *irrational beliefs* (14), and Seligman's theory of *learned helplessness* (15).

Behavioral Theories of Depression

Lewinsohn correlates depression with a lack of reinforcement from the environment. Reinforcement must follow behavior, and when it makes the person feel good, Lewinsohn calls it positive reinforcement. If people behave in a way that does not result in positive reinforcement or if they live in an environment that does not provide positive reinforcement, they become depressed (16, 17). Depression is also caused by a high level of punishing or negative reinforcement (in other words, effects that make the person feel bad).

Based on his theoretical formulation of depression, Lewinsohn developed a short-term, time-limited treatment approach that focuses on increasing the amount of positive reinforcement a person receives by changing behaviors. One central element to his approach is the "Pleasant Events Schedule," which is a listing of several hundred events in which a person might find pleasure (16). Patients go through this list and identify those items that they find pleasurable. Next the frequency of participation in these events is charted (it is usually very low in depressed persons), and a plan is developed to incorporate some of them into the regular daily schedule. This is carried out as a homework assignment that includes monitoring and recording feelings. Lewinsohn incorporates a number of cognitive and behavioral assignments into his treatment, which is usually conducted in an educational (classroom) manner. He has also published a self-help version of his treatment as a book (18).

Lewinsohn has supported both his theory of depression and the efficacy of this treatment approach with research. Once again, the research is looking at people who are already identified as being depressed, so cause and effect are hard to sort out. Because his subjects can be treated with this approach as outpatients, it is possible that their symptoms are less severe than those of a person hospitalized with major depression.

This discussion has not begun to cover all theories of depression, nor does it provide any detail or depth for those discussed. It is meant to illustrate the diversity of ways that this disease is conceptualized and to give some exposure to leading theoretical perspectives. Other perspectives and approaches in use include the interpersonal approach and approaches based upon stress. Many of the therapeutic approaches in use today combine aspects of several of these perspectives.

SIGNS AND SYMPTOMS OF DEPRESSION

Depression is defined by its symptoms. There is no blood test nor other laboratory means at the present time to determine whether or not a person has depression. DSM-III-R establishes a minimum of five of nine possible symptoms to diagnose a major depressive episode (which then becomes a major depression). These symptoms are listed in Table 6.1. There are also a group of associated symptoms that may be exhibited by depressed persons.

As you would expect, a depressed or sad mood is one of the major symptoms of depression. This obvious change in mood does not always occur in patients, and children and adolescents may display an irritable, rather than depressed, mood (1). People may say that they feel sad all the time or hopeless. They may say they are "down" or "feeling blue," or they may complain of always feeling tired. Children may not be able to describe their feelings very clearly.

Another major, and more frequent, indicator of a depression is a loss of interest or pleasure in most activities (1, 19). People who are seriously depressed do not want to do the things that they normally enjoy. If they do engage in these activi-

ties, it is without pleasure. Bowling with friends may seem more obligation than fun. The garden grows weedy as its owner neglects what was her major source of leisure enjoyment for the past 5 years. A grown daughter may no longer be able to convince her widowed mother to go on their monthly antique hunting and lunch expedition. Grandfather may not feel any joy in a fishing trip with his grandson. Even in the absence of any depressed feelings, the loss of interest and pleasure should be a strong indicator that a person may be depressed (19).

Decreased appetite is another common symptom of depression. This may not be evident until the person shows a notable weight loss without having consciously cut back on food. Conversely, a depressed person may overeat, though this is less common.

People who are depressed frequently complain of problems with sleeping. They may have a great deal of difficulty falling asleep at night. Sometimes they will report not sleeping at all, but this usually is not true. When sleep comes late in the night, depressed people have a great deal of trouble getting out of bed in the morning. Sometimes depression is characterized by awakening very early, typically around 4 AM, and not being able to return to sleep. Occasionally, depressed people sleep much more than normal.

Family and friends may notice that the depressed person moves much more slowly than usual or that he or she seems agitated and may pace or have trouble sitting still. These psychomotor symptoms are often accompanied by extreme fatigue. A man who routinely jogs may report that he just doesn't have the energy to do it anymore. Physical symptoms often cause the individual and concerned family members to look for physical causes and may be the reason for a visit to the family doctor. A focus on physical symptoms may obscure the diagnosis of depression. Gold et al., in a study of chronic fatigue (CF) and Epstein-Barr virus (EBV) found that "patients with CF had a strikingly higher

Table 6.1.
Diagnostic Criteria for Major Depression[a]

Diagnostic criteria for Major Depressive Episode

Note: A "Major Depressive Syndrome" is defined as criterion A below.

A. At least five of the following symptoms have been present during the same two-week period and represent a change from previous functioning: at least one of the symptoms is either (1) depressed mood, or (2) loss of interest or pleasure. (Do not include symptoms that are clearly due to a physical condition, mood-incongruent delusions or hallucinations, incoherence, or marked loosening of associations.)

   (1) depressed mood (or can be irritable mood in children and adolescents) most of the day, nearly every day, as indicated either by subjective account or observation by others
   (2) markedly diminished interest or pleasure in all, or almost all, activities most of the day, nearly every day (as indicated either by subjective account or observation by others of apathy most of the time)
   (3) significant weight loss or weight gain when not dieting (e.g., more than 5% of body weight in a month), or decrease or increase in appetite nearly every day (in children, consider failure to make expected weight gains)
   (4) insomnia or hypersomnia nearly every day
   (5) psychomotor agitation or retardation nearly every day (observable by others, not merely subjective feelings of restlessness or being slowed down)
   (6) fatigue or loss of energy nearly every day
   (7) feelings of worthlessness or excessive or inappropriate guilt (which may be delusional) nearly every day (not merely self-reproach or guilt about being sick)
   (8) diminished ability to think or concentrate, or indecisiveness, nearly every day (either by subjective account or as observed by others)
   (9) recurrent thoughts of death (not just fear of dying), recurrent suicidal ideation without a specific plan, or a suicide attempt or a specific plan for committing suicide

B. (1) It cannot be established that an organic factor initiated and maintained the disturbance
   (2) The disturbance is not a normal reaction to the death of a loved one (Uncomplicated Bereavement)

   Note: Morbid preoccupation with worthlessness, suicidal ideation, marked functional impairment or psychomotor retardation, or prolonged duration suggest bereavement complicated by Major Depression.

C. At no time during the disturbance have there been delusions or hallucinations for as long as two weeks in the absence of prominent mood symptoms (i.e., before the mood symptoms developed or after they have remitted).

D. Not superimposed on Schizophrenia, Schizophreniform Disorder, Delusional Disorder, or Psychotic Disorder NOS.

Major Depressive Episode codes: fifth-digit code numbers and criteria for severity of current state of Bipolar Disorder, Depressed, or Major Depression:
   1—**Mild:** Few, if any, symptoms in excess of those required to make the diagnosis, **and** symptoms result in only minor impairment in occupational functioning or in usual social activities or relationships with others.

   2—**Moderate:** Symptoms or functional impairment between "mild" and "severe."

   3—**Severe, without Psychotic Features:** Several symptoms in excess of those required to make the diagnosis, **and** symptoms markedly interfere with occupational functioning or with usual social activities or relationships with others.

Table 6.1.   (Continued)

4—**With Psychotic Features:** Delusions or hallucinations. If possible, **specify** whether the psychotic features are *mood-congruent* or *mood-incongruent.*

Mood-congruent psychotic features: Delusions or hallucinations whose content is entirely consistent with the typical depressive themes of personal inadequacy, guilt, disease, death, nihilism, or deserved punishment.

Mood-incongruent psychotic features: Delusions or hallucinations whose content does *not* involve typical depressive themes of personal inadequacy, guilt, disease, death, nihilism, or deserved punishment. Included here are such symptoms as persecutory delusions (not directly related to depressive themes), thought insertion, thought broadcasting, and delusions of control.

5—**In Partial Remission:** Intermediate between "In Full Remission" and "Mild," **and** no previous Dysthymia. (If Major Depressive Episode was superimposed on Dysthymia, the diagnosis of Dysthymia alone is given once the full criteria for a Major Depressive Episode are no longer met.)

6—**In Full Remission:** During the past six months no significant signs or symptoms of the disturbance.

0—**Unspecified.**

Specify chronic if current episode has lasted two consecutive years without a period of two months or longer during which there were no significant depressive symptoms.

Specify if current episode is **Melancholic Type.**

Diagnostic criteria for Melancholic Type

The presence of at least five of the following:

   (1) loss of interest or pleasure in all, or almost all, activities
   (2) lack of reactivity to usually pleasurable stimuli (does not feel much better, even temporarily, when something good happens)
   (3) depression regularly worse in the morning
   (4) early morning awakening (at least two hours before usual time of awakening)
   (5) psychomotor retardation or agitation (not merely subjective complaints)
   (6) significant anorexia or weight loss (e.g., more than 5% of body weight in a month)
   (7) no significant personality disturbance before first Major Depressive Episode
   (8) one or more previous Major Depressive Episodes followed by complete, or nearly complete, recovery
   (9) previous good response to specific and adequate somatic antidepressant therapy, e.g., tricyclics, ECT, MAOI, lithium

Diagnostic criteria for seasonal pattern

A. There has been a regular temporal relationship between the onset of an episode of Bipolar Disorder (including Bipolar Disorder NOS) or Recurrent Major Depression (including Depressive Disorder NOS) and a particular 60-day period of the year (e.g., regular appearance of depression between the beginning of October and the end of November).
   Note: Do not include cases in which there is an obvious effect of seasonally related psychosocial stressors, e.g., regularly being unemployed every winter.

B. Full remissions (or a change from depression to mania or hypomania) also occurred within a particular 60-day period of the year (e.g., depression disappears from mid-February to mid-April).

C. There have been at least three episodes of mood disturbance in three separate years that demonstrated the temporal seasonal relationship defined in A and B; at least two of the years were consecutive.

D. Seasonal episodes of mood disturbance, as described above, outnumbered any nonseasonal episodes of such disturbance that may have occurred by more than three to one.

[a]From American Psychiatric Association. Diagnostic and statistical manual of mental disorders. 3rd ed. revised. Washington, D.C.: American Psychiatric Association, 1987:222–224. With permission.

rate of lifetime and current major depression than controls." They found "no significant differences in the prevalence of active EBV infection" between subjects and controls (20). Chronic fatigue or EBV may be a more socially acceptable diagnosis than depression, but accurate diagnosis will help the individual get correct treatment. Further work on CF may identify another cause or causes, but the similarity of symptoms to those of depression is striking.

People who are depressed often feel useless and unworthy. They may be preoccupied with guilt over some real or delusional occurrence in the past. Having others worry about them or do kind things for them increases their sense of guilt and/or worthlessness. They may often think of death or suicide, and frequently plan and/or attempt suicide. William Styron writes of the relentlessness of depression, the lack of hope, and the physical pain. "And so, because there is no respite at all, it is entirely natural that the victim begins to think ceaselessly of oblivion" (2). Ann's failed suicide attempt may be the factor that brings her into treatment. Joe's suicide may be the first indication to his family and friends that he was experiencing depression, and it may forever leave them trying to understand what happened. Sometimes the individual's preoccupation with death is focused on others (e.g., the woman who reads obituaries and recites the recent deaths of all her friends as the major content of her conversation).

Depressed people often have difficulty thinking and problem solving, even in areas where they are usually quite skilled. In children this may show up in school performance: Amy "daydreams" and doesn't get her work done, and she no longer "tries" in math. Adults may start to have difficulty handling their work. Making decisions is often extremely difficult. Mrs. Smith agonizes over whether to shop before or after lunch, and it takes her half the day to select a menu for dinner.

A number of symptoms may occur with depression that are not central to its diagnosis. These include such things as crying a great deal, high levels of anxiety, preoccupation with the state of one's health, brooding over minor incidents, and panic attacks. Depressed persons may be delusional and/or experience hallucinations, usually related to their unworthiness or to being persecuted or punished for something they have done.

Depressed persons exhibit these symptoms to varying degrees. Although not symptoms, per se, the feelings of family and friends may also help identify people with depression. Families may worry and feel that they need to take care of the individual. The family may be angry because depressed people are no fun to be around and furthermore resist all attempts by the family to cheer them.

Some symptoms vary according to age. In addition to school problems, children may show more psychomotor agitation and hallucinations than adults. Adolescents may engage in antisocial behavior, including substance abuse. Withdrawal from the family and school difficulties are common. Elderly adults with depression may be misdiagnosed as having dementia. In fact, a number of symptoms of Alzheimer-type dementia are also symptoms of depression, e.g., decreased interest, poor concentration, fatigue, and changes in psychomotor activity (21). Careful diagnosis is important, since depression is usually reversible with appropriate treatment. When physical symptoms of depression predominate, the person may undergo many unnecessary diagnostic procedures if depression is not considered.

Progression and Prognosis

Depression may be acute or chronic, but even in acute cases there is a typical duration of 6 months and at least 2 weeks of symptoms are required to diagnose a major depressive episode (1). For people with a chronic depression, some symptoms may persist, even when the major symptoms have lifted. A person may have a single episode of depression or may have recurring episodes over a lifetime.

Depression may lift without treatment, but there is no reason for a person to go through the pain and disruption of a major depression, waiting for it to go away by itself. This is a very treatable disorder, at least in terms of alleviating symptoms, but people often go without treatment because they and others around them do not recognize that they are experiencing a depression, or they fail to seek help because they fear the stigma of having a mental illness. Knowledge of the biologic causes of depression may make seeking treatment more acceptable.

Until recently, few studies were done of the long-term prognosis for depression. It was assumed that people returned to normal functioning once the symptoms of depression had subsided. Studies now show that this is not universally true. About 20% of persons who have major depression may develop chronic depression (22), and about the same proportion may have a recurrence during the first year. It is not yet clear how patients function over time in their daily occupational performance following major depression.

The major complication of depression is the high risk of suicide. It is estimated that over half the suicides in the United States are related to depression. Ten to 15% of people who are hospitalized with depression will eventually commit suicide (3, 5). The risk of suicide is high for persons who are in the hospital for medical conditions and also suffer from depression and for people in the months following discharge from a psychiatric unit.

Potential suicide should always be a consideration when working with an individual who is depressed. Clinicians should observe closely for signs that persons might be thinking of hurting themselves or have a suicide plan. All such suggestions must be taken very seriously. Patients considered to be acutely suicidal are usually placed on a one to one staffing

ratio or are on ward restrictions with 15-minute checks. In occupational therapy careful counts are kept of any potentially dangerous implements, and toxic materials are kept locked up when not in use. Use of any dangerous tools or substances is closely monitored. Suicide may be a risk with other conditions, and similar precautions should be followed.

Another common complication of depression is substance abuse. Depressed people may turn to alcohol or drugs and a means of "self-medication," or the depression may be secondary to the substance abuse problem.

Diagnostics

As stated earlier, depression is diagnosed on the basis of symptoms. In addition to meeting criteria for symptoms, the person must have had the symptoms for at least 2 weeks and must not be going through a normal reaction to a bereavement. The clinician must be sure that there is no organic cause for the symptoms and must rule out other disorders with similar characteristics, such as schizophrenia, delusional disorder, and anxiety disorder.

There are some scales and inventories that are used to help diagnose depression, such as the Beck depression inventory (23), the Hamilton rating scale (24), the schedule of affective disorders and schizophrenia (SADS) (25), and the research and diagnostic criteria (19). These seem most useful in classifying subtypes of depression or in ensuring homogeneity of subjects for research purposes. They have demonstrated concurrent validity with each other and with other diagnostic criteria.

No laboratory or other medical tests are able to diagnose depression reliably at this time.

Medications

Antidepressant medications fall into three categories, the heterocyclics (tricyclics until fairly recently), the monoamine oxidase inhibitors (MAOIs) (26), and those chemically unrelated to either of those categories. Antidepressant medications are summarized in Appendix 6.2.

The most commonly used drugs are the heterocyclics. They take several weeks to reach full therapeutic benefits. No particular type is more effective than any other, but they vary in their side effects. Physicians often choose a particular drug because of such factors as side effects and patient preference. For example, a person with a cardiac problem would be prescribed a medication with no known cardiovascular side effects, and a person with an agitated depression might be given a drug that had sedative side effects. If a patient reports good results with a particular medication in the past, it will usually be the first thing tried. Some antidepressants (e.g., amoxapine) are antipsychotic as well, and may be a good choice for treatment of a person with psychotic symptoms in addition to the depression (i.e., delusions and/or hallucinations) or with schizophrenia and depression, but the risk of extrapyramidal side effects is added to those typical for antidepressants alone.

MAOIs are used less frequently than heterocyclics in the treatment of depression because they require more careful management and are somewhat less effective. They work by inhibiting the production of monoamine oxidase, a normally occurring enzyme that breaks down certain amines in the body, including serotonin and norepinephrine. When the levels of monoamine oxidase are reduced, the levels of serotonin and norepinephrine rise, effecting a remission of the depression. Unfortunately, the effects of monoamine oxidase are quite general, and some of the amines it breaks down become toxic. These substances that break down into dangerous products come from a wide variety of food, much of it aged or fermented, including aged cheese, pickled herring, red wine, beer, and cured meats as well as some over-the-counter and prescribed medications. Patients must be well educated in what foods to avoid

and be motivated to follow the dietary restrictions. (Therapists should check with the dietician or nurse before any use of food in occupational therapy treatment groups.) If dietary restrictions are not followed, the person taking MAOIs may develop increased blood pressure, headaches, and intracranial bleeding resulting in death. In spite of the care that must be followed when taking MAOIs, they are the only effective type of medication for some people.

Antidepressants that don't fit into either of the above categories have been developed recently. Fluoxetine hydrochloride (Prozac) is now in common use. While this medication appears to be very effective for many people, there is concern that it may increase the risk of suicide. At the time of this writing, this relationship has not been clearly established.

Antidepressant medications are quite toxic, with lethal doses being only a few times greater than the normal daily dose. Thus suicidal patients must be carefully monitored to be sure that they are taking medication as prescribed (not saving pills), and outpatients should not be given large supplies of medication until the risk of suicide has declined.

Antidepressants usually take 3 to 4 weeks to alleviate depression, and even after the obvious symptoms of depression begin to lift, the individual may still *feel* very depressed. The period after treatment begins and before effects are felt can be very difficult for depressed patients; the lack of immediate relief adding to their feeling of hopelessness. Much reassurance and education is needed during this time, and care givers and family should watch for signs of potential suicide. If a heterocyclic is not helpful, at least 2 weeks without medication should occur before introducing an MAOI, because of possible toxic interactions.

Electroconvulsive Therapy (ECT)

Electroconvulsive therapy (ECT) is "the brief application of an electrical stimulus to the brain to produce a generalized seizure" (27). ECT can be very effective in short-term treatment for some people who have depression, notably when the depression includes delusions, when it has no known antecedents, or when the person is at extremely high risk for suicide (27). Effects of treatment are seen more rapidly than with antidepressant medication.

Unfortunately, ECT has received a "bad press" because it was massively misused in treatment of psychiatric patients in the past. Public reaction to this abuse continues to limit access to this treatment. ECT is also frightening, and why it works is not understood. Thus, it is probably not used as much as it could be, and often it is considered only as a last resort, when medications have not been effective or the patient's depression is considered life-threatening.

When ECT is used, strict protocols are followed, including consultation with other physicians and careful attention to informed consent for the patient and family. A thorough medical screening is completed before use of ECT.

ECT is given on an inpatient or outpatient basis by a physician, with a professional anesthetist and nursing personnel in attendance. Treatment is usually given in the morning after 8 to 12 hours of fasting. Before treatment, the patient is given an anticholinergic agent, a brief anesthetic, and a muscle relaxant. Oxygen is administered throughout the procedure, and the electrocardiogram (ECG), blood pressure, and pulse rate are continuously monitored. A brief electrical stimulus is given to the brain through one or two electrodes, using the lowest amount of electrical energy needed to produce a seizure (as evidenced by electroencephalogram [EEG] monitoring and/or physical evidence of a seizure). Usually a patient has 6 to 12 of these treatments at the rate of 3 per week.

After treatment, patients are monitored in the recovery room for a period and then returned to the patient ward or home to rest. Often they can engage in activity in the afternoon, although they may still feel tired.

The major adverse effect of ECT is memory loss, which is seen in almost all cases. The severity of the memory deficit varies according to the individual and the degree of treatment. For many patients, memory problems relate to the time around the treatment and persist for as long as 3 years. During the time patients are receiving treatment and for a few weeks after its completion, they may have transient difficulty learning and retaining new information (27). The treatment does carry some risk of complications such as cardiorespiratory problems, severe confusion, and falls (28).

In addition to medication or ECT, psychotherapy is often helpful for people with depression. While such therapy might not alleviate symptoms or prevent relapse, it can enhance social functioning (29).

DEPRESSION AND OCCUPATIONAL PERFORMANCE

All occupational performance areas may be affected by this condition, a fact reflected in the number of symptoms that relate directly to functioning. In a very large study of functioning and well-being of depressed patients, Wells et al. demonstrated that depression is associated with limitations in functioning (physical, social, and role) and well-being. They also concluded that depressed people have comparable or worse functioning than patients with chronic medical conditions, with the exception of current heart conditions (30). Table 6.2 highlights the performance components where dysfunction is most likely to be seen.

The typical symptoms of depression affect occupational performance according to each individual's characteristics (e.g., age, sex, life situation, roles) and environmental expectations (e.g., family responsibilities, support systems, roles). There is no single "typical" depressed person, but the following case study shows how occupational performance is affected for one person with a major depression.

CASE STUDY

M.K. is a 38-year-old married woman with two children, aged 14 and 16. For 2 months prior to admission M.K. complained of constant fatigue and not being able to sleep at night. She began to stay up late to avoid tossing and turning and to decrease the chance that her husband would want to have sex, something she no longer enjoyed. M.K. works part-time in the grade school library, a job she always said she loved. She now says that "the job hasn't been the same lately"

Table 6.2.
Effects of Depression on Occupational Performance Components[a]

Sensory Motor Component	Cognitive Integration & Cognitive Components	Psychosocial Skills & Psychological Components

1. Sensory integration
  a. Sensory awareness
  b. Sensory processing
    1. Tactile
    2. Proprioceptive
    3. Vestibular
    4. Visual
    5. Auditory
    *6. **Gustatory**
    7. Olfactory
  c. Perceptual skills
    1. Stereognosis
    2. Kinesthesis
    3. Body scheme
    4. Right-left discrimination
    5. Form constancy
    6. Position in space
    7. Visual-closure
    8. Figure ground
    9. Depth perception
    10. Topographic orientation
	*1. **Level of arousal**
	2. Orientation
	3. Recognition
	*4. **Attention span**
	5. Memory
	  a. Short-term
	  b. Long-term
	  c. Remote
	  d. Recent
	6. Sequencing
	7. Categorization
	*8. **Concept formation**
	9. Intellectual operations in space
	*10. **Problem solving**
	*11. **Generalization of learning**
	*12. **Integration of learning**
	*13. **Synthesis of learning**
		1. Psychological
		  *a. **Roles**
		  *b. **Values**
		  *c. **Interests**
		  *d. **Initiation of activity**
		  e. Termination of activity
		  *f. **Self-concept**
		2. Social
		  *a. **Social conduct**
		  *b. **Conversation**
		  *c. **Self-expression**
		3. Self-management
		  *a. **Coping skills**
		  *b. **Time management**
		  c. Self-control

2. Neuromuscular
  a. Reflex
  b. Range of motion
  c. Muscle tone
  *d. **Strength**
  *e. **Endurance**
  f. Postural control
  g. Soft tissue integrity		

3. Motor
  *a. **Activity tolerance**
  b. Gross motor coordination
  c. Crossing the midline
  d. Laterality
  e. Bilateral integration
  f. Praxis
  g. Fine motor coordination
  h. Visual-motor integration
  i. Oral-motor control		

Table 6.2.   (Continued)

Occupational Therapy Performance Areas (any of these areas <u>may</u> be affected)

Activities of Daily Living	Work Activities	Play/Leisure Activities

1. Grooming
2. Oral hygiene
3. Bathing
4. Toilet hygiene
5. Dressing
6. Feeding and eating
7. Medication routine
8. Socialization
9. Functional communication
10. Functional mobility
11. Sexual expression
	1. Home management
	  a. Clothing care
	  b. Cleaning
	  c. Meal preparation and cleanup
	  d. Shopping
	  e. Money management
	  f. Household maintenance
	  g. Safety procedures
	2. Care of others
	3. Educational activities
	4. Vocational activities
	  a. Vocational exploration
	  b. Job acquisition
	  c. Work or job performance
	  d. Retirement planning
		1. Play or leisure exploration
		2. Play or leisure performance

*Asterisks indicate areas affected.

and reports that she called in sick frequently over the past 2 months and knows her work performance has deteriorated. Lately she has been preoccupied with thoughts that she will be fired, although her supervisor has always been pleased with her work.

M.K.'s interests in the past were broad, including doing things with her husband and children such as attending church, going on picnics, and participating in school social events. She bowled in a neighborhood league with her husband and socialized with a group of friends on a regular basis. M.K. also enjoyed cooking and playing cards. When she started feeling tired all the time she discontinued all of these interests except attending church, explaining to everyone that she was not feeling well and had to save her energy for work.

At home, M.K. started to pay less and less attention to her usually immaculate house and carried out only those chores necessary to keep the home functioning. When her husband or children offered help, she reacted with tears and accusations that they didn't think she was able to do anything. M.K. tells the occupational therapist that she feels terribly guilty about not taking care of her family.

M.K. used to dress stylishly and wear carefully applied makeup. Lately her clothes have not always matched, and she rarely applies makeup or bothers to style her hair. She says it doesn't matter anyway because nobody cares how she looks.

M.K.'s usual "sunny" relationships with her family and friends have also changed. She no longer participates in mutual activities, and her concerns with her own feelings override concern for others. Her children complain openly that she is not fun like she used to be. They no longer bring friends to the house and avoid spending time there. Her husband has gently tried to discuss the situation, but each time that he tries, M.K. starts crying and accuses him of not loving her anymore, of having an affair, and/or of not understanding her. He, too, is starting to stay away from the home, often working late. M.K. has cut off all contact with friends, many of whom have stopped calling after repeated failed attempts to involve M.K. in some activity. M.K.'s job performance has probably suffered least, but lately she has had difficulty handling unusual situations, has stopped taking time to talk with the children, and has difficulty managing the physical demands of the job.

For 2 weeks before coming to the hospital, M.K. often found herself crying for no apparent reason. She was unable to get out of bed for several mornings and only went to work twice. Her husband brought her to the hospital emergency room because she said she couldn't breathe and felt like she was dying.

M.K. was given a diagnosis of major depression and started on a treatment program that included antidepressant medication, group and individual therapy, and occupational therapy. The occupational therapist's assessment of M.K.'s occupational performance is summarized in Table 6.3.

To summarize, M.K.'s performance of activities of daily living is affected with respect to grooming, socialization, and sexual expression. In work activities, almost all areas of home management are affected, as is care for her family and job performance. Neither leisure exploration nor performance occurs.

With appropriate treatment (antidepressant medication and psychotherapy), it is highly likely that M.K.

will return to her previous lifestyle. She may have a recurrence of the depression in the future, but her psychotherapist has educated her and her family to recognize the early symptoms and seek treatment as soon as she feels that she may be becoming depressed.

BIPOLAR DISORDER

Etiology

Bipolar disorders, often referred to as manic-depressive disease, have been clearly linked to heredity. About 50% of people with bipolar disorder have a parent with the disease (6). Evidence that this disorder is genetic has been found in studies of family incidence, twin studies, and adoption studies. Scientists have now identified a genetic marker for the disease. The existence of any blood relative with a history of bipolar disorder, depression, or for that matter, mental illness, lends support to this diagnosis for persons meeting other diagnostic criteria. Where there is doubt about presenting symptoms, the family history often provides sufficient support for the physician to prescribe lithium, a medication known to treat the symptoms of bipolar disorder effectively. In a roundabout way, good response to lithium confirms the diagnosis.

Although the genetic component of bipolar disorders is well established, it is not clear what triggers individual episodes. In some cases there appears to be a correlation with levels of psychosocial stress in the individual's environment, but this is not universally true. Often there does not seem to be any relation between episodes and life circumstances.

Incidence and Prevalence

"The lifetime expectancy of developing bipolar disorder is about 1% in both men and women" (6). Variations in rates between the United States and other countries suggest differences in patterns of diagnosis by physicians, rather than a difference in prevalence. The onset of manic episodes occurs in the early 20s on average, but people may develop a bipolar disorder at any age.

Signs and Symptoms

A person with bipolar disorder will, at the least, experience manic episodes and may also have periods of major depression. (See Table 6.4.) The symptoms of the depression are the same as those described earlier, and they will not be described again here.

Persons in the manic phase of a bipolar disorder are often easy to spot, especially if their illness is severe enough to require hospital treatment. There is an "excessive" quality about everything they do. They may start sleeping very little, without experiencing fatigue (a trait many of us would like to have when studying for exams!); become unusually euphoric, expansive, "high," or irritable; and become more active in work or school. The unusually elevated mood is recognized by those close to the individual. However, the euphoric outlook may explode into rage with little provocation. During a manic episode, the individual may speak rapidly and loudly, expressing intense enthusiasm for everything planned or accomplished. Sometimes people with this disorder believe they are very powerful or special. People with mania may take risks in their activities because they feel invincible. For example, a businessman may start a number of new ventures with very little capital, or a student may party the night before an examination because she "knows" that she will "ace" the test. If the individual is delusional, the content of the delusions is usually grandiose: a patient may tell you that he owns the hospital and will see to it that you receive a big bonus. John repeatedly told me that all of the women in the world were his wives, including me in this category!

Many of the symptoms may be enjoyed by the individuals and those around them, as long as they do not get out of hand. Some symptoms, at controlled levels, may be an asset in certain jobs. For example, not needing much sleep may benefit the long-distance truck driver, or increased goal-directed activity might help

Table 6.3.
Occupational Performance Profile[a]—M.

		Performance Areas			
		Work Activities			
		Vocation	Education	Home Management	Care of Others
SENSORIMOTOR	**SENSORY INTEGRATION** Intact				
	NEUROMUSCULAR	Fatigue limits		Fatigue limits	
	MOTOR Intact				
COGNITIVE	**COGNITIVE**	Difficulty with unusual situations		Misinterprets others' offers to help	
PSYCHOSOCIAL	**PSYCHOLOGICAL**	Role behaviors diminished; no longer enjoys or has interest; questions her abilities		Decreased engagement in roles; no longer meets previous standards	Unable to initiate caring activities
	SOCIAL	All social activities severely limited			
	SELF-MANAGEMENT	Not able to cope with unusual situations; often unable to get to work			

(left margin: PERFORMANCE COMPONENTS)

EXTERNAL FACTORS WHICH INFLUENCE PERFORMANCE

ENVIRONMENT   Her response to others has "turned them off." They are avoiding her, thus environment is less interesting and stimulating.

[a]Grid adapted from Uniform Terminology (2nd ed.). Developed by the occupational therapy faculty at Eastern Michigan University.

Client initials: **M.K.**
Diagnosis: **Major depression**
Age: **38**

Play or Leisure Activities		Activities of Daily Living				
Exploration	Performance	Self-Care	Socialization	Functional Communication	Functional Mobility	Sexual Expression
Fatigue limits	Fatigue limits					Fatigue limits
		Believes it does not matter				
All roles eliminated; does not initiate	Feels that no one cares how she looks	Does not initiate social interaction; most social roles have been given up; misinterprets others' motives				No longer interested
						Does not directly express lack of interest
	"Saves" energy for work		Concerns about self limit concern for others; tearful when others try to help			

Table 6.4.
Diagnostic Criteria for Manic Episode and Bipolar Disorders[a]

Diagnostic criteria for Manic Episode

Note: A "Manic Syndrome is defined as including criteria A, B, and C below. A "Hypomanic Syndrome" is defined as including criteria A and B, but not C, i.e., no marked impairment.

A. A distinct period of abnormally and persistently elevated, expansive, or irritable mood.
B. During the period of mood disturbance, at least three of the following symptoms have persisted (four if the mood is only irritable) and have been present to a significant degree:
   (1) inflated self-esteem or grandiosity
   (2) decreased need for sleep, e.g., feels rested after only three hours of sleep
   (3) more talkative than usual or pressure to keep talking
   (4) flight of ideas or subjective experience that thoughts are racing
   (5) distractibility, i.e., attention too easily drawn to unimportant or irrelevant external stimuli
   (6) increase in goal-directed activity (either socially, at work or school, or sexually) or psychomotor agitation
   (7) excessive involvement in pleasurable activities which have a high potential for painful consequences, e.g., the person engages in unrestrained buying sprees, sexual indiscretions, or foolish business investments

C. Mood disturbance sufficiently severe to cause marked impairment in occupational functioning or in usual social activities or relationships with others, or to necessitate hospitalization to prevent harm to self or others.
D. At no time during the disturbance have there been delusions or hallucinations for as long as two weeks in the absence of prominent mood symptoms (i.e., before the mood symptoms developed or after they have remitted).
E. Not superimposed on Schizophrenia, Schizophreni Disorder, Delusional Disorder, or Psychotic Disorder NOS.
F. It cannot be established that an organic factor initiated and maintained the disturbance. **Note:** Somatic antidepressant treatment (e.g., drugs, ECT) that apparently precipitates a mood disturbance should not be considered an etiologic organic factor.

Manic Episode codes: fifth-digit— code numbers and criteria for severity of current state of Bipolar Disorder, Manic or Mixed:
   1—**Mild:** Meets minimum symptom criteria for a Manic Episode (or almost meets symptom criteria if there has been a previous Manic Episode).
   2—**Moderate:** Extreme increase in activity or impairment in judgment.
   3—**Severe, without Psychotic Features:** Almost continual supervision required in order to prevent physical harm to self or others.
   4—**With Psychotic Features:** Delusions, hallucinations, or catatonic symptoms. If possible, **specify** whether the psychotic features are *mood-congruent* or *mood-incongruent.*
   Mood-congruent psychotic features: Delusions or hallucinations whose content is entirely consistent with the typical manic themes of inflated worth, power, knowledge, identity, or special relationship to a deity or famous person.
   Mood-incongruent psychotic features: Either *(a)* or *(b):*
   (a) Delusions or hallucinations whose content does *not* involve the typical manic themes of inflated worth, power, knowledge, identity, or special relationship to a deity or famous person. Included are such symptoms as persecutory delusions (not directly related to grandiose ideas or themes), thought insertion, and delusions of being controlled.
   (b) Catatonic symptoms, e.g., stupor, mutism, negativism, posturing.
   5—**In Partial Remission:** Full criteria were previously, but not currently, met; some signs or symptoms of the disturbance have persisted.
   6—**In Full Remission:** Full criteria were previously met, but there have been no significant signs or symptoms of the disturbance for at least six months.
   0—**Unspecified.**

Table 6.4.   (Continued)

Diagnostic criteria for Bipolar Disorders

296.6x Bipolar Disorder, Mixed

For fifth digit, use the Manic Episode codes (p. 218) to describe current state.
A. Current (or most recent) episode involves the full symptomatic picture of both Manic and Major Depressive Episodes (except for the duration requirement of two weeks for depressive symptoms) (p. 217 and p. 222), intermixed or rapidly alternating every few days.
B. Prominent depressive symptoms lasting at least a full day.

Specify if seasonal pattern (see p. 224).

296.4x Bipolar Disorder, Manic
For fifth digit, use the Manic Episode codes (p. 218) to describe current state.
Currently (or most recently) in a Manic Episode (p. 217). (If there has been a previous Manic Episode, the current episode need not meet the full criteria for a Manic Episode.)

Specify if seasonal pattern (see p. 224).

296.5x Bipolar Disorder, Depressed
For fifth digit, use the Major Depressive Episode codes (p. 223) to describe current state.

A. Has had one or more Manic Episodes (p. 217).

B. Currently (or most recently) in a Major Depressive Episode (p. 222). (If there has been a previous Major Depressive Episode, the current episode need not meet the full criteria for a Major Depressive Episode.)

Specify if seasonal pattern (see p. 224).

---

*a*Reproduced with permission from DSM-111-R. Washington, D.C.: American Psychiatric Association, 1987: 217–218, 225–226.

the employee in an advertising firm when a new campaign is being developed. Individuals who experience their symptoms as pleasurable may reject treatment.

The occupational therapy clinic is often very exciting for the patient in a manic episode. Plans are stated enthusiastically to make every available project bigger and more complex than ever before. A simple project is described as a "masterpiece," and accepted rules and standards of performance are rejected as "not creative" or "too restrictive." On the hospital unit, the patient in a manic episode will keep things stirred up, and more than one person with this diagnosis may create chaos! Mental health professionals often describe manic patients as being extremely intrusive.

Until symptoms are partially controlled by medication and by the natural course of the illness, management of the patient with mania is focused on avoiding stimulation (thus you might not see this patient in the occupational therapy clinic during the early stages of hospitalization) and providing a firm and consistent structure.

Course and Prognosis

Manic episodes usually develop rapidly over a few days and may last for a few days to a few months (1). Symptoms generally respond well to pharmacologic intervention, and people who receive prophylactic medication may function well for years. As with depression, few studies of functioning over time have been completed for people with this diagnosis. Harrow et al. completed a prospective follow-up study of patients with bipolar disorder and found that many had moderately impaired or poor functioning in the period following hospitalization. Very poor outcomes were found in 30% (31). People with bipolar disease should be carefully monitored as outpatients, to ensure that medication levels are sufficiently high and to identify stressful life circumstances that might lead to relapse or a reoccurence.

Some people with bipolar disorder experience rapid cycling of moods from manic to depressed. Others never experience a clear depression. For some the intervals between episodes are brief, for others relatively long, stretching into years without clinically significant symptoms.

Common "complications" for persons with bipolar disorders result from behaviors during manic episodes. The incidence of "risky" behaviors, such as substance abuse, sexual promiscuity, and reckless driving, is high. Thus persons may experience effects on their physical and mental well-being, work performance, and social relationships. Even with remission of symptoms, occupational performance may not improve (32), perhaps because the social structures that support this performance were destroyed by the person's behavior while manic. Potential complications during depressive episodes are the same as for major depression.

Diagnostics and Medications

Persons who experience symptoms of mania without marked impairment in occupational performance or risk of harming themselves or others are said to have a *hypomanic* syndrome. When occupational performance is markedly impaired, the symptoms are called a *manic* syndrome.

According to DSM-III-R, a person may have intermixed manic and major depressive episodes or an alteration of the two fairly rapidly (every day or two) (1). This is called *bipolar disorder, mixed.* If the individual is currently experiencing a manic episode, the diagnosis is *bipolar disorder, manic.* A person who is in a major depressive episode, *and has previously experienced a manic episode,* receives the diagnosis of *bipolar disorder, depressed.* Note that a depressed person must have experienced a manic episode to be diagnosed with a bipolar disorder, but a person with a manic episode need not have ever had a depressed episode to receive the bipolar diagnosis (1).

Bipolar disorders are diagnosed according to the symptoms using the DSM-III-R criteria (Table 6.4). In addition, presence of mood disorders or any history of mental illness in blood relations indicates the possibility of this diagnosis. Possible organic causes such as use of psychoactive substances or brain disorders must be ruled out. Sometimes it is difficult to distinguish between paranoid schizophrenia and manic episodes, especially when onset occurs in young males and involves irritability and delusions of grandeur and persecution, but usually the person with a bipolar disorder has a better premorbid level of functioning in social and vocational areas (1). Again, family history supports a bipolar diagnosis. Bipolar disorders usually respond well in both manic and depressive episodes to treatment with a compound of lithium (a carbonate or citrate), and people may be maintained on this medication for many years with few side effects. Lithium is metabolized differently by different persons and over time by the same person. Because it is highly toxic, patients receive a careful medical screening before administration, and monitoring of blood levels is essential for safe and effective use. Initially, blood is drawn for analysis several times a week, then tapered off over time. On maintenance doses, blood levels are determined as infrequently as once a year. A level between 0.8 and 1.2 mEq/liter is considered therapeutic (33). Anything lower is not effective, and higher levels are dangerous and potentially fatal.

Side effects of lithium treatment include a fine tremor of the hands, nausea, and vomiting. These usually occur in the first few days of treatment. Signs of possible toxicity include drowsiness, blurred vision, fatigue, thirst, dizziness, gait problems, coarse tremor, and muscle twitching. Moderate toxicity may be indicated with more severe neuromuscular symptoms, seizures, and confusion. Severe toxicity can result in coma and death.

At this time, lithium is believed to be an extremely effective method of treating bipolar disorders and preventing reoccurrences. It is not, however, a panacea. Some people discontinue taking it because of weight gain, polyuria, and fine hand tremor. It is also known to be teratogenic, so use with women of childbearing age must be approached with caution (34). Further, only about 20% of those taking it have no further recurrences, although it probably moderates the rate of occurrence and severity of manic or depressed episodes. Research is being conducted on alternatives to lithium, with the anticonvulsive carbamazepine showing promise (34).

Bipolar Disorder and Occupational Performance

The sensorimotor components of occupational performance are not likely to be affected by this disorder, except as side effects of medications. Any cognitive or psychologic component may be disturbed, according to the individual, the severity of the episode, and the manner in which symptoms are manifested.

The following case shows how a person's occupational performance may be affected by this illness.

CASE STUDY

P.J. is a 32-year-old college graduate who owns a small business. He is married and has two children. His wife describes him as usually fun to be around, well liked, and good with the children. Once in college, and again just prior to his marriage 7 years ago, P.J. went through periods of several weeks when he hardly slept at all. The first time he was planning a fraternity party, which he was determined would be the best ever held, and was working extra hours to have money for a summer vacation. He says he felt as if he was invincible and on a "natural high." At first all of his friends were eager to be with him, but as the episode went on he became irritable, and friends dropped away. One night he began to shout that he was the leader of the universe and no one could tell him what to do. He fought off those who tried to quiet him down. He was taken by police to the campus clinic and was hospitalized for 2 weeks on a psychiatric unit. His psychiatrist was unsure of a diagnosis, and when symptoms cleared spontaneously, P.J. was discharged with the recommendation that he receive counseling.

P.J. successfully completed college and took a job in business. He used a small inheritance to make some investments, and made enough money to buy a small retail business. Usually P.J. put in a 12-hour day at work. He spent a great deal of time contacting new customers, putting together new product lines, developing displays, and supervising a small staff. After 2 years, he and his live-in girlfriend from college decided to get married. Two months before the wedding, P.J. started talking constantly about how great it was to be single, how much women liked him, plans he had to develop a retail chain, plans to return to school for a degree in law, and other diffuse and generally grandiose ideas he had for his immediate and future life. He started staying up late and often left home for hours in the evening. One night his fiancée received a call from the jail where P.J. had been taken after a fight over a woman at a bar. When she went to the jail to bail him out, P.J. told her not to bother, he knew the judge and would be out the next day. He yelled at her loudly, telling her he was the best thing that had ever happened to her and she ought to appreciate him more.

P.J. was taken to a psychiatric hospital and given the diagnosis of acute intoxication and bipolar disorder, manic. After he became sober, he continued to exhibit a state of euphoria for several days until the medication (lithium carbonate) took effect. After P.J. returned home, he continued to take the lithium, returned to work, and got married as planned. At work he noticed that some of his old customers had not returned and that his financial records were in disarray. Bills had not been paid for many months, and his stock inventory was at an unusually high level, reflecting excessive ordering he had done during his hypomanic episode.

From then until this episode, P.J. worked hard and put his business back in order. He and his wife enjoyed an active social life together that included bowling, softball, and card playing with friends. Such activities often included heavy drinking and occasional use of marijuana. Sometimes P.J. would become loud and "obnoxious," but often he was the life of the party, and the couple was sought out by others.

Six weeks ago, P.J. started to talk about adding new lines to his stock and took out several bank loans to buy large orders. He began to stay late at work and sometimes would go home with one or another of the female employees. He contacted local business leaders to propose partnerships, bought himself a luxury car, and planned to take his wife on a trip to the Riviera to gamble. His wife, however, was more concerned about his not coming home at night, and when she objected, P.J. became verbally abusive toward her. Two weeks ago she told him she'd had enough, and she and the children went to her parents to stay. P.J. called her frequently, telling her that he had changed, reminding her of the fun they had together, and then becoming angry again when she refused to move back.

Table 6.5.
Occupational Performance Profile[a]—P.J.

		Performance Areas			
		Work Activities			
		Vocation	Education	Home Management	Care of Others
SENSORIMOTOR	**SENSORY INTEGRATION**				
SENSORIMOTOR	**NEUROMUSCULAR**	High and low endurance during episodes have had good and bad effects			
SENSORIMOTOR	**MOTOR** Intact				
PERFORMANCE COMPONENTS — COGNITIVE	**COGNITIVE** Short attention span	Past errors in judgment have ruined his business; unable to plan job search		Appears unable to see need to perform in this area with wife working	Does not plan for family
PERFORMANCE COMPONENTS — PSYCHOSOCIAL	**PSYCHOLOGICAL**	No present worker role; values owning business		Has not developed role; money management poor in manic episodes	Few current roles
PERFORMANCE COMPONENTS — PSYCHOSOCIAL	**SOCIAL**	Conduct at work has not always been appropriate			
PERFORMANCE COMPONENTS — PSYCHOSOCIAL	**SELF-MANAGEMENT**	Inability to control self in work; situations in the past			

EXTERNAL FACTORS WHICH INFLUENCE PERFORMANCE
ECONOMIC FACTORS: Financial situation poor due to past actions.
ENVIRONMENT: Current environment affected by P.J's past bahavior while manic. Family and friends are cautiously supportive.

[a]Grid adapted from Uniform Terminology (2nd ed.). Developed by the occupational therapy faculty at Eastern Michigan University.

Client initials: **P.J.**
Diagnosis: **Bipolar disorder (in remission)**
Age:

Play or Leisure Activities		Activities of Daily Living				
Exploration	Performance	Self-Care	Socialization	Functional Communication	Functional Mobility	Sexual Expression
High arouisal						Poor judgment in sexual behavior caused family & work problems
Many interests; initiates activity						
Does well in social activities						Problems with self-control in the past

One week ago, P.J. started to feel very tired and overwhelmed. He says it was like a black cloud, a weight, descending on his head. He could hardly bring himself to go to work in the morning, and when he got there would often find himself crying for no apparent reason. He decided that there was no reason to go on—his marriage was in trouble, he was heavily in debt, and one of his female employees was threatening to sue him for harassment if he didn't give her a raise. P.J. purchased a gun and wrote a suicide note, but decided to give his wife a last call. The tone of his voice was so different that she became worried and called the police to go to the house. They found P.J. with the gun in his hand, easily disarmed him, and took him to the psychiatric emergency room. This time the diagnosis was bipolar disorder, depressed.

P.J. again responded well to medication, but the effects of his illness on his life were not so easy to mend. With individual and couple counseling his wife agreed to return to the home on a trial basis. The business was in such a bad state that P.J. had to declare bankruptcy and sell it at a loss. In addition, he discovered that one of the employees with whom he'd had sexual relations is an IV drug user, and he worries about the possibility that he might have contracted AIDS. Because P.J. has very little work experience in anything but his own business he has not been able to find work, and his wife has returned to work to make ends meet. Still, P.J. talks of the big plans he has to succeed, and he continues to be enjoyable company most of the time.

P.J.'s occupational performance areas have all been affected by his bipolar disorder. These effects have varied over time. His present occupational performance is analyzed in Table 6.5.

In summary, P.J. shows dysfunction in the area of activities of daily living in socialization. In the occupational performance area of work activities, he does not manage money well, and has failed to take appropriate safety precautions in his sexual activity. His ability to care for others is questionable. P.J.'s work performance in the past has been both excellent and horrible. At this time he is not managing vocational exploration and job acquisition, both necessary to rebuilding his life. In leisure performance there does not seem to be any present problem, but in the past P.J. has engaged in leisure activities that were dangerous and/or destructive to his family life.

P.J.'s prognosis is unclear. He is now taking lithium, which controls the symptoms of his bipolar disorder, but his behavior during past manic episodes has severely eroded his support systems. P.J. is a good candidate for psychotherapy, which should focus on setting and working toward realistic goals to get his life back in order. P.J. and his wife might also benefit from marital counseling.

REFERENCES

1. American Psychiatric Association. Diagnostic and statistical manual of mental disorders. 3rd ed. revised. Washington, D.C.: American Psychiatric Association, 1987.
2. Styron W. Why Primo Levi died. New York Times, Dec 19, 1988.
3. Doherty K. The good news about depression. Business Week 1989; (Mar): 39–42.
4. Sinaikin PM. A clinically relevant guide to the differential diagnosis of depression. J Nerv Ment Dis 1985;173:199–211.
5. Regier DA, Hirshfeld RMA, Goodwin FK, Burke JD, Lazur JB, Judd LL. The NIMH depression awareness, recognition, and treatment program: structure, aims and scientific basis. Am J Psychiatry 1988;145:1351–1357.
6. Kaplan HI, Sadock BJ. Synopsis of psychiatry, 5th ed. Baltimore: Williams & Wilkins, 1988.
7. Andreasen NC. Concepts, diagnosis and classification. In: Paykel ES, ed. Handbook of affective disorders. New York: Guilford Press, 1982:24–44.
8. Akiskal HS, Tashjian R. Affective disorders: II. Recent advances in laboratory and pathogenetic approaches. Hosp Community Psychiatry 1983;34:822–830.
9. Wehr TA, Rosenthal NE. Seasonality and affective illness. Am J Psychiatry 1989;146:829–839.
10. Karasu TB. Toward a clinical model of psychotherapy for depression, I: Systematic comparison of three psychotherapies. Am J Psychiatry 1990;147:133–147.
11. Beck AT. Depression: causes and treatment. Philadelphia: University of Pennsylvania Press, 1967.
12. Sackeim HA, Wegner AZ. Attributional patterns in depression and euthymia. Arch Gen Psychiatry 1986;43:553–560.
13. Silverman JS, Silverman JA, Eardley DA. Do maladaptive attitudes cause depression? Arch Gen Psychiatry 1984;41:28–30.
14. Ellis A, Harper, RA. A guide to rational living. Hollywood, CA: Wilshire, 1973.
15. Seligman, MEP. Helplessness: on depression, development, and death. San Francisco: WH Freeman, 1975.
16. Lewinsohn PM, Libet J. Pleasant events, activity schedules and depression. J Abnorm Psychol 1972;79:291–295.
17. Lewinsohn PM, Youngren MA, Grosscup SJ. Reinforcement and depression. In Depue RA, ed. The psychobiology of the depressive disorders: implications for the effects of stress. New York: Academic Press, 1979.
18. Lewinsohn PM, Munoz RF, Youngren MA, Zeiss, AM. Control your depression. Englewood Cliffs, NJ: Prentice-Hall, 1978.
19. Spitzer RL, Endicott J, Robins E. Research diagnostic criteria: rationale and reliability. Arch Gen Psychiatry 1978;35:773–783.
20. Gold D, Bowden R, Sixbey J, Riggs R, Katon WJ, Ashley R, Obrigewitch RM, Corey L.

Chronic fatigue: a prospective clinical and virologic study. JAMA 1990;264:48–53.

21. Rubin EH, Zorumski CF, Burke WJ. Overlapping symptoms of geriatric depression and Alzheimer-type dementia. Hosp Community Psychiatry 1988;39:1074–1079.

22. Sargeant JK, Bruce ML, Florio LP, Weissman MM. Factors associated with 1-year outcome of major depression in the community. Arch Gen Psychiatry 1990;47:519–526.

23. Beck AT, Ward CH, Mendelson M, Mock JE, Erbaugh J. An inventory for measuring depression. Arch Gen Psychiatry 1961;4:561–571.

24. Hamilton MA. A rating scale for depression. J Neurol Neurosurg Psychiatry 1960;23:56–62.

25. Endicott J., Skpitzer RL. A diagnostic interview: the schedule for affective disorders and schizophrenia. Arch Gen Psychiatry 1978;35:837–844.

26. Bowden CL. Current treatment of depression. Hosp Community Psychiatry 1985;36:1192–1200.

27. National Institutes of Health. Electroconvulsive therapy. Consensus Development Conference statement. U.S. Department of Health and Human Services 1985;5(1).

28. Zorumski-CF, Rubin EH, Burke WJ. Electroconvulsive therapy for the elderly: a review. Hosp Community Psychiatry 1988;39:643–647.

29. Weissman MM, Klerman GL, Paykel ES, Prusoff BP. Treatment effects on the social adjustment of depressed patients. Arch Gen Psychiatry 1974;30:771–778.

30. Wells KB, Stewart A, Hays RD, Bornam MA, Rogers W, Daniels, M, Berry S, Greenfield S, Ware J. The functioning and well-being of depressed patients. JAMA 1989;262:914–919.

31. Harrow M, Goldberg JF, Grossman LS, Meltzer HY. Outcome in manic disorders. Arch Gen Psychiatry 1990;47:665–671.

32. Dion GL, Tohen N, Anthony WB, Waternaux CS. Symptoms and functioning of patients with bipolar disorder six months after hospitalization. Hosp Community Psychiatry 1988;39:652–657.

33. O'Connell RA. Lithium update. In: Flach F, ed. Affective disorders. New York: WW Norton, 1988.

34. Prien RF, Gelenberg AJ. Alternatives to lithium for preventive treatment of bipolar disorder. Am J Psychiatry 1989;146:840–848.

Glossary

Affective disorders: A term sometimes used in place of *mood disorders*.

Affect: The external expression of emotional content.

Antidepressant: A drug used for relief of symptoms of depression.

Cognition: That operation of the mind process by which we become aware of objects of thought and perception, including all aspects of perceiving, thinking, and remembering.

Dementia: An organic mental disorder characterized by a general deterioration of intellectual abilities involving impairment of memory, judgment, and abstract thinking as well as changes in personality without clouding of consciousness (delirium).

Disorder: A derangement or abnormality of function; a morbid physical or mental state.

Epidemiology: The science concerned with the study of the factors influencing and determining the frequency and distribution of disease, injury, and other health-related events and their causes in a defined human population for the purpose of establishing programs to prevent and control their development and spread.

Episode: A noteworthy happening occurring in the course of a continuous series of events. Mood episodes: Mood syndromes that have no known cause other than the mood disorder.

Epstein-Barr virus (EBV): A herpesvirus that may be the etiologic agent of infectious mononucleosis. Also called EB virus. EBV has been implicated in cases of chronic fatigue.

Existentialism: A philosophical movement of the 20th century which emphasized immediate individual existence as the focus of reality and meaning.

Extrapyramidal system: A functional, rather than anatomic, unit comprising the nuclei and fibers (excluding those of the pyramidal tract) involved in motor activities; they control and coordinate especially the postural, static, supporting, and locomotor mechanisms. It includes the corpus striatum, subthalamic nucleus, substantia nigra, and red nucleus, along with their interconnections with the reticular formation, cerebellum, and cerebrum; some authorities include the cerebellum and vestibular nuclei.

Hallucinations: Sensory perceptions not associated with real external stimuli. Hallucinations indicate a psychotic disturbance only when associated with impairment in reality testing.

Hypomania: An abnormality of mood resembling mania (persistent elevated or expansive mood, hyperactivity, inflated self-esteem) but of lesser intensity.

Monozygotic: Pertaining to or derived from a single zygote (fertilized ovum); identical twins.

Mood: "A pervasive and sustained emotion" (1), subjectively experienced and reported by an individual; examples include depression, elation, and anger. *Mood syndrome:* Symptoms of depression or mania that can occur separately as part of another disorder.

Neuroendocrine: Pertaining to neural and endocrine influence, and particularly, to the interaction between the nervous and endocrine systems.

Neurotransmitter: A substance (e.g., norepinephrine, acetylcholine, dopamine) that is released from the axon terminal of a presynaptic neuron on excitation, and that travels across the synaptic cleft to either excite or inhibit the target cell.

Norepinephrine: A neurotransmitter.

Paradigm: An example or model; a means for organizing thinking.

Psychodynamic theories: The study of mental forces and motivations that influence human behavior and mental activity, including recognition of the role of unconscious motivation in human behavior.

Psychomotor agitation: Motor restlessness or excessive overactivity, usually nonproductive and in response to inner tension.

REM (rapid eye movement): A phase of sleep associated with dreaming, mild involuntary muscle jerks, and rapid movements of the eyes.

Serotonin: A hormone and neurotransmitter.

Syndrome: A combination of symptoms resulting from a single cause or so commonly occurring together as to constitute a distinct clinical picture.

Medications

Note: Information has been excerpted from the Physician's Desk Reference, 44th ed. Oradell, NJ: Medical Economics Company

Antidepressants—General information

Action: Exact action unknown. Act on neurotransmission in the central nervous system.

Indication: Used for treatment of depression.

Available by prescription only

Common side effects: Anticholinergic effects such as dry mouth, blurred vision, hypotension, and urinary retention. Some have cardiovascular effects. Sedation. May interact with other medications.

Dosage: See PDR.

Generic Name	Brand Name	Action	Indication	Potential Side Effects	Usual Adult Dose	Comments
HETEROCYCLIC ANTIDEPRESSANTS (TRICYCLICS, TETRACYCLICS)						
Imipramine	Imipramine hydrochloride (HCl) Janimine Tofranil			Potential cardiac effects; should not be given with MAO inhibitors	See Physician's Desk Reference	The original tricyclic antidepressant; now manufactured by several companies
Amitriptyline HCl	Amitriptyline HCl Chlordiazepoxide and Amitriptyline HCl Elavil Endep Limbitrol (combined with antianxiety agent)			Potential cardiac effects; Limbitrol may cause withdrawal symptoms		

Generic Name	Brand Names	Side Effects	Comments
	Etrafon Perphenazine & Amitriptyline HCl Triavil (previous 3 brands are combined with perphenazine, have some of the potential side effects of antipsychotic medications)		
Desipramine	Desipramine HCl Norpramin Pertofrane	Same as other tricyclics	
Doxepin	Adapin Doxepin HCl Sinequan	Drowsiness	
Nortriptyline HCl	Pamelor		
Protriptyline	Vivactil		Lacks sedative effects
Trimipramine maleate	Surmontil		
Amoxapine	Asendin	Possible anticholinergic effects, may produce tardive dyskinesia	Mild sedative action, neuroleptic activity
Maprotiline	Ludiomil	May potentiate seizures	Tetracyclic; useful for depression with associated anxiety

Generic Name	Brand Name	Action	Indication	Potential Side Effects	Usual Adult Dose	Comments

MONOAMINE OXIDASE INHIBITORS (MAOI)

Precautions: All MAO inhibitors must be used with strict control of diet and other drug use. Foods high in tryptophan (e.g., broad beans) and tyramine (e.g., aged cheese, beer, wine, pickled herring, chicken liver, yeast extract) must be avoided. May cause hypertensive crisis if restrictions are not followed.

Contraindicated for persons with impaired liver function, congestive heart failure or phenochromocytoma.

Avoid use with other psychotropic medications.

Avoid use with elderly persons and with persons with cardiovascular or cerebrovascular disease or hypertension.

Avoid high intake of caffeine.

Generic Name	Brand Name	Action	Indication	Potential Side Effects	Usual Adult Dose	Comments
Isocarboxazid	Marplan					
Phenelzine sulfate	Nardil					
Tranylcypromine sulfate	Parnate					

CHEMICALLY UNRELATED ANTIDEPRESSANTS

Generic Name	Brand Name	Action	Indication	Potential Side Effects	Usual Adult Dose	Comments
Trazodone	Desyrel	Unknown; may act on serotonin		Associated with priapism		
Fluoxetine HCl	Prozac	Inhibits uptake of serotonin		May cause anxiety and nervousness; weight loss		

7

Traumatic Brain Injury

GERRY E. CONTI

It had been a hot summer day, the work hard, and the boss kept hanging around the garage. At last it was over. John picked up Kathy, his girlfriend of 4 years, and headed for the beach. Five hours and as many beers later, they sped home on familiar secondary roads. John negotiated the first part of an S-curve fine, but his reflexes were too slow to manage the second. Overcompensating, he lost control of the car, slamming it up against a tree.

Kathy was killed. John D., age 20, survived, with a traumatic brain injury.

EPIDEMIOLOGY

Traumatic brain injury (TBI), or head injury, involves a traumatic insult to the brain, capable of producing a complex matrix of physical, intellectual, emotional, social, and vocational changes. Many functions are compromised, including the ability to move in a coordinated manner, speak, remember, reason, and alter behavior (1). The combination of these changes makes the total disability far greater than any sum of individual deficits (2).

While they vary, most estimates suggest that there are now between 1 and 1.8 million cases of TBI in the United States (3–6). It is the most common cause of death and disability for persons under age 38. At greatest risk are young men between 15 and 24; they are twice as likely as women to sustain a head injury. Other groups that show an increased incidence of traumatic brain injury include adults over age 75, and children below the age of 5. Motor vehicle accidents are the cause for more than half of all traumatic brain injuries, and alcohol is a prominent contributing factor. Gunshot wounds and falls are the next most common causes of TBI, with falls being the major cause for the elderly and the very young (3, 7–8).

Severity of injury is related to cause. Motor vehicle accidents are more likely to result in death or more severe disability; falls are more often associated with mild injury. When all head injuries are considered, 70% result in mild injury, 20% in moderate-to-severe injury, and 10% are fatal (8). Factors most correlated with outcome include age, length of coma, length of posttraumatic amnesia, and the area and extent of brain damage.

The costs, both individually and for society, are staggering; 50,000 to 70,000 TBI victims are discharged annually from acute-care hospitals with little chance of resuming their previous social or economic lives. Another 50,000 to 70,000 begin the months-long process of rehabilitation, as a group incurring approximately $4 billion in hospitalization and treatment expenses. To this is added $75 to $100 billion per year because of the loss of productive work skills for many persons with TBI (7).

ETIOLOGY

Brain injury may be caused in three different ways. Primary damage occurs at the time of injury and is caused by impact. It may be either focal or diffuse. Focal damage is associated with direct impact of short duration and is typically related to acceleration/deceleration forces. Such forces occur with the high-speed impact of a motor vehicle accident and result in a coup-countercoup injury. (Direct damage is done to the brain as it is hurled against the skull, then richochets in the opposite direction to hurl against the skull.) This continues until the force of impact has been absorbed. In addition to actual brain damage, the force may fracture the skull, injure the scalp, block the ventricles and blood vessels, and cause contusions or hematomas. The frontal lobes and temporal lobes are particularly sensitive to contusion, hematoma, and other effects of direct damage.

Diffuse damage, called diffuse axonal injury (DAI), occurs with the shearing of white brain cells from each other at the time of impact. While cell death usually does not occur, the transmission of normal neural impulses is disrupted. The cerebral hemispheres, mesencephalon, and brainstem are sensitive to DAI (3, 9–10).

Secondary damage occurs shortly after impact. Factors causing secondary damage include increased intracranial pressure, brain swelling, hemorrhage or infarction, and oxygen deprivation.

Physiologic changes occurring after injury are the third cause of brain injury. These changes include hyperthermia, electrolyte disturbances, hyperventilation, and damage to the hypothalamus or pituitary gland (1, 9).

SIGNS AND SYMPTOMS

The most obvious sign of recent traumatic brain injury is coma, or prolonged loss of consciousness. During this time, the patient may respond only minimally to cues from the external environment and does not obey commands, speak, or demonstrate eye opening (10).

As consciousness and cognition return, the patient displays a variety of symptoms and signs, which have been identified in the Rancho Los Amigos (RLA) cognitive scale (see Table 7.1). This scale presents a typical progression pattern for the recovery of cognitive skills.

Level I is a period of dense unresponsiveness. In level II, the patient begins to respond ineffectively to pain. For example, a leg may extend in response to a pinch of the triceps tendon in the arm. Eye movement may be present, but the eyes do not appear to focus. Sounds and words may occur, but often seem meaningless. With further recovery to RLA level III, the patient may be successful in moving an arm from pain, and may now respond to a simple request to squeeze the therapist's hand. Verbal communication is still limited. The patient may respond unintelligibly or with automatic cursing. Self-initiation of a verbal or motor response is limited. Action occurs only in response to strong cues from either the external environment (e.g., the therapist providing upper extremity range of motion) or the internal environment (e.g., an irritating urinary catheter).

At RLA level IV, the patient becomes confused and agitated. This phase may now involve intentional gross movement of the arms, legs, head, and even trunk. Confusion and agitation predominate. The patient appears to have heightened sensations and responds to routine stimuli in an explosive, exaggerated, and agitated manner. A disorientation to person, place, time, and circumstance is apparent. Retrograde amnesia, or memory loss for events immediately prior to injury, is apparent. Brief conversations can be held, as basic speech patterns are now present; however, speech may be frequently interrupted by perseverative or profane phrases. At best, the patient can attend to any stimulus for only a short time. Physical discomfort and physical or men-

Table 7.1.
Rancho Los Amigos Cognitive Scale[a]

I. No response: Unresponsive to any stimulus

II. Generalized response: Limited, inconsistent, nonpurposeful responses, often to pain only

III. Localized response: Purposeful responses; may follow simple commands; may focus on presented object

IV. Confused, agitated: Heightened state of activity; confusion, disorientation; aggressive behavior; unable to do self-care; unaware of present events; agitation appears related to internal confusion

V. Confused, inappropriate: Nonagitated; appears alert; responds to commands; distractable; does not concentrate on task; agitated responses to external stimuli; verbally inappropriate; does not learn new information

VI. Confused, appropriate: Good directed behavior, needs cueing; can relearn old skills as activities of daily living (ADLs); serious memory problems; some awareness of self and others.

VII. Automatic, appropriate: Appears appropriate, oriented; frequently robot-like in daily routine; minimal or absent confusion; shallow recall; increased awareness of self, interaction in environment; lacks insight into condition; decreased judgment and problem solving; lacks realistic planning for future.

VIII. Purposeful, appropriate: Alert, oriented; recalls and integrates past events; learns new activities and can continue without supervision; independent in home and living skills; capable of driving; defects in stress tolerance, judgment, abstract reasoning persist; many function at reduced levels in society.

[a] Prepared by Professional Staff Association, Rancho Los Amigos Hospital, Inc., Downey, California. Reprinted with permission from Duncan PW. Physical therapy assessment. In: Rosenthal M, Griffith ER, Bond MR, Miller JD, eds. Rehabilitation of the adult and child with traumatic brain injury. 2nd. ed. Philadelphia: FA Davis, 1990: 265.

tal fatigue occur quickly and may trigger an aggressive physical response (1).

With further improvement and movement through levels V through VIII, the patient changes from a confused state to an aware, intentional state and from random selection of behaviors, appropriate or inappropriate, to consistently more appropriate behavior (1).

With an increased cognitive and communicative capacity, additional deficits become apparent, including deficits of vision, perception, sensation and movement, and cognition. Abnormal or inappropriate behavioral responses may also appear. Visual deficits may include double or blurred vision, visual field loss, and decreased oculomotor skills. Visual convergence and smooth-scanning abilities may be impaired (11). Perceptual deficits are apparent. Apraxia, or the inability to perform purposeful movement despite normal coordination, muscle function, and sensation, may be present. The patient may be unaware of a personal body scheme (i.e., the internal physical model of one's body). Unilateral inattention or neglect is common and indicates a parietal lobe lesion, with the patient unaware of sensation coming from one side of the body. Visual discrimination and spatial relations deficits are also common and can be seen in disorders of form perception and constancy, topographical orientation, figure ground perception, position in space, and spatial relations (11).

Abnormal postural reflexes, abnormal muscle tone, and decreased sensation are signs of ongoing motor dysfunction. Hypertonicity and movement disorders are frequently present. Hypertonicity appears as either rigidity or spasticity. The two types of rigidity most frequently seen in the early stages of recovery are decorticate and decerebrate posturing. In decorticate posturing, the lower extremities are intermittently or constantly held in a rigidly extended posture, while the upper extremities are tightly flexed. With decerebrate posturing, all extremities are rigidly extended. When spasticity is present, it presents as an increased involuntary resistance to passive range of motion and voluntary movement. Head and total body control are impaired. Movement is uncoordinated and reflex-bound and may include ataxia, tremors, and myoclonus (12, 13).

As early cognitive signs of confusion and disorientation begin to decrease, underlying cognitive deficits appear. The ability to pay attention, sustain attention, and focus it selectively or in an alternating manner is impaired (1). Retrograde amnesia typically continues to improve, but short-term and long-term memory problems become apparent. These ongoing memory deficits contribute significantly to ongoing disorientation and confusion (1, 14). Higher-level cognitive skills, such as those needed to select and execute plans, manage time, and regulate personal behavior, are impaired. These deficits are apparent as the patient shows difficulty identifying a goal, initiating a plan of action, and selecting appropriate steps and their sequence. Altering a plan in the face of new and conflicting feedback is difficult. Response time is slowed. Symptoms of limited time management include difficulty estimating time, scheduling time, and changing schedules when necessary.

The psychosocial problems caused by deficits in higher-level cognitive skills are of major concern. Impulsiveness, perseveration, or the use of repetitive behaviors, and a limited awareness of self and the effect of personal behavior on others are frustrating symptoms of a self-management deficit. Irritability, impatience, childlike behavior, lability, apathy, or an altered sexual drive may be seen. An unrealistic self-appraisal and a lack of insight make these problems particularly difficult to manage (15–17).

MEDICAL MANAGEMENT

Medical management in the acute phase centers around the preservation of life and the prevention of secondary damage.

Maintenance of an effective airway and continuing circulatory function are critical life-preservation steps immediately after injury. An endotracheal tube may be placed. Upon arrival at the hospital and medical stabilization, diagnostic tests are begun and the location and severity of all injuries identified. The patient typically receives a computerized axial tomography (CT or CAT) scan. If this reveals an intracranial hematoma, immediate surgical decompression is needed. Constant monitoring of consciousness occurs, as the duration and depth of coma are significant indicators of both mortality and morbidity (18).

The Glasgow coma scale (GCS) is the most frequently used measure of consciousness. It evaluates three simple responses: eye opening, best motor response to stimulation, and best verbal response (6, 18, 19). Research has shown this scale to be a good predictor of both mortality and outcome. For outcome prediction, individual scores in the three areas are summed (Table 7.2). A total GCS rating of 8 or below correlates with an outcome of severe injury, 9–12 with moderate injury, and 13–15 with mild impairment. Of the three factors, the strongest predictor is the patient's motor response. Patients who can at least withdraw from a painful stimulus in a normal manner are significantly more likely to have only mild-to-moderate residual impairment (18, 19).

Additional factors are also used to estimate outcome. Posttraumatic amnesia of less than 1 hour suggests a mild injury, while amnesia lasting more than 1 day indicates a severe injury. A younger age at injury improves both chance of survival and overall outcome. The absence of pupillary light responses and abnormal eye movements indicates brainstem dysfunction, with an increased risk of death. Prolonged increased intracranial pressure is associated with death and severe disability (18, 19).

Physicians from neurology, neurosurgery, internal medicine, or orthopaedics

Table 7.2.
Assessment of Conscious Level (Glasgow Coma Scale)[a,b]

	Examiner's Test	Patient's Response	Assigned Score
EYE OPENING	Spontaneous	Opens eyes on own	E4
	Speech	Opens eyes when asked to in a loud voice	3
	Pain	Opens eyes upon pressure	2
	Pain	Does not open eyes	1
BEST MOTOR RESPONSE	Commands	Follows simple commands	M6
	Pain	Pulls examiner's hand away upon pressure	5
	Pain	Pulls a part of body away upon pressure	4
	Pain	Flexes body inappropriately to pain (decorticate posturing)	3
	Pain	Body becomes rigid in an extended position upon pressure (decerebrate posturing)	2
	Pain	Has no motor response to pressure	1
VERBAL RESPONSE (talking)	Speech	Carries on a conversation correctly and tells examiner where he/she is, who he/she is, and the month and year	V5
	Speech	Seems confused or disoriented	4
	Speech	Talks so examiner can understand victim but makes no sense	3
	Speech	Makes sounds that examiner cannot understand	2
	Speech	Makes no noise	1

[a] Reprinted with permission from Miller JD, Pentland B, Berroll S. Early evaluation and management. In: Rosenthal M, Griffith ER, Bond MR, Miller JD, ed. Rehabilitation of the adult and child with traumatic brain injury, 2nd ed. FA Davis, 1990: 36.
[b] Coma score (E + M + V) = 3 to 15.

may direct overall medical management in the acute phase. Over one-half of patients with a severe head injury have associated injuries. Hydrocephalus, or the abnormal accumulation of cerebrospinal fluid in the brain, is a serious complication for up to 75% of patients; 82% of patients with TBI have one or more extracranial fractures as well, and 10% of these may be cervical spinal cord injuries. The patient then requires management for both a brain injury and a high-level spinal cord injury (20, 21). Due to rigid abnormal posturing and other motor disturbance,

up to 84% of patients develop contractures of the neck, trunk, arms, and legs. The longer the coma, the greater is the potential for abnormal body posturing and the development of contractures. About one-third of patients aspirate food into their lungs, causing pneumonia. These patients usually have a delayed or absent swallowing reflex (20, 21).

Medical management at the intensive-care level is constant. An indwelling urinary catheter is placed and closely monitored. A nasogastric tube is also placed and is used for high caloric feeding. Close

Table 7.3.
Occupational Performance Components

Sensory Motor Components	Cognitive Integration & Cognitive Components	Psychosocial Skills & Psychological Components

1. Sensory integration
  a. Sensory awareness
  b. Sensory processing
    1. Tactile
    2. Proprioceptive
    3. Vestibular
    4. Visual
    5. Auditory
    6. Gustatory
    7. Olfactory
  c. Perceptual skills
    1. Stereognosis
    2. Kinesthesis
    3. Body Scheme
    4. Right-left discrimination
    5. Form constancy
    6. Position in space
    7. Visual-closure
    8. Figure ground
    9. Depth perception
    10. Topographic orientation
	1. Level of arousal
	2. Orientation
	3. Recognition
	4. Attention span
	5. Memory
	  a. Short-term
	  b. Long-term
	  c. Remote
	  d. Recent
	6. Sequencing
	7. Categorization
	8. Concept formation
	9. Intellectual operations in space
	10. Problem solving
	11. Generalization of learning
	12. Integration of learning
	13. Synthesis of learning
		1. Psychological
		  a. Roles
		  b. Values
		  c. Interests
		  d. Initiation of activity
		  e. Termination of activity
		  f. Self-concept
		2. Social
		  a. Social conduct
		  b. Conversation
		  c. Self-expression
		3. Self-management
		  a. Coping skills
		  b. Time management
		  c. Self-control

2. Neuromuscular
  a. Reflex
  b. Range of motion
  c. Muscle tone
  d. Strength
  e. Endurance
  f. Postural control
  g. Soft tissue integrity
	Note: All occupational performance components and areas are affected: degree depends on level of coma, severity of injury, and progress during rehabilitation.	

3. Motor
  a. Activity tolerance
  b. Gross motor coordination
  c. Crossing the midline
  d. Laterality
  e. Bilateral integration
  f. Praxis
  g. Fine motor coordination
  h. Visual-motor integration
  i. Oral-motor control		

attention to skin integrity is essential, and the patient's total body position is changed frequently. Twice-daily range of motion of all extremities helps prevent contractures. Suctioning of the endotrachial tube and vigorous respiratory therapy treatments help prevent additional pulmonary problems. Monitoring of the level of consciousness occurs frequently (18).

Rehabilitation in the intensive care unit may begin as soon as neurologic stability is achieved. Early rehabilitation centers around a program of graded and specific sensory stimulation, with the assumption that selective sensory bombardment may speed or improve neurologic recovery.

Medical stability, cognitive level, and the ability to benefit from intensive re-

Occupational Performance Areas

Activities of Daily Living	Work Activities	Play/Leisure Activities

1. Grooming
2. Oral hygiene
3. Bathing
4. Toilet hygiene
5. Dressing
6. Feeding and eating
7. Medication routine
8. Socialization
9. Functional communication
10. Functional mobility
11. Sexual expression
	1. Home management
	  a. Clothing care
	  b. Cleaning
	  c. Meal preparation and cleanup
	  d. Shopping
	  e. Money management
	  f. Household maintenance
	  g. Safety procedures
	2. Care of others
	3. Educational activities
	4. Vocational activities
	  a. Vocational exploration
	  b. Job acquisition
	  c. Work or job performance
	  d. Retirement planning
		1. Play or leisure exploration
		2. Play or leisure performance

habilitation are commonly used to identify the appropriate time for transfer to the rehabilitation phase (18). The patient's rehabilitation is typically directed by a physiatrist, a physician specializing in medical rehabilitation. The goals of the intensive rehabilitation program are to restore the persons to their optimal level of function in all areas, as well as to minimize additional physical or psychosocial disability (18). The core rehabilitation team includes specialists in occupational therapy, physical therapy, speech and language pathology, nursing, neuropsychology, social work, and the physician. Typical occupational therapy long-term rehabilitation goals are to reestablish sensorimotor integration and control, basic self-care skills and activities of daily living, and basic cognitive and communication skills. Where remediation is not possible or when maximal neurologic recovery can be assumed to have occurred, compensation strategies are taught. As these goals are accomplished, the patient may be discharged from the hospital, to meet higher-level goals on an outpatient basis. Outpatient occupational therapy long-term goals include all activities of daily living, community reintegration, and vocational rehabilitation (1).

MEDICATIONS

Medications used with the traumatically brain-injured individual must be carefully selected and closely monitored because of the potential for negative interactions with an already injured central nervous system. Tegretol and phenobarbitol are frequently used to prevent or reduce seizure activity, but they further depress already slowed central nervous system responses. Increased muscle tone, or spasticity, may be treated with Dilantin, Dantarium or baclofen. Sleep disorders may be regulated by Valium, which may also help moderate behavior (4, 5, 21). Appendix 7.2 lists common medications and their side effects.

EFFECT ON OCCUPATIONAL PERFORMANCE

The deeply comatose patient, Rancho Los Amigos levels I through III, shows depressed function in all occupational performance components and is dependent in all occupational performance. With further recovery, improvement in all performance components occurs, and basic function within the self-care, home management, vocational activity, leisure activity, and community reintegration occupational performance areas may become

Table 7.4.
Occupational Performance Profile[a]—J.D.

| | | Performance Areas | | |
| | | Work Activities | | |
	Vocation	Education	Home Management	Care of Others
SENSORY INTEGRATION Sensory processing delayed; poor topographic orientation	UNABLE TO PERFORM ALL ROLES			
NEUROMUSCULAR Abnormal tone; poor postural control; low endurance	UNABLE TO PERFORM ALL ROLES			
MOTOR Poor gross coordination; poor oculomotor control	UNABLE TO PERFORM ALL ROLES			
COGNITIVE Level IV; agitated; disoriented; poor short-term memory; decreased attention span; delayed processing of information	UNABLE TO PERFORM ALL ROLES			
PSYCHOLOGIC Self-concept limited to name; unaware of deficits	UNABLE TO PERFORM ALL ROLES			
SOCIAL Limited response to any social activity	UNABLE TO PERFORM ALL ROLES			
SELF-MANAGEMENT Disinhibited	UNABLE TO PERFORM ALL ROLES			

SENSORIMOTOR / COGNITIVE / PSYCHOSOCIAL — PERFORMANCE COMPONENTS

EXTERNAL FACTORS WHICH INFLUENCE PERFORMANCE; CULTURE, ECONOMY, ENVIRONMENT

[a] Grid adapted from Uniform Terminology (2nd ed.). Developed by the occupational therapy faculty at Eastern Michigan University.

Client initials: J.D.
Diagnosis: TBI
Age: 19

Play or Leisure Activities		Activities of Daily Living				
Exploration	Performance	Self-Care	Socialization	Functional Communi-cation	Functional Mobility	Sexual Expression
		Requires moderate assistance for bathing, dressing, feeding			Requires moderate assistance for transfer	
		Requires moderate assistance for bathing, dressing, feeding			Nonambulatory; uses wheelchair	
			Does not tolerate group treatment	Gives short phrases with slowed response time		
				Swears frequently		

Table 7.5.
Occupational Performance Profile[a]—C.R.

		Performance Areas			
		Work Activities			
		Vocation	Education	Home Management	Care of Others
PERFORMANCE COMPONENTS — SENSORIMOTOR	**SENSORY INTEGRATION**				
	NEUROMUSCULAR Decreased endurance				
	MOTOR Decreased visual-motor control, poor visual convergence, decreased coordination in RUE & hand, ambulation slowed	Able to type for no more than 10 minutes before complaining of eye strain			
PERFORMANCE COMPONENTS — COGNITIVE	**COGNITIVE** Level VII: decreased short term memory, decreased problem solving, decreased sequencing, decreased cognitive flexibility	Difficulty problem solving new approaches to work problems		Safety problems due to short-term memory deficits	
PERFORMANCE COMPONENTS — PSYCHOSOCIAL	**PSYCHOLOGIC** Decreased self awareness, decreased initiation, frustrated by limitations				
	SOCIAL Conversation limited; responds pleasantly, but seldom initiates other than basic social remarks				
	SELF-MANAGEMENT Self-centered			Difficulty initiating home-care tasks	

EXTERNAL FACTORS WHICH INFLUENCE PERFORMANCE; CULTURE, ECONOMY, ENVIRONMENT

[a] Grid adapted from Uniform Terminology (2nd ed.). Developed by the occupational therapy faculty at Eastern Michigan University.

Client initials: J.D.
Diagnosis: TBI, Outpatient rehab
Age:

Play or Leisure Activities		Activities of Daily Living				
Exploration	Performance	Self-Care	Social-ization	Functional Communica-tion	Functional Mobility	Sexual Expression
		Independent	Appropriate but slowed			
		Independent	Appropriate but slowed			
	Unable to read more than 15 minutes	Independent		Decreased coordination for typing	Limited walking en-durance	
				Forgets con-versation within 20 minutes	Unable to drive due to visual cogni-tive deficits	
No expres-sion of in-terest in re-suming activities or developing new activi-ties			Decreased initiation			
			Decreased interactions			
Conversa-tion self-centered; does not ex-press inter-est in others						

possible. Table 7.3 lists all performance components, as all performance components are dramatically affected by a traumatic brain injury.

CASE STUDIES

Case 1

J.D., age 20, survived an automobile accident, with a moderate traumatic brain injury. Following 2 weeks in intensive care and 4 weeks in an acute medical unit, he is to begin intensive rehabilitation. His occupational therapist cannot get reliable information from him, so she relies on a medical record review for his medical history, and a discussion with his mother to identify his previous occupational performance levels.

The medical record review reveals that J.D. sustained a right tibia-fibula fracture with the TBI. Following 3 days of general unresponsiveness, he began to obey simple commands (RLA level III). From there he moved quickly to the agitated, confused state of level IV. At this point speech became intelligible and perseverative swearing was noted. Soft restraint of his arms became necessary, as he persisted in pulling out both his urinary catheter and his nasogastric tube.

The agitation has lessened somewhat, but he continues to be intermittently disoriented. He responds to therapeutic requests more quickly and positively in the morning. He persists in incorrectly calling the occupational therapist, "Kathy." Moderate-to-severe spasticity is present, and J.D. demonstrates poor sitting postural control. Right upper extremity movement is limited by spasticity, while the left upper extremity is slowed but functional. His eyes do not appear to focus, and he performs any activity better with an eye patch on.

His mother is very vague about his activities. She states that he has had three garage mechanic's jobs in the last 2 years. She says he seemed to get tired of routine and didn't get along well with his bosses. He moved into her two-bedroom apartment about 6 months ago, so he could start saving money for a new car. He does not participate in any home-care tasks but does help with the rent. Leisure activities included fixing up his old car and "hot-rodding" around. J.D.'s mother does not care for many of his friends, but becomes tearful when asked about his relationship with Kathy. She says they were planning to be married in the fall.

At this time, J.D. is dependent in all areas of occupational performance. See Table 7.4 for J.D.'s deficit profile at the start of intensive rehabilitation. His greatest strength lies in the occupational performance categories of self-care and functional mobility. He requires moderate assistance and verbal cuing for showering seated in a shower chair and for donning and removing his shirt. He can eat with verbal cuing needed only for task completion. Bed-to-wheelchair

transfers now require only moderate physical assistance because of his fracture.

J.D. has come a long way, but there is a longer way yet to go.

Case 2

C.R.'s-family had the misfortune to be in the wrong place at the wrong time. Returning late one night, tanned and happy from 2 weeks at the lake, her husband could not avoid the oncoming car that went through a red light and sideswiped them. All family members were hurt, but C.R. most of all.

At the hospital, she was initially responsive to request, then became unresponsive during the third hour after injury. Following surgical intervention for increased intracranial pressure, she regained awareness, and achieved a RLA level IV within 2 weeks, at which time intensive rehabilitation began.

Surprisingly, she had no broken bones, and her sensorimotor status improved rapidly. By the time of discharge from the hospital, she was walking in a slow but stable manner. Her primary physical problems involved decreased right upper extremity coordination and decreased endurance. Cognitively, she improved quickly to level VI. At the time of discharge, she had trouble with organization, sequencing, and task initiation. C.R. was delighted to leave the hospital and return home. She did not anticipate any problems in resuming her roles as wife, mother, and homemaker. She did not think that she could return to being a secretary at present.

At the time of admission to an outpatient rehabilitation program, she had deficits in a number of occupational performance areas (Table 7.5). She can now type only 20 words per minute, and complains of eyestrain after 10 minutes of copy work. This does not bother her as she states she no longer plans to return to work in the near future, if at all.

She is neat and clean in appearance at all times. However, her clothes are all quite tight, as she gained 15 pounds during her rehabilitation stay, despite a strict diet. She has always been proud of her clean home, but now does not clean it thoroughly. When pressed, she also admits that she has trouble organizing her day to accomplish all the tasks she previously did. Many tasks have been assumed by other family members. She is able to prepare simple meals, but the family has learned that she is often unable to read her recipe card correctly and that her memory problems make stove use a safety hazard.

C.R. was outgoing, assertive, and pleasant prior to injury. Presently she seems content just to stay at home. She expresses no interest in going out with the family or in resuming any of her previous activities. When not involved, she tends to sit in front of the television. Conversation is limited. She responds pleasantly, politely, but slowly, to questions. She seldom initiates conversation, other than basic social remarks. When she speaks, it tends to be of herself, and she no longer actively asks after others. Occasionally the noise created by two healthy children and their friends bothers her, and she becomes very angry. Her children now spend more time at their friends' homes than previously. C.R. recognizes that she is different and blames her change on her memory and vision problems. While she cannot identify just how she is different, she does recognize those differences when they are pointed out. She would like to get better.

Comments on Case Studies

J.D. and C.R. are each just one person at one point in the extended continuum of recovery. Each patient with TBI has a very personal psychosocial background, an individual mechanism of injury, specific factors affecting recovery, and individualized timelines for recovery. At any point recovery may slow or stop. The occupational therapist working with brain-injured patients must first identify and evaluate the many occupational performance roles and performance components affected by injury. Goals must be established either to remediate or maintain skills or to compensate for lost skills. Treatment is then prioritized, emphasizing performance skills initially, then gradually adding areas of occupational performance when improved skill levels make success feasible. All treatment must be established within the boundaries of the patient's physical endurance, cognitive endurance, and frustration tolerance.

For the occupational therapist, patients with TBI represent a formidable, but highly rewarding, challenge. Principles of neurologic recovery must be understood and applied, and effective treatment techniques identified and incorporated into meaningful activity. Despite the challenge, the rewards are great, as a brain-injured person returns to a prized occupational role.

REFERENCES

1. Sohlberg MM, Mateer CA. Introduction to cognitive rehabilitation. Theory and practice. New York: Guilford Press, 1989.
2. Jennett B, Bond M. Assessment of outcome after severe brain damage. *Lancet* 1975; March 1:480–484.
3. Rimel RW, Jane JA, Bond MR. Characteristics of the head-injured patient. In: Rosenthal M, Griffith ER, Bond MR, Miller JD, eds. *Rehabilitation of the adult and child with traumatic brain injury.* 2nd ed. Philadelphia: FA Davis, 1990:8–16.
4. Manzi DB, Weaver PA. *Head injury. The acute care phase.* Thorofare, NJ: Slack, 1987.
5. Slater B. *A positive approach to head injury. Guidelines for professionals and families.* Thorofare, NJ: Slack, 1987.
6. Jennett B. Teasdale G. *Management of head injuries.* 6th ed. Philadelphia: FA Davis, 1984.
7. Levati A, Farina M. Vecchi G, Rossanda M, Marrubini MB. Prognosis of severe head injuries. *J Neurosurg* 1982;57:779–783.
8. Horn LJ. Garland DE. Medical and orthopedic complications associated with traumatic brain injury. In: Rosenthal M, Griffith ER, Bond MR, Miller JD, eds. *Rehabilitation of the adult and child with traumatic brain injury.* 2nd ed. Philadelphia: FA Davis, 1990:107–126.
9. Jennett B. Scale and scope of the problem. In: Rosenthal M, Griffith ER, Bond MR, Miller JD, eds. *Rehabilitation of the adult and child with traumatic brain injury.* 2nd ed. Philadelphia: FA Davis, 1990:3–7.
10. Bond MR. Standardized methods of assessing and predicting outcome. In: Rosenthal M. Griffith ER, Bond MR, Miller JD, eds. *Rehabilitation of the adult and child with traumatic brain injury.* 2nd ed. Philadelphia: FA Davis, 1990:59–74.
11. Zoltan B. Remediation of visual-perceptual and perceptual-motor deficits. In: Rosenthal M. Griffith ER, Bond MR, Miller JD, eds. *Rehabilitation of the adult and child with traumatic brain injury.* 2nd ed. Philadelphia: FA Davis, 1990:351–365.
12. Griffith ER, Mayer NH. Hypertonicity and movement disorders. In: Rosenthal M, Griffith ER, Bond MR, Miller JD, eds. *Rehabilitation of the adult and child with traumatic brain injury.* 2nd ed. Philadelphia: FA Davis, 1990:127–147.
13. Brooks DN. Cognitive deficits. In: Rosenthal M, Griffith ER, Bond MR, Miller JD, eds. *Rehabilitation of the adult and child with traumatic brain injury.* 2nd ed. Philadelphia: FA Davis, 1990:163–178.
14. Goethe KE, Levin HS. Behavioral manifestations during the early and long-term stages of recovery after closed head injury. *Psychiatr Ann* 1984:14(7):540–546.
15. Livingston MG. Effects on the family system. In: Rosenthal M, Griffith ER, Bond MR, Miller JD, eds. *Rehabilitation of the adult and child with traumatic brain injury.* 2nd ed. Philadelphia: FA Davis, 1990:225–235.
16. Rosenthal M, Bond MR. Behavioral and psychiatric sequelae. In: Rosenthal M, Griffith ER,

Bond MR, Miller JD, eds. *Rehabilitation of the adult and child with traumatic brain injury.* 2nd ed. Philadelphia: FA Davis, 1990:179–192.

17. Miller JD, Pentland B, Berroll S. Early evaluation and management. In: Rosenthal M, Griffith ER, Bond MR, Miller JD, eds. *Rehabilitation of the adult and child with traumatic brain injury.* 2nd ed. Philadelphia: FA Davis, 1990:21–51.

18. Mack A, Horn LJ. Functional prognosis in traumatic brain injury. In: Horn LJ, Cope DN, eds. *Physical medicine and rehabilitation: state of the art reviews.* Philadelphia: Hanley & Belfus, 1989:3(1):13–26.

19. Sandel ME. Rehabilitation management in the acute care setting. In: Rosenthal M, Griffith ER, Bond MR, Miller JD, eds. *Rehabilitation of the adult and child with traumatic brain injury.* 2nd ed. Philadelphia: FA Davis, 1990:27–41.

20. Hanscom DA. Acute management of the multiply injured head trauma patient. J Head Trauma Rehabil 1987:2(2):1–12.

21. Eames P, Haffey WJ, Cope DN. Treatment of behavioral disorders. In: Rosenthal M, Griffith ER, Bond MR, Miller JD, eds. *Rehabilitation of the adult and child with traumatic brain injury.* 2nd ed. Philadelphia: FA Davis, 1990:410–432.

Glossary

Amnesia: Pathologic impairment of memory usually resulting from physical damage to areas of the brain from injury, disease, or alcoholism. Anterograde: Inability to learn new material in an individual demonstrating a normal state of consciousness; a short-term memory deficit. Posttraumatic: Amnesia resulting from concussion or other head trauma. Retrograde: Inability to recall material that was well known in the past; a long-term memory deficit. Also refers to memory loss for events immediately prior to injury.

Apathy: Dulled emotional tone associated with detachment or indifference.

Apraxia: A disorder of skilled purposeful movement that is neither caused by deficits in primary motor skills nor comprehension problems. It can affect the praxic components of ideation and concept formation, as well as programming and planning of movement. Apraxia can include loss of the ability to use objects correctly. Disturbances of motor execution, on the contrary, are usually related to primary motor skills.

Aspiration: The act of inhaling or withdrawal of fluid by a method of suction. Pathologic inhalation of mucus into the respiratory tract may occur when a person is unconscious or under effects of general anesthesia.

Ataxia: Failure of muscular coordination; irregularity of muscular action.

Coma: A state of unconsciousness from which the patient cannot be aroused, even by powerful stimuli.

Contractures: Abnormal shortening of muscle tissue, rendering the muscle highly resistant to stretching, which can lead to permanent disability. In many cases contractures can be prevented by range-of-motion exercises (active or passive) and by adequate support of the joints to eliminate constant shortening or stretching of the muscles and surrounding tissue.

Convergence: The coordinated inclination of the two lines of sight toward their common point of fixation, or the point itself.

Decerebrate: Abnormal extensor posturing; in response to painful stimuli, the extremities extend rigidly and the palms turn outward. Decerebrate rigidity indicates damage to the brain stem and as a rule is a sign of greater cerebral impairment than is decorticate rigidity.

Decorticate: Abnormal flexor posturing, i.e., the arms, wrists, and fingers are drawn up; the legs may be extended with plantar flexion. Decorticate rigidity usually indicates a lesion in the cerebral hemispheres or a disruption of the corticospinal tracts.

Diffuse axonal injury (DAI): Shearing of white brain matter at time of impact during a traumatic brain injury so that transmission of normal neural impulses is disrupted. A rotational component during impact injuries to the head is believed essential for diffuse brain injury. Diffuse: Not definitely limited or localized; usually involving several areas of the brain.

Endotracheal: Within the trachea. Endotracheal tube: An airway catheter inserted in the trachea during intubation to assure patency of the upper airway by allowing for removal of secretions and maintenance of an adequate air passage.

Figure ground: The ability to determine the shape or outline of an object against a background environment; differentiate between foreground and background forms and objects.

Focal: The chief center of a morbid process; usually involving one area of the brain. Linear movement of the head leads to focal lesions at the site of impact (coup) or the opposite side of the brain (countercoup).

Form constancy: The ability to recognize forms and objects as the same in various environments, positions, and sizes.

Hematoma: A localized collection of extravasated blood, usually clotted, in an organ, space, or tissue. Hematomas are almost always present with a fracture and are especially serious when they occur inside the skull, where they may produce local pressure on the brain. Epidermal hematoma: occurs above the dura mater, between it and the skull, usually the result of rupture of a relatively large meningeal artery by a heavy blow to the head. There is rapid leakage of blood, causing increased intracranial pressure (ICP) that can be fatal in a short time. Subdural hematoma: Occurs between the dura mater, between the tough casing and the more delicate membranes covering the tissue of the brain, the pia-arachnoid. This kind of injury is often caused by the head striking an immovable object, such as the floor. The brain moves violently, tearing blood vessels and forming a swelling that may include fluid from the brain tissue.

Hydrocephalus: A condition characterized by enlargement of the cranium caused by abnormal accumulation of cerebrospinal fluid within the cerebral ventricular system; also called "water on the brain."

Hyperthermia: Greatly increased temperature.

Hypertonicity: The state or quality of having abnormally increased tension in the muscles.

Impulsive: A tendency to obey internal drives, without regard for acceptance by others or pressure from society. Impulse: A sudden uncontrollable act often seen in posttraumatic brain injured individuals.

Infarct: A localized area of ischemic necrosis produced by occlusion of the arterial supply or the venous drainage of the part.

Lability: The quality of being labile (i.e., unstable, fluctuating, moving from point to point). In psychiatry, emotional instability; a tendency to show alternating states of gaiety and somberness.

Mesencephalon: The midbrain.

Myoclonus: Shocklike contraction of part of a muscle, an entire muscle, or a group of muscles.

Perception: The process of transferring physical stimulation into psychologic information; mental process by which sensory stimuli are brought to awareness.

Perseveration: The persistence or repetition of a response after the causative stimulus has ceased or in response to different stimuli; for example, a patient answers a question correctly but gives the same answer to succeeding questions. Perseveration is most often associated with organic brain lesions such as TBI but is also seen in schizophrenia.

Position in space: The ability to determine the spatial relationships of figures and objects to self or other forms and objects.

Rigidity: Difficulties initiating movements and slow performance of active movements as well as increased resistance to passive movements because of increased muscle tone. There are different types of rigidity, including cogwheel (seen in Parkinson's disease) and clasp-knife rigidity.

Spasticity: Continuous resistance to stretching by a muscle because of abnormally increased tension, with heightened deep tendon reflexes.

Spatial relations: Ability to determine the relationship of one object to another in space. Spatial relation dysfunction: Difficulties in relating objects to each other, or to the self. When due to visual-spatial impairment, this term becomes synonymous with spatial-relations dysfunction. Spatial relations syndrome: Defects common to apraxias and agnosias, with related difficulties in areas such as constructional apraxia, figure-ground differentiation, interpretation of concepts related to spatial positioning of objects, spatial relations, impaired spatial memory, perceptual deficits related to depth and distance, and topographic disorientation.

Topographic orientation: The ability to adjust or become adjusted to the surface features of the environment or any changes therein; to determine the location of objects and settings and the route to the location, usually as a result of amnestic and/or agnostic problems.

Tremors: An involuntary trembling of the body or limbs, occurring either at rest or during activity, depending on the origin of the lesion.

Unilateral body inattention (neglect): Failure to report, respond, or orient to a unilateral stimulus presented to the body side contralateral to a cerebral lesion. It can be a result of either defective sensory processing or an attention deficit, resulting in ignorance or impaired use of the extremities.

Unilateral spatial neglect: Inattention to or neglect of visual stimuli presented in the extrapersonal space on the side contralateral to a cerebral lesion, as a result of visual perceptual deficits or impaired attention. It may occur independently of visual deficits or with hemianopsia.

Medications

Generic Name	Brand Name	Action	Indication	Potential Side Effects	Usual Adult Dose & Avail-ability
Diazepam	Valium	Inhibits muscle contraction; enhances inhibition; depresses reticular activating system	To sedate; to decrease muscle spasticity	Sedation, dizziness, ataxia, muscle weakness, decreased attention & memory; habit-forming	24 mg q.d. or b.i.d. to start, with gradual increase if needed Prescription
Phenobarbitol	—	Anticonvulsant	To eliminate or prevent seizure activity	Sedation, ataxia, rash; habit-forming	Prescription
Dantrolene sodium	Dantrium	Decreases muscle spasticity	To decrease alpha spasticity	Drowsiness, muscle weakness, liver toxicity, gastrointestinal complaints	25 mg q.d. gradually increasing to 400 mg q.d. Prescription
Lioresal	Baclofen	Decreases muscle spasticity	To decrease spasticity; mediated at all levels	Sedation, dizziness, nausea/vomiting, constipation, decreased attention & memory, possible liver toxicity	5 mg t.i.d. with gradual increase to 20 mg q.i.d. Prescription
Tegretol	Dilantin	Anticonvulsant	To eliminate or prevent seizure activity; to decrease spasticity	Rash, nystagmus, ataxia, gum hyperplasia	100 mg t.i.d. initially; gradual increase if needed Prescription

8

Chronic Pain

CATHERINE HECK EDWARDS

Valerie has worked at the hospital for the past 8 years. She had started as a dishwasher and worked her way up to being a food server on the tray line, then to salad and dessert preparation, and is now a cook. She enjoys her job and hopes her next promotion will be to kitchen supervisor.

Six months ago, Valerie gained custody of her 4-year-old nephew who has cerebral palsy. Her own son, who is 17, has been watching the young nephew after school until Valerie gets home from work. In 2 months, however, her son will be going away to college on a scholarship, and Valerie has been concerned about the afterschool child care costs that she'll incur when her son leaves.

During a busy morning rush, Valerie slipped on a wet floor and fell, straining her back. She has tried returning to her job several times, but each time has experienced an increase in back pain after 2 or 3 days back at work. Her job requires standing for 7 hours a day, as well as frequent lifting, carrying, and bending. Recovery has also been hampered by the custodial needs of her nephew, whom she needs to lift and carry frequently. Valerie's accident occurred over a month ago, and the concerns around her son's departure, combined with her back pain, are weighing heavily on her.

Pain is best described as a subjective response to distress which cannot be quantitatively measured. There are three components to pain: physiologic, pathologic, and psychologic. Pain may result from one or any combination of the three. The degree to which each component contributes to the individual's experience of pain is difficult to assess. However, to provide effective treatment, every attempt must be made to accurately evaluate all three, keeping in mind that no matter what the cause, the effects can be equally disabling.

There are three types of pain: acute, chronic, and that associated with malignancy. The emphasis of this chapter is on chronic pain, most particularly, pain associated with soft tissue injuries. Individuals with this complaint are being seen more frequently in occupational therapy settings.

Chronic pain is defined as pain that lasts 6 months or longer or pain that lasts 3 to 4 weeks after "normal" healing should have occurred, in the absence of any objective pathologic findings. Early identification and treatment of this problem increases the likelihood that the person can either overcome or learn to manage the pain effectively, thus minimizing the chance of prolonged disability.

ETIOLOGY OF PAIN

The literature on chronic pain is extensive, complicated, and often conflicting. Scientists and researchers have yet to determine how the human body and mind communicate, interpret, and respond to pain. As a consequence, there are numerous theories about the etiology of pain in general and, specifically, about the true nature of chronic pain.

This section of the chapter contains a review of some possible causes of pain that are specifically related to human anatomy and physiology. The major emphasis is on the transmission of acute pain. This is followed by a description of some of the major pathologic and psychologic factors in chronic pain. These theories provide a framework for understanding the general characteristics of chronic pain. (For more detailed information see the references and recommended readings at the end of the chapter.)

Anatomy and Physiology of Acute Pain

The exact pathways by which pain is transmitted have not been clearly identified nor is there any clear correlation between the amount of tissue damage and the degree of pain and disability. A recently developed theory about the physiology and anatomy of pain poses the following explanation (1). At the time of injury, the peripheral nerves respond to the noxious or nociceptive (painful) stimulus. When the peripheral, somatic nerve endings receive a painful impulse, an afferent cue is transmitted through specific nerve fibers and pathways. The small-diameter nerve fibers appear to be the primary transmitters of pain, and they are able to selectively respond to either high- or low-intensity pain stimuli. Also, certain nociceptors may play a role in further differentiating the intensity and the type of stimulus (e.g., heat).

With the onset of acute pain, the type of noxious stimulus (e.g., electrical shock, pin prick, laceration or contusion) is usually obvious. Once the pain threshold has been reached, a pain signal is sent to warn the individual that tissue damage is occurring. Tissue damage usually begins at the same time the pain threshold is reached. Because of the tissue damage, acute pain is often accompanied by inflammation.

When nerve endings receive a painful stimulus, amines and peptides such as prostaglandin (1, 2) and substance P (1–4), among others, are released by the nerve cells. These neurotransmitters trigger the firing of an electrical impulse by the nerves. This impulse travels through designated pathways in the central nervous system (CNS). The dorsal horn, spinothalamic tract (1–5), and spinoreticular tract (1, 3) are commonly identified as the primary conduits for pain transmission in the spinal column. As the fibers enter the brain and divide, information is sent to different areas. The first supraspinal receptors of pain seem to be the reticular formation (1, 3, 4) and the thalamus (1–4). The thalamus interprets the signal as pain and relays messages to the limbic system, where an immediate emotional awareness is generated. Impulses are also sent to the somatosensory cortex (1–4), which consciously evaluates and locates the pain. The final transmission is to the frontal cortex (3), where emotional and physical responses are organized and carried out.

Descending analgesic pathways suppress the pain sensations through a linking mechanism in the brain that activates the body's natural defenses against pain. Studies using electrical stimulation reveal that descending pathways transmit analgesics (1, 2) produced at the midbrain level (2–4). Specifically, the periaqueductal, periventricular gray matter in the midbrain has been identified as having a large concentration of opiate receptor cells, thus playing a key role in producing analgesia (5). Some research suggests that the body's natural analgesic abilities are enhanced as the descending messages pass through opiate neurotransmitters in the spinal column, which in turn block ascending pain messages (1). At the spinal cord level, the substantia gelatinosa, with a high concentration of opiate receptors, assists in the modulation of pain (1, 2, 5).

The fact that pain pathways seem capable of self-activating their own modulatory systems (1) may yet lead researchers to more effective means of controlling pain.

Another conceptualization of pain transmission is the "gate theory" of Melzack and Wall (6). Although subsequent research has disproven parts of the theory, the concept of "gating" is still considered valid (1). While a painful stimulus triggers the small fibers to fire, Melzack and Wall believe that nonpainful stimuli trigger the firing of large nerve fibers. Thus, the perception of pain depends on the balance between the transmissions by the two types of fibers. The final effect is based on the networking of these different sensory nerves (large and small) converging in the substantia gelatinosa of the dorsal horn in the spinal cord (5, 7). If more large than small fibers are firing, the gate is closed and there is no pain perception. Facilitating a dominance of large fibers is done by either decreasing the noxious stimulus or applying a nonnoxious stimulus. The old remedy of rubbing a bump or bruise to make it feel better is a good illustration of increasing nonnoxious stimuli to decrease pain. Similarly, the basis for the use of transcutaneous electrical nerve stimulation (TENS) is that it induces competitive inhibition by stimulating the large nerve fibers.

A further review of current literature suggests that multiple sites and mechanisms affect both the transmission and modulation of pain and that these mechanisms may have either selective or multiple functions. The individual's response will differ, depending on the type or intensity of the pain. It is clear from this brief discussion that much is still unknown about how the body and the brain receive, analyze, and respond to pain.

Pathology of Chronic Pain

The models that have been developed to describe chronic pain are fewer and generally less advanced that those for acute pain. Chronic pain is often explained by the pathologic changes in the nervous or musculoskeletal system, including prolonged muscle spasm, trigger points, radiculopathy, peripheral neuropathy, and causalgia.

One theory (1) proposes that in the absence of a tissue-damaging stimulus, neuronal elements may cause inappropriate firing of the nerve fibers. For example, a damaged nociceptive terminal may produce chemicals that lower the threshold of other nociceptive fibers (1, 2). This causes typically nonnoxious stimuli to be interpreted as painful. A second hypothesis suggests that damaged axons may regenerate by forming abnormal nerve sprouts (1, 2). These sprouts may fire in the absence of any stimuli or may be hypersensitive. The CNS is then inappropriately signaled that tissue damage is occurring. A third is the theory of dysfunctional gating (1). For some reason the CNS becomes unable to differentiate the sensory information from nerves. Signals become garbled like a poor telephone connection and result in an erroneous pain message being sent. This may happen without any stimulus being applied or may cause the sensation of pain in locations distant from the stimulus.

Pathology of Soft Tissue Pain. Included in the category of soft tissue are muscles, tendons, connective tissue, nerves, bursae, and blood vessels. Common diagnoses in this category are provided in Appendix 8.2.

One of the leading scholars in this field, Rene Cailliet, believes that the primary causes of soft tissue pain are muscle spasm and decreased circulation. He believes that prolonged muscle contraction or spasm may result from an imbalance of the agonist-antagonist muscles, nerve malfunction, and/or internal changes in the muscle (8). These spasms cause catabolites to accumulate in the muscle, producing pain. Catabolites are the by-products of muscle metabolism and are normally removed from the muscle by capillary action. With a prolonged contraction, however, the catabolites build up. Once this happens, it is difficult to remove them. Even after the muscle contraction has stopped, an accompanying reflexive vasospasm still exists. The presence of concentrated catabolites, combined with a lack of efficient capillary action, affects the proximal nociceptors and triggers a pain signal. A cyclical response may begin with the prolonged muscle contraction, a build-up of catabolites, pain signal, emotional tension, and further muscle contraction.

Ischemia may also be a cause of soft tissue pain (8). Changes in arterial pressure may quicken the onset of pain and cause it to be more severe (8). An example is shoulder or upper back pain caused by activity that requires reaching overhead for extended periods of time, as when painting a ceiling.

Another explanation used by Dr. Cailliet and others is called myofascial pain, myalgia, or myofascitis. One of the primary concepts of myofascial pain is the trigger point, a hypersensitive point within a muscle or its fascia (8, 9), which may be accompanied by inflammation. A trigger point is speculated to be caused or perpetuated by muscle loading or emotional stress (8, 9). It is very painful when pressure is applied (9). The location of these trigger points is very similar from individual to individual. Each trigger point has an area of referred pain that is also generally consistent from person to person (9). Pressure to the trigger point reproduces pain in the referred pain area. Researchers have been able to draw a map of common trigger points and their associated areas of referred pain.

A spasm in a segment of the muscle with a trigger point is another identifying trait. When palpated or "strummed," a localized twitch response is seen. There may also be a palpable "ropy" feeling to the muscle, as when you roll a thick cord back and forth between your index finger and thumb. The muscle may be locally "hard" to palpation, and there is always extreme local tenderness when deep pressure is applied to the trigger point. Relief may be achieved through injection of the trigger point with a local anesthetic or a steroid. The effects may not be permanent, however (8, 9).

Psychology of Chronic Pain

A third component of chronic pain is psychologic. Emotional distress such as anxiety, depression, or hysteria can intensify pain (7, 10). Ultimately, there is a psychogenic component to all chronic pain, if not as a primary cause, then as a result of the pain's duration and debilitating effects. If a patient experiences a muscle spasm after an injury, there may be an unconscious increase in muscle tension. This increase in muscle tension produces a state of emotional tension that further aggravates the spasm and pain (Fig. 8.1). Thus, a psychophysiologic cycle is established which perpetuates the pain. This is commonly seen in muscles of the spine, especially the neck and trunk, where a flexion/extension injury has occurred (7).

However, psychologic distress alone can heighten the perception of pain. This can occur in the absence of a painful stimulus or can cause nerve signals to be misinterpreted. Pain tolerance can be influenced by psychologic factors such as emotional tension, stress, or fatigue. A person with chronic pain is likely to have a lowered pain tolerance and, as a result, functions less effectively (7).

Significant, predisposing factors for persons with chronic pain are associated with their childhood experiences. Often they have been verbally or physically abused as a child, had a family member with a physically debilitating condition, and/or were unable to deal with significant losses, such as death of a family member, in a normal and timely manner (11). Other common characteristics include previous psychiatric illness; psychosocial problems, such as a poor work history or family problems; or a history of frequent medical problems that the person perceives as responding poorly to medical care (12).

Examples of psychologic disturbances that may precede or follow chronic pain

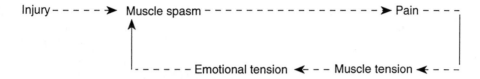

Figure 8.1. Cycle of psychophysical response to pain.

include depression, anxiety disorder, hypochondriasis, hysterical neurosis, somatization disorder, malingering, and substance abuse disorder (7, 10, 12). These disturbances may exist prior to chronic pain or may develop as its result. Regardless of their etiology, such disorders will certainly affect the pain the individual experiences and their response to treatment.

Organic complaints sometimes accompany psychologic problems. They may be a result of treatment, such as failed surgery or postsurgical scar tissue. Other problems may be the effect of medications. Common side effects of medication include gastrointestinal distress, loss of appetite, swelling, and drowsiness, among others. It is important to differentiate psychologic issues and organic causes of pain in order to provide effective treatment.

Beliefs about health and illness can also play a role in the perpetuation of chronic pain. In our society, the expectation is that most illnesses and injuries can be cured. On the other hand, a sick person is expected to be dependent and exempt from certain social responsibilities (7, 11). The intertwining of these perceptions can lead to the following expectations:

"If I have pain, I must be sick; the pain will go away when I am better."
"Too much activity will only make me sicker."
"I need to rest if I am going to heal."
"I am in pain, therefore, something is wrong."

With medical and pharmacologic advances, society has come to expect a "cure" for most ailments. Within this context it is not surprising that many people with chronic pain view themselves as disabled.

Most individuals with chronic pain are earnestly seeking relief. A small minority, however, complain of chronic pain to receive unwarranted financial remuneration through workers' compensation or Social Security benefits. These individuals are labeled as malingerers. They will exaggerate their pain and are often very dramatic in their verbal and nonverbal communication about their pain. However, it is important to remember that persons who have genuinely high levels of emotional distress will often respond in a similar fashion. Along with an incongruence between the malingerers' complaints and medical findings, they also have normal physical abilities. Experienced clinicians estimate that only 2 to 5% of persons with chronic pain are malingerers (13).

Another challenge when working with individuals with chronic pain are those who achieve secondary gains from their disability. Secondary gains are events or responses that result from the pain/disability and serve to reinforce the problem's existence. These gains may be subtle or obvious. An example of secondary gain is the individual who initially injures himself at his factory job and during the course of his recovery is able to devote more time to his college studies and get better grades. Another example is a mother with young children who no longer has to struggle with the conflict of spending too much time away from home, working to supplement the family income. Secondary gains are the "silver lining" to the "cloud" of pain. As time progresses, the individual may become consciously aware of the secondary gains and try either to eliminate or perpetuate them.

Conclusion

As mentioned earlier, there are differences between acute and chronic pain. A common medical management problem is that persons with chronic pain are treated like those with acute pain. It is important to distinguish not only the cause(s) of the pain, but whether it is acute or chronic, since chronic pain does not respond to conventional acute pain treatments. Refer to Table 8.1 for a summary of some of the major differences between acute and chronic pain.

INCIDENCE AND PREVALENCE

Chronic pain is a condition that affected an estimated 75 to 80 million Americans in 1983 and resulted in estimated annual costs of $65 to $70 billion for medical care, lost wages, and legal fees (14). The Social Security Administration has estimated that "about 150,000 applicants per year (10% of the total) have pain as their primary complaint without clinical findings to fully substantiate it" (15). There are no precise statistics, however, on the *actual* prevalence and costs associated with chronic pain because there is no systematic record keeping and data collection.

It is hard to obtain precise data on the numbers of individuals with chronic pain for three main reasons. One is the lack of a common pool of data because information is not shared among medical providers, insurance carriers, and governmental agencies. A second problem is the way the data are collected. Existing data are organized according to the type of problem and body part affected (e.g., low back pain) and do not indicate the degree of chronicity. Finally, much of the data details on-the-job injuries only and disregards injuries for example, that happen at home.

Difficulty in determining the exact cost of chronic pain can be largely attributed to the inability to estimate indirect costs such as lost productivity, hiring and training of replacement employees, and increased insurance premiums. Ultimately, these increased costs are passed on to the consumer and the public.

The remainder of this chapter focuses on two conditions that are commonly associated with chronic pain: lower back pain and cumulative trauma disorder. Both are seen frequently in occupational therapy settings.

Lower back pain is a pervasive disability. It is estimated in the literature that 80% of the U.S. population will experience back pain at some time during their

Table 8.1.
Overview of Differences between Acute and Chronic Pain

Acute	Chronic
• Provides warning of tissue damage occurrence	• Has no known function
• Fast, sudden, sharp followed by dull ache	• Ache, cramp, or burn; constant or intermittent
• Initially discrete, well-localized, then more diffuse	• Generally more diffuse and may have radiating component
• Usually has identifiable cause such as injury, pathology or disease	• May or may not have associated injury, pathology or disease
• Pain pattern follows known dermatomes and nerve distributions	• May stray from known dermatomes and nerve distributions
• Usually accompanied by objective findings	• May or may not be accompanied by objective findings
• Responds to analgesics or narcotics	• Analgesics have little to no effect; narcotics become addictive

lives. One study suggests that 5% of the U.S. population has experienced chronic low back symptoms that have permanently disabled 2.6 million individuals and temporarily disabled another 2.6 million (16). A second study (17) reports that chronic back problems will disable 1% of Americans on a total and permanent basis and partially disable many more. A third study reported that approximately 74% of workers with back injuries return to work within a month, while 7% are unable to return for more than 6 months (18). This latter group incurs over 75% of medical costs and overall compensation for low back injuries (18). The likelihood of these individuals returning to work after a 6-month absence is 50%. After 1 year, the rate of return is reduced to 25%, and those absent for more than 2 years never return to gainful employment (18). The estimated costs for those with back pain range from $5 billion per year for medical costs (19) to $56 billion when compensation costs are included (20).

The other primary type of soft tissue disability associated with chronic pain is cumulative trauma disorder. In 1989, there were 147,000 cases of cumulative trauma disorder reported to the Bureau of Labor Statistics; these disorders are the leading cause of increases in job-related occupational illnesses (21).

It has been estimated by the American Academy of Orthopedic Surgeons that national costs for cumulative trauma disorders, including medical care and lost wages, approximate $27 billion per year (22). Carpal tunnel syndrome, one type of cumulative trauma disorder, occurs at the average rate of 0.8 cases per 1000 workers in general industry (21). These figures are as high as 15 to 20% for workers in high-risk occupations (21).

A company at high risk for cumulative trauma injuries, will spend an estimated $250,000 per year per 100 employees for costs associated with the problem (23). To illustrate, only 5% of individuals who are diagnosed with carpal tunnel require surgery. In a study of meat cutters, however, of those who had surgery, 50% had not returned to their original jobs 1 year later (24).

Data seem to indicate that cumulative trauma disorders occur more frequently in certain occupations and that in severe cases (i.e., those that don't respond to conservative treatment), a high percentage of individuals are unable to return to work because of chronic pain.

SIGNS AND SYMPTOMS

It is important to reiterate that, at the present time, there is no objective way to measure pain. Pain is a subjective response that can be substantiated through observation and possibly by the results of clinical tests/assessments. The signs and symptoms of chronic pain vary, depending on such factors as the presence or absence of an underlying pathology; the type and location of pathology; physical fitness; and psychologic state. Table 8.2 lists some common signs and symptoms associated with soft tissue chronic pain of the upper extremity and lower back. Signs and symptoms listed in the table may be present because of pathology, a psychologic problem, or a combination of the two. The only universal measure of chronic pain is its presence over time.

The individual's personal and medical history are often good predictors of dysfunction from chronic pain and should be given careful consideration. The person's psychosocial history (refer to the previous section on psychology of pain) and the course of previous events and treatment for the condition are important aspects of the total clinical picture.

Many share a common experience or series of events that led to their disability. Frequently the individual has undergone a significant amount of testing to rule out various disorders and pathologies. There is a history of unsuccessful treatments, surgeries, and/or medications with poor pain control. The person may have consulted a number of physicians and therapists, seeking alternative methods of

Table 8.2.
Signs and Symptoms of Chronic Pain

SIGNS
A. **Objective**
Asymmetry—structural or postural
Atrophy
Autonomic discharge—sweating, flushing, tachycardia, elevated blood pressure
Crepitus
Edema
Erythema
Incoordination
Inflammation
Muscle spasm, tightness, hardness, ropiness, or twitch response
Reflex exaggerated, diminished, or absent
Skin temperature increased or decreased
Spinal irregularities—misalignment, flattening, general asymmetry
Vascular abnormalities—discoloration, diminished or absent hair growth and/or pulses, ulcerations
B. **Objective but requiring accurate patient report or cooperation**
Balance
Gait abnormalities
Fluidity of motion
Muscle cramps or weakness
Numbness
Pain—usually poor localized
Paresthesias (tingling)
Projected pain
Radiculopathy
Range-of-motion limitation, passive and/or active
Sensory impairment
Sudden motor loss, (e.g., dropping things or falling without warning)
Trigger points

SYMPTOMS
Antalgic movement and postures
Eating pattern changed—increased or decreased
Emotional distress—anger, irritability, depression, anxiety, emotional lability, etc.
Fatigue
Functional capacity diminished
Glove anesthesia
Muscle weakness observed as a sudden, giving way to applied resistance
Pain behaviors—guarding, grimacing, sighing, holding or rubbing body parts, etc.
Preoccupation with pain
Referred pain
Tenderness to palpation
Tolerance to pain diminished
Sexual activity diminished
Sleeping disturbances
Social withdrawal

treatment for relief. This is sometimes referred to as "doctor shopping" and it can significantly inflate medical care costs. Having seen a variety of medical providers, the patient is often confused about the cause of the pain, the diagnosis, appropriate treatments, and safe activity level. With contradictory advice, it is not surprising that the patient becomes confused, suspicious, or defensive.

As pain persists, the person becomes more and more distressed, especially when no medical cause is found for the continuing pain. The distress may manifest itself in a number of ways depending upon such factors as premorbid personality, cultural influences, and financial incentives or disincentives. Distress may result in anger directed at self or others, depression, anxiety, and guilt. These responses can heighten emotional tension and, thus, the perception of pain.

Drug dependency can be another result of frequently changed or mismanaged care (7). The patient finds that narcotic medication helps "take the edge off," even though it doesn't cure the pain. In extreme situations, the person will change doctors or see several concurrently to maintain drug dependence.

Some individuals find it necessary to "prove" that they have a disability. Insurance carriers/employers often require an independent medical evaluation (IME). The intent is to provide an objective, impartial physician's opinion. This is not unusual when the employee has been unable to return to work and has a history of chronic pain of unknown origin. In some states, if the IME reveals no objective findings to substantiate the patient's continued complaints of pain, it is possible, particularly in workers' compensation cases, that the patient will be asked to return to work or risk losing benefits. In this situation, the person may concentrate on proving that the disability is real.

In summary, some of the precipitating factors leading to the diagnosis of chronic pain are:

1. Pain that extends beyond the normal course of healing;
2. Lack of objective physical signs or fluctuating physical findings;
3. Significant functional disability as a result of the pain;
4. Psychological dysfunction;
5. Multiple failed treatments and/or surgeries;
6. Use of many different medications;
7. Inability to be gainfully employed;
8. Receiving financial remuneration for disability or involvement in litigation to determine disability.

DIAGNOSTICS AND MEDICATIONS

The diagnosis of chronic pain is made when pain lasts beyond the normal healing period. Underlying pathology and psychologic factors may be present or absent. Chronic pain is considered dysfunctional when it interferes with performance.

Chronic pain can be present in an unlimited number of diagnoses. This section focuses on diagnostic tests done to determine if an underlying pathology can be identified for lower back or upper extremity conditions associated with chronic pain. Positive test results substantiate the likelihood of a pathologic condition and associated chronic pain. A negative test result, however, does not rule out the existence of chronic pain. Psychologic tests are used to determine whether or not there is an underlying affective disorder, to gain an understanding of how the patient perceives pain, and how the pain affects the individual both personally and socially. Appendix 8.3 lists some of the common medical diagnostic tests used with lower back and upper extremity pain, as well as psychological tests.

The use of medication will vary according to the presence of an underlying organic pathology, the type of pathology, and its stage. If no organic pathology is identified, medications are prescribed according to the duration of the pain. Selection of appropriate medication depends upon a specific diagnosis. For example, medications prescribed for an inflammatory flare-up are different than those prescribed to manage on-going pain.

Information on medications (25–30) is presented in Appendix 8.4. Dosages and daily maximum levels are approximate guidelines. Potential side effects that are common and may affect occupational performance are listed. A word of caution: narcotic analgesics are generally not used for chronic pain because they are addictive. In some situations, they are prescribed on a limited basis for short-term bouts of increased pain.

In addition to the drugs listed in Appendix 8.4, such medications as Zantac or Cytotec are used to inhibit the secretion of gastric acid and relieve problems of secondary gastrointestinal distress caused by other medications. Antihistamines can be prescribed (50–100 mg dosage) to help induce sleep, in place of a sedative with addictive properties.

Diagnostic or therapeutic nerve blocks, which are an injection of local anesthetics, are used to: identify or relieve pain in the peripheral nerves, nerve roots, or viscera; decrease trigger point pain; interrupt reflex sympathetic activity; and improve vascular supply (25). Steroid injections are given to reduce inflammation.

EFFECT ON PERFORMANCE COMPONENTS AND OCCUPATIONAL PERFORMANCE AREAS

As previously discussed, chronic pain can be, in itself, a disabling condition, regardless of the etiology. The person who is experiencing chronic pain encounters limitations in a number of performance components and performance areas. These factors may be present or absent for any particular individual, or may be experienced to varying degrees by different people.

Performance Components

Sensorimotor. Neuromuscular disruptions are common. There is usually a limitation in active and sometimes passive range of motion. Patients have pain when they attempt to use the muscles, tendons, etc. that have been damaged. For example, in lateral epicondylitis ("tennis elbow"), the patient experiences pain at the muscle's points of origin when attempting to forcefully extend and sometimes supinate the wrist. This condition is caused by forcefully snapping the wrist into extension as with a tennis stroke or by mechanical overload of the muscle(s) through repetitive work. To minimize the pain, the person will avoid wrist extension, especially

to maximum range or against force. Initially, passive range of motion is normal; however, it may diminish with prolonged inactivity over time. Pain is reproduced when the involved muscles are put on maximum stretch. In this example, pain may occur when the wrist is passively placed in full flexion. In less severe cases, this may only be referred to as "tightness" by the patient.

Loss of strength and endurance are significant and common problems for chronic pain patients. They often result from prolonged inactivity due to pain avoidance or overuse of orthotic devices. Extended periods of inactivity will cause muscle weakness and then atrophy. Generalized deconditioning can also affect activity tolerance.

If the patient continually avoids using the body part (either actively or passively), the muscles can shorten, and the connective tissues lose their "glide" quality. This, in turn, can cause secondary pain. In addition, inflammation and crepitus compromise the soft tissue integrity and can also cause pain.

In sum, there is a self-perpetuating cycle established as a result of initial pain, later sustained by secondary pain (Fig. 8.2). Also, because chronic pain is diffuse and poorly localized, there may be a tendency to protect areas of referred pain. This draws additional soft tissues/muscle groups into the chronic pain syndrome, and there is an additive effect on limitations in activities as more and more muscles are involved.

Postural control is another potential area of dysfunction. As a guarding mechanism, the patient may hold the body part in a protective, abnormal position. This is particularly common with upper extremity injuries. The extremity is held close to the body with slight elevation of the shoulder. Holding the arm in this position for long periods can cause prolonged static muscle contraction and referred pain in the upper back, particularly the trapezius and levator scapulae. This results in fatigue and loss of symmetry. A person with

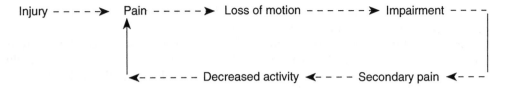

Figure 8.2. Secondary pain cycle.

low back pain can be observed shifting weight to the unaffected side or leaning to the painful side to avoid stretching muscles of the lower back. Greater energy demands are made when maintaining a position against gravity, such as holding the injured arm in slight abduction or laterally flexing the trunk. Unnatural weight distribution can also reduce normal range of motion because of muscle shortening.

Proprioception is associated with postural control. The areas of particular concern are the shoulders, scapulae, and smaller joints of the spine. Normally, a person is aware of the gross position of these structures, but fine positioning, such as slight flexion of C3 or shoulder rounding, is often not perceived. Poor proprioception may play a cumulative role in chronic pain (5).

Finally, sensory awareness and processing may be impaired with chronic pain. This impairment may manifest itself as tactile hyposensitivity or hypersensitivity to noxious stimuli. For example, pain messages may be sent to the brain when no stimulus is present. Also, the person who has chronic pain may not be able to differentiate various stimuli and may have exaggerated responses.

Cognitive. The individual with chronic pain often becomes very focused on the pain, and as a result, cognitive function may be affected. Perceptions, capacities, and processing are distorted or inhibited because of the emotional stress and/or fatigue caused by the pain. Some typical changes in cognitive function follow.

Attention span becomes limited. The pain distracts the patient by interrupting concentration. This is seen in tasks that are monotonous or repetitious, where there is little cognitive challenge or emotional interest. When the perceived pain overrides concentration on the activity, the quality of performance may suffer.

Similarly, increased focus on the pain may decrease the patient's ability to attend to things in the surrounding environment. Therefore, secondary to the attention deficit, short-term or recent memory may be affected. This may be further compounded by the effects of depression, which also contributes to poor attention and short-term memory.

Issues of dependency and fear of additional pain or injury can influence problem solving, particularly that related to managing the pain in order to maintain function. In a dependent role, allowing others to do the work until they are "better," patients may not take the initiative, for example, to analyze everyday activities that are aggravating the pain. This is more common when there is no incentive for the patient to learn to function independently, such as when there is someone else available to perform the task or it is associated with a role that the patient is willing to give up.

Patients often fail to use good problem-solving skills or judgment when they are "having a good day." Often, in this instance, patients will try to do too much. In failing to properly pace activities, they may experience a subsequent increase in pain, which will help perpetuate their misconceptions about their actual abilities and tolerances.

Finally, patients frequently have a hard time learning new strategies to manage the pain. This is particularly evident in the psychophysical response to pain, that is, learning to relax muscles when pain occurs instead of increasing muscle tension. It is often difficult for patients to learn to associate relaxation with the pain response.

Psychosocial. Chronic pain often has a strong psychologic component that limits functional capacities and perpetuates the pain cycle. The person experiences dramatic changes or even losses of societal roles. Self-concept is inevitably affected, as are values, interests, and social interactions. The loss of familiar roles and activities affects the patients' management of self, since there has been a loss of control over their daily lives.

A role change or loss may be the single and most apparent effect with which the patient must deal. Subsequent psychologic components may be directly affected by role interruption. Chronic pain can affect a large number of performance components, therefore, any number of roles can similarly be affected. Since the sense of identity and worth are largely defined by an individual's roles and multiple roles can be affected, there may be substantial feelings of loss, grief, and anger in every aspect of the patient's daily life. In some cases, familiar roles may even be reversed, further complicating the sense of self.

Values may change, as roles and perspectives are modified or reversed. Typically, if a new role is assumed, the person assumes the values associated with that role. A threat to personal or familial security may also intensify the focus on some values and diminish it on others. There may also be an increased awareness of mortality, causing patients to reassess what is important.

As a result of changes in performance components over time, patients may experience a change in interests. If there is an activity in which they can no longer participate, there may be a resulting loss of interest. An increase in unstructured time, as a result of limitations in roles, may go unchanneled, demonstrating poor time-management skills, or the patient may

develop new interests or routines to fill the time.

A change in self-concept almost always follows a significant or long-standing change in roles. As the role definition changes, so does a person's self-concept. These changes may be interpreted by the patient as either good or bad. The interpretation depends on how closely the changes match the patient's long-term goals and/or motivations. There may be perceptions of oneself as worthless or a failure, or the perception may be one of success in shedding an unwanted role.

Social skills are often affected. Patients' conduct may not be appropriate to the situation when their focus on pain overrides the discussion or issues at hand. Nonverbal communication such as sighing or grimacing may send signals to others about the patient's state of mind. These behaviors can guide or otherwise affect the patient's interpersonal relationships in very significant but subtle ways.

As a result of the emotional effects of long-term pain, changes, and loss of control among others, coping skills are invariably affected. In the long run, the effects can be positive or adverse. A formerly shy, introverted patient may learn to express herself openly and assertively. Conversely, others may become withdrawn and dependent. New coping skills are developed in response to the situations in which patients find themselves. Very often, however, feelings of anger, loss, fear, and inability to sleep soundly impair a person's ability to cope with day-to-day stresses on top of the pain. As a result, sudden, angry outbursts, crying, blaming of others, and personal distancing are seen. The patient perceives a loss of control and often demonstrates a personal loss of self control.

PERFORMANCE AREAS

Work. Since chronic pain primarily affects adults, work is the most commonly affected performance area. Working requires some level of activity tolerance whether it involves standing for long periods or frequent handling of small objects. The inability to sustain activity over time is why many people with chronic pain conditions are unable to work, particularly outside of the home. In other cases, particular tasks associated with their jobs cause an increase in pain. If the employer can provide work that is within their physical abilities, and the patient feels able to do the job, the patient may be able to continue working. Otherwise, long-term or permanent restrictions may prevent them from returning to their job. These same restrictions may also require the patient to look at alternative or transferrable work skills to find a new job. A role reversal may even occur if, for example, a husband is no longer able to work outside of the home. He may stay home with the children while his wife takes a job to ensure an adequate income.

Educational activities may be affected in the same way. In other instances, however, individuals with chronic pain use the change in their work capacity to return to school and obtain new skills. This is particularly common when an individual can no longer perform a manual occupation and must learn job skills that involve higher level cognitive skills.

Work activities that involve home management or caring for others may also be limited by physical and emotional tolerances to the pain. A mother may find that she has a shorter temper with her children or she may become more reliant on her children for performing tasks around the house. If there is no one else to assist with the work, patients with chronic pain may find that they do less work and/or pace themselves so that they can do the essential chores. For example, cleaning may become less important so the patient can save energy for shopping, cooking, and laundry.

Activities of Daily Living. Activities that require either endurance or motion can be affected. Persons with lower back pain may modify the way they dress, to avoid the pain associated with bending. Chronic

hip pain can be managed by using a tub seat instead of climbing in and out of the tub. A woman with hand pain may be unable to use her curlers or blow dryer without aggravating her pain.

More pervasive, however, are problems encountered with mobility. Lower back pain can impair an individual's ability to walk or ride long distances. Similarly, chronic hand pain can impair tolerance for driving. Limitations in mobility may further affect a person's ability to get to and from work, to get around on the job, to visit friends, or to attend leisure events.

Finally, impaired mobility and flexibility can affect sexual expression. The capacity for sexual interaction may be impaired both physically and psychologically, though adaptation and modification of physical expression can be satisfying.

Leisure Activities. Involvement in leisure activities may also change. This can be solely the result of physical limitations (e.g., the father who cannot play football with his son because of chronic back pain) or it can be limited by psychologic function (e.g. the depressed individual who has withdrawn from club activities). Finally, an increased focus on the pain may draw on the attention span so a person may no longer enjoys the activity, (e.g., crocheting or doing crossword puzzles).

A summary of occupational performance components and performance areas commonly seen in chronic pain patients is provided in Table 8.3. From the preceding discussion it is apparent that each of the three primary performance components and areas can be affected by chronic pain. While the table provides an overview, the following case studies provide some specific examples of chronic pain and its impact on occupational performance.

CASE STUDIES

Case 1

C.S. is a 43-year-old man employed as a manual laborer at a small chrome plating plant. He has been employed there for 12 years, has a good work record,

Table 8.3.
Occupational Performance Areas and Performance Components Commonly Affected by Chronic Pain

Sensory Motor Component	Cognitive Integration & Cognitive Components	Psychosocial Skills & Psychological Components

1. Sensory integration
  a. **Sensory awareness**
  b. Sensory processing
    1. **Tactile**
    2. **Proprioceptive**
    3. Vestibular
    4. Visual
    5. Auditory
    6. Gustatory
    7. Olfactory
  c. Perceptual skills
    1. Stereognosis
    2. Kinesthesia
    3. Body scheme
    4. Right-left discrimination
    5. Form constancy
    6. Position in space
    7. Visual-closure
    8. Figure ground
    9. Depth perception
    10. Topographic orientation
 	
2. Neuromuscular
a. Reflex
b. **Range of motion**
c. Muscle tone
d. **Strength**
e. **Endurance**
f. **Postural control**
g. **Soft tissue integrity**
 	
3. Motor
  a. **Activity tolerance**
  b. Gross motor coordination
  c. Crossing the midline
  d. Laterality
  e. Bilateral integration
  f. Praxis
  g. Fine motor coordination
  h. Visual-motor integration
  i. Oral-motor control
	1. Level of arousal
	2. Orientation
	3. Recognition
	4. **Attention span**
	5. **Memory**
	  a. **Short-term**
	  b. Long-term
	  c. Remote
	  d. **Recent**
	6. Sequencing
	7. Categorization
	8. Concept formation
	9. Intellectual operations in space
	10. **Problem solving**
	11. Generalization of learning
	12. Integration of learning
	13. **Synthesis of learning**
		1. Psychological
		  a. **Roles**
		  b. **Values**
		  c. **Interests**
		  d. Initiation of activity
		  e. Termination of activity
		  f. **Self-concept**
		2. Social
		  a. **Social conduct**
		  b. Conversation
		  c. Self-expression
		3. Self-management
		  a. **Coping skills**
		  b. **Time management**
		  c. **Self-control**

Table 8.3 **(Continued)**

Occupational Therapy Performance Areas

Activities of Daily Living	Work Activities	Play/Leisure Activities
1. **Grooming**	1. Home management	1. **Play or leisure exploration**
2. Oral hygiene	a. **Clothing care**	2. **Play or leisure performance**
3. **Bathing**	b. **Cleaning**	
4. Toilet hygiene	c. **Meal preparation and cleanup**	
5. **Dressing**	d. **Shopping**	
6. Feeding and eating	e. Money management	
7. Medication routine	f. **Household maintenance**	
8. **Socialization**	g. Safety procedures	
9. Functional communication	2. **Care of others**	
10. **Functional mobility**	3. **Educational activities**	
11. **Sexual expression**	4. Vocational activities	
	a. **Vocational exploration**	
	b. **Job acquisition**	
	c. **Work or job performance**	
	d. Retirement planning	

and is well liked by supervisors and co-workers. He has only one previous workers' compensation claim, for an incident 6 years ago when he was exposed to toxic chemical fumes.

He is married with three children, ages 7, 9, and 11 and has a good relationship with his wife and children. His wife works as a waitress at a hotel. C.S. is illiterate. In his spare time, he enjoys playing basketball and riding motorcycles. He belongs to a motorcycle club and is active in their volunteer work to raise money for a local charity. He also assists with his sons' Little League, driving the team to games, handling the equipment, and cheering the team on. In the winter, he spends a lot of time working on his motorcycle and pickup truck in a neighbor's heated garage.

C.S. injured his lower back while lifting at work. He was taken to the hospital's emergency department; x-ray films showed no structural damage, and examination found no neurologic deficits. A severe muscle spasm in the right, lower back was the only positive finding. A diagnosis of severe lumbosacral strain was made. He was given prescriptions for antiinflammatory agents and muscle relaxants and told to go home to bed for 3 days and then follow up with his family doctor.

After 3 days of bedrest, he still had difficulty getting up and down from a seated position, standing, and walking. His family doctor noted a paravertebral spasm in the right low back. Further examination revealed trunk flexion limited by pain to 30° and full extension at −10°. When he straightened from standing, C.S. used his hands on his thighs to "walk" himself back up. Side bending was normal on the right but limited by 20° on the left. Rotation was limited in both directions. Straight leg raising was negative on the left and pos-

itive at 25° on the right. His stance and gait showed a pain scoliosis on the right. Sensory and reflex testing were normal. Bowel and bladder function were reported to be normal. Muscle strength appeared good, although he had "give away" response (sudden release of a muscle contraction when resistance is applied) in his right hip flexors and extensors. The doctor confirmed the diagnosis of back strain and renewed his prescriptions. He told C.S. to stay home and rest for a week but to gradually begin increasing his activities. The doctor would run some laboratory tests to rule out organic pathologies. The doctor asked him to return in a week.

C.S. again went home and tried to resume some of his activities. He dressed each day but found it very painful to get into his pants, shoes, and socks. He was most comfortable in his recliner chair and spent significant time watching television. His wife and children were very concerned and tried to help him as much as possible.

When he returned to the doctor, C.S. was very concerned about new pain that had developed in his right buttock and anterior thigh. A few of the same tests were quickly repeated, but little change was found. The laboratory results had all been normal. C.S. told the doctor he wasn't ready to go back to work. The following week, when C.S. did feel ready, his employer was unable to offer him restricted work.

C.S. returned to his doctor several more times. He was growing restless and bored at home, and the constant pain made him irritable. The doctor, who had observed little improvement, felt there was nothing more he could do. He referred C.S. to an orthopaedic specialist. The orthopaedist reviewed his x-ray films and conducted a detailed examination and inter-

Table 8.4.
Occupational Performance Profile[a]—C.S.

		Performance Areas			
		Work Activities			
		Vocation	Education	Home Management	Care of Others
PERFORMANCE COMPONENTS — SENSORIMOTOR	**SENSORY INTEGRATION** Increased sensitivity to touch or palpation in the lower back				
	NEUROMUSCULAR Limited range of motion in trunk; strength & endurance for gross motor activities diminished; postural control decreased as result of pain postures; shortening of trunk muscles	Unable to perform physical demands of job due to limited range of motion and pain			
	MOTOR Activity tolerance diminished for gross motor tasks, e.g., stand, walk, lift, carry, push, pull	Unable to tolerate being on feet for 8 hrs or doing heavy lifting		Unable to perform many household maintenance tasks	
PERFORMANCE COMPONENTS — COGNITIVE	**COGNITIVE** Decreased ability to attend to tasks; difficulty problem-solving how to perform activities without aggravating the pain; responds to pain with emotional & muscular tension		Unable to read (premorbid)	Spends most of the time in recliner rather than scheduling/pacing activities at home	
	PSYCHOLOGICAL Experienced change in roles, values and interests; diminished self-concept	Has lost role as worker; anger toward employer, wife has had to increase her working hours			Role as nurturing father & loving husband affected
PERFORMANCE COMPONENTS — PSYCHOSOCIAL	**SOCIAL** Expresses pain behaviors; often angry in communication with family	Has communicated questionable motivation to his employer			Easily loses temper with family members
	SELF-MANAGEMENT Coping skills are diminished time management unbalanced; self-control decreased	Loss of 8–10 hr day as worker		Spends increased time in recliner watching TV	

EXTERNAL FACTORS WHICH INFLUENCE PERFORMANCE; CULTURE, ECONOMY, ENVIRONMENT

[a]Grid adapted from Uniform Terminology (2nd ed.). Developed by the occupational therapy faculty at Eastern Michigan University.

Client initials: C.S.
Diagnosis: Chronic Pain
Age: 43

Play or Leisure Activities		Activities of Daily Living				
Exploration	Performance	Self-Care	Social-ization	Functional Communi-cation	Functional Mobility	Sexual Expression
						Hypersitivity to physical contact has limited intimacy
	Difficulty bending forward to work on truck	Difficulty dressing lower extremities				Experiences pain when engaging in sexual intercourse
	Unable to tolerate standing to work on motorcycle; vibration intolerance limits ability to ride the motorcycle				Decreased walking tolerance	
	Has been unable to problem-solve method for working on his vehicles					
Poor self-concept interferes with exploration of new, physically tolerable activities	Has lost interest in motorcycle club activities		Has lost social contact with club members and neighbors			Feels he has lost some of his masculine identity
			Demonstrates pain behaviors when around others			
	Loss of 2–4 hr per week in leisure interests					

Table 8.5.
Occupational Performance Profile[a]—B.A.

		Performance Areas		
		Work Activities		
	Vocation	Education	Home Management	Care of Others
SENSORIMOTOR — **SENSORY INTEGRATION** Increased sensitivity to touch or palpation of the arm				Protects arm from touch when around her children
NEUROMUSCULAR Strength & endurance for UE tasks diminished; soft tissue integrity has been compromised	Unable to perform physical demands of job			Difficulty carrying her youngest child
MOTOR Activity tolerance diminished for gross motor tasks: handle, lift, carry, push, pull			Decreased tolerance for cleaning, meal preparation, and household maintenance	
COGNITIVE — **COGNITIVE** Problem-solving limited to areas where motivation is high; responds to pain with increased emotional & muscular tension				
PSYCHOSOCIAL — **PSYCHOSOCIAL** Change in role; value role as mother reinforced	Lost role as worker; fear of further injury if she returns to work reinforced by mother			More relaxed and enjoys time spent with children as a result of decreased work demands
SOCIAL Expresses pain behaviors				
SELF-MANAGEMENT Coping skills diminished; time management affected, self-control decreased	Loss of 8 hrs as worker; feelings of conflict; worry about financial security			

EXTERNAL FACTORS WHICH INFLUENCE PERFORMANCE; CULTURE, ECONOMY, ENVIRONMENT

[a]Grid adapted from Uniform Terminology (2nd ed.). Developed by the occupational therapy faculty at Eastern Michigan University.

Client initials: B.A. (Case 2)
Diagnosis: Pain
Age: 27

| Play or Leisure | | Activities of Daily Living | | | | |
Exploration	Perform-ance	Self-Care	Social-ization	Functional Communi-cation	Functional Mobility	Sexual Expression
	Increased leisure time with children					
				Cries easily when discussing her problems		

views, including whether C.S. had been experiencing any personal problems at home or at work. He began to wonder if the doctor thought he was faking. During the examination, the doctor repeated many of the tests the family doctor had done. Other tests included standing on one leg, walking on his heels and then his toes, reflex testing, and measuring the lengths and circumferences of his legs. Upon completing his examination, the doctor told C.S. there was nothing structurally wrong. He suggested physical therapy to ease the pain, relax the muscles, and stretch out tightened muscles.

It was now 8 weeks since the injury and his discontent and concern were growing. Why wasn't the pain going away? Were the doctors missing something? He was anxious and confused. He continued with the therapy, working hard under his physical therapist's direction. He saw an occupational therapist for several sessions who showed him how to do things like put on his pants and get out of bed without aggravating the pain. He began to feel that he had some control over the pain and that he was making progress.

Then he reinjured his back at home. He returned to the emergency department and was again told there was no structural damage but that he should follow up with his doctor as soon as possible. The pain was worse than before. He returned to his orthopaedic physician, very upset and agitated. The doctor noted that C.S.'s posture again listed to the right and his trunk range-of-motion was limited by pain. The muscle spasm was back. C.S. reported that the buttock and thigh pains were worse, going all the way down into his calf. MRI results were normal. C.S. asked the doctor what *exactly* was causing the pain. The doctor again told him it was muscle spasm. C.S. wondered why a back spasm caused leg pain, but he didn't ask the doctor.

Weeks passed and C.S. experienced more and more problems at home. His family was beginning to tire of his short temper and dependency. They were also feeling the financial strain of reduced income. He felt guilty about his wife having to work more and about being so short tempered, but he couldn't help it. This increased his irritability; he felt rejected. He was also frustrated by the limits his back pain had put on his sexual life. As his depression grew, so did his withdrawal from the motorcycle club's activities. He no longer went to his neighbor's, even to talk, because it angered him that he couldn't work on his truck, something that had always helped him relax.

His employers wanted to know when he was coming back to work. They were short of help and needed him. C.S., angry that his boss didn't even ask how he was doing, yelled, "When I'm ready!" and hung up the phone. The employer wondered if C.S. was really trying.

It's now 8 months since the initial injury, and C.S. is still at home. He has good and bad days, but is fearful of reinjuring his back. He also doubts his ability to keep up with the other guys at work. The problems he has at home are at least familiar to him; he doesn't know if he can handle returning to work. Table 8.4 summarizes C.S.'s occupational performance deficits.

Case 2

B.A. is the single mother of two children, ages 3 and 6. She is 27 years old and was divorced 6 months ago, after a difficult marriage to an abusive husband. She lives in a rented trailer.

She works in a large manufacturing plant where plastic components for car dashboards are made. She has worked there for 9 months. Her mother took a medical retirement from the same plant because of carpal tunnel syndrome in both wrists. Her mother had worked there for 17 years.

For the last 3 months B.A. has been cutting off the "flash" (i.e., seams on plastic that has been hot molded) with a razor knife. She began to notice an aching in her right, dominant forearm at the end of her shift one Friday. By Saturday morning it was gone, and she didn't think twice about it. As the weeks passed, however, the aching developed earlier in her shift and lasted into the next day. Then it became constant. The pain runs from her elbow into the dorsum of her forearm.

She was sent to a doctor frequently used by the company. He asked about the pain: what it felt like, where it was and what seemed to make it worse. B.A. noted that cutting the plastic flash seemed to bother it the most. The doctor palpated the arm, and checked for tender spots. He asked about any numbness or tingling, touched the arm for hot spots, and looked at the color. He noted that she was extremely tender at the lateral epicondyle and, less so, in her dorsal forearm. He told her she had epicondylitis and gave her a wrist splint to wear at work. She wore the splint at work for a few days, but it interfered with her cutting. She discarded it and the pain persisted.

She then began to have difficulty doing household chores (e.g., cutting food, opening jars, and lifting her toddler). Keeping up with production at work became more and more difficult. B.A. returned to the doctor, and when asked how things were going, she broke into tears and said that the splint hadn't helped, her pain had increased, and she didn't think she could keep on working. He gave her several days off work. Without the rigorous work demands, the pain decreased. She felt more relaxed and enjoyed the time at home with her children.

When she went back to work, the pain quickly returned. At the doctor's suggestion, her supervisor moved her to a job that required removing duct tape from components that had just been painted. This job also bothered her arm.

She asked to see a doctor of her own choice who specialized in industrial injuries. She explained the problem and how it had developed, adding that she now had a generalized numbness and tingling in her fingers. Tearfully, she requested she be given time off work as it had helped before. The doctor agreed after noting a significant amount of crepitus in the common extensor tendon and suggested that B.A. have an electromyelogram (EMG).

Again, with rest, she improved. Her mother was concerned and sympathetic. She warned her daughter not to let "them" ruin her, as they had her mother.

Over the next 6 months, with intermittent therapy, B.A. was on and off work. She found she could tolerate some light-duty jobs, but her employer insisted that she be able to return to her regular job before they could approve her for another job on a permanent basis. Each time she returned to the cutting job, her pain grew worse. Her EMG results were negative.

At this point, B.A. got angry with her employers, blaming them for what had happened to her. She sought out various specialists, received injections, and went to therapy. Nothing seemed to help the pain. Eventually she had surgery to debride the tendon, but the pain did not subside.

B.A. feels she can never go back to work at the plant because the work increases her pain. The employer sent her for an IME, which showed "no objective findings." Her employer maintains that she can return to work and has cut off her workers' compensation benefits. She has filed a dispute and it will be 6 to 8 months before the matter is legally settled. In the meantime, she is handicapped. Table 8.5 summarizes the impact of B.A.'s disability on her occupational performance.

CONCLUSION

Pain is a multifaceted phenomenon with many varied components. We are still learning much about the way pain works. Its presence, over time, affects sensory motor, physical, cognitive, and psychologic performance, yet often no cause is found. Since chronic pain can affect all aspects of a person's life, it can cause the individual to feel "out of control." Occupational therapists can analyze an individual's deficits in specific performance components and determine how these deficits affect the person's occupational performance. The occupational therapist works with clients to improve occupational performance, giving them back a sense of control over both the pain and their lives.

REFERENCES

1. Collins JG. Pain mechanisms. In: Wu W, ed. Pain management: assessment and treatment of chronic and acute syndromes. New York: Human Sciences Press, 1987:23–43.
2. Iggo A. Physiology of pain. In: Burrows GD, Elton D, Stanley GV, eds. Handbook of chronic pain management. New York: Elsevier, 1987:7–18.
3. Smith GC. The anatomy of pain. In: Burrows GD, Elton D, Stanley GV, eds. Handbook of chronic pain management. New York: Elsevier, 1987:1–5.
4. Fessler RG. Physiology, anatomy and pharmacology of pain perception. In: Camic PM Brown FD, eds. Assessing chronic pain, a multidisciplinary clinic handbook. New York: Springer-Verlag, 1989:5–19.
5. Zohn DA. Musculoskeletal pain, diagnosis and physical treatment, 2nd ed. Boston: Little, Brown and Co, 1988.
6. Melzack R, Wall PD. Pain mechanism: a new theory. Science 1965;150:971–979.
7. Gildenberg PL, DeVaul RA. The chronic pain patient: evaluation and management. Pain and headache, vol 7. New York: Karger, 1985.
8. Cailliet R. Soft tissue pain and disability. Philadelphia: FA Davis, 1977.
9. Travell JG, Simons DG. Myofascial pain and dysfunction, the trigger point manual. Baltimore: Williams & Wilkins, 1983.
10. Benca RM. In: Camic PM, Brown FD, eds. Assessing chronic pain, a multidisciplinary clinic handbook. New York: Springer-Verlag, 1989:148–160.
11. Grzesiak RC, Perrine KR. In: Wu W, ed. Pain management: assessment and treatment of chronic and acute syndromes. New York: Human Sciences Press, 1987:44–69.
12. Savitz D. Medical evaluation of the chronic pain patient. In: Aranoff GM, ed. Evaluation and treatment of chronic pain. Baltimore: Urban & Schwarzenberg, 1985:39–60.
13. Jerome J.; unpublished data. Ingham Medical Center, Lansing, MI.
14. Bonica JJ. Importance of the problem. In: Aranoff GM, ed. Evaluation and treatment of chronic pain. Baltimore: Urban & Schwarzenberg, 1985:xxxi–xliv.
15. Institute of Medicine: Committee on Pain, Disability and Chronic Illness Behavior. Pain and disability: clinical, behavioral and public policy perspectives. Washington, D.C.: National Academy Press, 1987.
16. Frymoyer JW, Gordon SL. Research perspectives in low-back pain. Spine 1989;14:1384–1388.
17. Mayer TG, Gatchel RJ, Mayer H, Kishino ND, Keeley J, Mooney V. A prospective two-year study of functional restoration in industrial low back injury. JAMA 1987;258:1763–1767.
18. VanOort G, Frederick M, Pinto D, Ragone D. Back injuries require integration of aggressive and passive treatment. Occup Health Saf 1990;59(1):22–24.

19. Morris A, Randolph JW. Back rehabilitation programs speed recovery of injured workers. Occup Health Saf 1984;53(7):53–68.

20. Bauer WI. Scope of industrial low back pain. In: Wiesel SW, Feffer HL, Rothman RH, eds. Industrial low back pain, a comprehensive approach. Charlottesville, VA: The Michie Co, 1985:1–35.

21. AOTA. Repetitive motion disorders lead increase in job illness. OT Week, 12/13/90:12.

22. Joyce M. Ergonomics will take center stage during 90s and into the new century. Occup Health Saf 1991;60(1):31–37.

23. Barrer S. Gaining the upper hand on carpal tunnel syndrome. Occup Health Saf 1991;60(1):38–43.

24. Field T. A rise in pain from repetitious work. USA Today, 7/23/90:4D.

25. Gourlay GK, Cousins MJ, Cherry DA. Drug therapy. In: Handbook of chronic pain management. New York: Elsevier, 1987:163–192.

26. Fessler RG. Pharmacologic treatment of chronic pain. In: Camic PM, Brown FD, eds. Assessing chronic pain, a multidisciplinary clinic handbook. New York: Springer-Verlag, 1989:115–147.

27. Physicians' Desk Reference. 44th ed. Oradell, NJ: Medical Economics Co, 1990.

28. Sunshine A, Olson NZ. Non-narcotic analgesics. In: Wall PD, Melzack R, eds. Textbook of pain. New York: Churchill Livingstone, 1984:670–685.

29. Twycross RG, McQuay HF. Opiods. In: Wall PD, Melzack R, ed. Textbook on pain. New York: Churchill Livingstone, 1984:686–701.

30. Monks R, Merskey H. Psychotropic drugs. In: Wall PD, Melsack R, ed. Textbook of pain. New York: Churchill Livingstone, 1984:702–721.

31. Thomas CL, ed. Taber's cyclopedic medical dictionary. 12th ed. Philadelphia: FA Davis, 1973.

Suggested Readings

Cromwell FS, ed. Occupational therapy and the patient with pain. New York: Haworth Press, 1984.

Hadler, NM. Medical management of the regional musculoskeletal diseases. Orlando: Grune & Stratton, 1984.

Hendler NH, Long DM, Wise TM, eds. Diagnosis and treatment of chronic pain. Boston: John Wright—PSG, 1982.

Kirkaldy-Willis WH, ed. Managing low back pain. 2nd ed. New York: Churchill Livingstone, 1988.

Pawl RP. Chronic pain primer. Chicago: Year Book Medical Publishers, 1979.

Philips HC. Psychological management of chronic pain: a treatment manual. New York: Springer, 1988.

Sternbach RA, ed. The psychology of pain. 2nd ed. New York: Raven Press, 1986.

Wall PD, Melzack R, eds. Textbook of pain. 2nd ed. New York: Churchill Livingstone, 1989.

Glossary

Analgesic: A substance that relieves pain.

Ankylosis: Immobility and consolidation of a joint because of disease, injury, or surgical procedure.

Anxiety disorder: A group of mental disorders in which anxiety is the most prominent disturbance or is experienced if the person attempts to control the symptoms. The person feels an emotional response similar to a normal response to a dangerous or unusual situation; however, the response has no apparent reason and the person cannot identify the source of the threat that produces the anxiety, which actually has its origin in unconscious fears or conflicts.

Catabolites: By-products of muscle metabolism normally removed from muscle by the capillaries; with prolonged contraction, catabolites build up.

Causalgia: A severe, burning pain often associated with trophic skin changes in the hand or foot, caused by peripheral nerve injury. The syndrome may be aggravated by the slightest stimulus or it may be intensified by emotions. Causalgia usually begins several weeks after the initial injury and the pain is described as intense, with persons sometimes taking elaborate precautions to avoid any stimulus they know to be capable of causing a flare-up of symptoms. In most cases, there has been some injury to the median or sciatic nerve.

Crepitus (crepitation): A dry, palpable trill in an a muscle or tendon as a result of inflammation, swelling, and loss of tissue glide quality.

Debridement: The removal of all foreign material and all contaminated and devitalized tissues from or adjacent to a traumatic of infected lesion until surrounding healthy tissue is exposed.

Dermatome: An area of skin innervated by various segments of spinal cord nerves; the area of skin supplied with afferent nerve fibers by a single posterior spinal root.

Discogenic: Caused by derangement of an intervertebral disc.

Facet joint syndrome: Facet: a small, plane surface on a hard body, such as a bone.

Fibrositis: Varied symptoms including deep muscle tenderness, generalized aching, and stiffness. Often accompanied by sleep disturbance. Characteristic of perfectionistic personality and chronicity.

Glove anesthesia: Pattern of numbness with glove-like distribution; does not correspond to documented dermatomes and is often a symptom of psychologic involvement.

Hypochondriasis: A mental disorder characterized by preoccupation with one's health and exaggeration of normal sensations and minor complaints into serious illness.

Hysterical neurosis (conversion disorder): A mental disorder in which the individual converts anxiety caused by a psychologic conflict into physical symptoms.

Indurated: Hardened; abnormally hard.

Ischemia: Deficiency of blood in part, caused by functional constriction or actual obstruction of a blood vessel, often leading to necrosis of surrounding tissue.

Macrotrauma: A large lesion or injury.

Malingerer: One who is guilty of willful, deliberate, and fraudulent feigning or exaggeration of the symptoms of illness or injury to attain a consciously desired end.

Microtrauma: A microscopic lesion or injury.

Muscle loading: Repeated or static contracture of a muscle, which results in inefficient metabolism.

Myalgia: Muscle pain or tenderness.

Myofascial pain: Regional musculoskeletal pain accompanying a trigger zone.

Neuralgia: Pain in a nerve or along the course of one or more nerves. Neuralgia is usually a sharp, spasm-like pain that may recur at intervals, caused by inflammation or injury to a nerve or group of nerves; paralysis can also result. Sciatica, or pain occurring along the sciatic nerve, is a form of neuralgia with pain felt in the back and down the back of the thigh to the ankle.

Neuritis: Inflammation of a nerve, which may affect different parts of the body, depending upon the location of the nerve causing pain, and possible paralysis, since both motor and sensory endings can be affected.

Neuroma: A cyst on a nerve or nerve ending, comprised of axis cylinders, Schwann cells, and fibrous tissue.

Neuropathy: Disease of the nerves.

Nociceptive: Pain sensation.

Nociceptors: Sensory receptors involved in the perception and transmission of noxious stimuli.

Noxious: Tissue damaging.

Pain: Chronic pain: Pain occurring for 6 months or longer; or 3–4 weeks after "normal" healing should have occurred.

Projected-pain: Caused by pain to a nerve or nerve root, which follows the anatom-

ical course of the nerve, or portion thereof projecting pain into another part of the anatomy. See Referred pain.

Proprioception: From the Latin word for "one's own." Interpretation of stimuli originating in muscles, joints, and other internal tissues, which give information about the position of one body part in relation to another. Perception is mediated by sensory nerve endings chiefly in muscles, tendons, and the labyrinth. Proprioceptive input tells the brain when and how muscles are contracting or stretching, and when and how the joints are bending, extending, or being pulled or compressed. This information enables the brain to know where each part of the body is and how it is moving.

Psychogenic: Having an emotional or psychologic origin.

Radiculopathy: Pathology related to the roots of the spinal nerves.

Referred pain: Experienced within the same dermatome as the injured area, in a distant area supplied by the same nerve, or in areas with no anatomical correlation.

Somatic: Pertaining to or characteristic of the body (soma).

Somatoform: Denoting psychogenic symptoms resembling those of physical disease.

Somatization disorder: Vague, multiply recurring somatic complaints that are not caused by any real physical illness.

Spondylolisthesis: Forward displacement of a vertebra over a lower segment, caused by a congenital defect or fracture in the pars interarticularis, usually of the fifth lumbar over the sacrum or of the fourth lumbar over the fifth.

Spondylosis: Ankylosis of a vertebral joint; also, a general term for degenerative changes in the spine.

Sprain: Wrenching or twisting of a joint, with partial rupture of its ligaments. There may also be damage to the associated blood vessels, muscles, tendons, and nerves. A sprain is more serious than a strain, which is simply the overstretching of a muscle, without swelling. Severe sprains are so painful that the joint cannot be used.

Strain: An overstretching or overexertion of some part of the musculature.

Tendon: A cord or band of strong white fibrous tissue that connects a muscle to a bone. When the muscle contracts, or shortens, it pulls on the tendon, which moves the bone.

Threshold: Intensity at which one becomes aware of pain; usually occurs when tissue damage is beginning.

Tolerance: The level of pain that one can endure while still maintaining control.

Trigger zone/point: Palpable, tender, indurated portion of muscle or fascia. Reflex neuromuscular irritability. Irritable focus within a muscle. Commonly accompanied by a patter of referred pain. May be residual to a macrotrauma or the result of faulty body mechanics.

APPENDIX **8.2**

Soft Tissue Disorders Associated with Chronic Pain

Carpal tunnel syndrome: Compression of the median nerve at the wrist

Chronic low back pain: Common diagnosis for undifferentiated pain in the lower back; frequently associated with an incident of sprain or strain

Cubital tunnel syndrome: Compression of the ulnar nerve at the elbow

Degenerative joint disease: osteoarthritis of vertebral joints causing an encroachment on nerve roots or spinal canal; most commonly associated with the cervical region

de Quervain's disease: A form of tenosynovitis of the abductor pollicus longus and the extensor pollicus brevis tendons

Epicondylitis: Periosteal tear of the muscles at the site of their epicondylar origin or ligament

  Lateral: (Tennis elbow) involving extensor muscles

  Medial: (Golfer's elbow) involving flexor muscles

Hand-arm vibration syndrome/Raynaud's disease/white finger: Condition primarily affecting peripheral neural and vascular structures; commonly caused by prolonged exposure to vibration

Reflex sympathetic dystrophy (RSD): Chronic, painful condition, usually affecting extremities after an injury; signs of localized autonomic dysfunction are present, with the hallmark being signs of abnormal sympathetic activity

Rotator cuff tear: Full or partial tear of muscles, which effectively limits active shoulder abduction

Tendonitis: Low-grade, inflammatory process; may be an acute strain or a chronic process and may be degenerative

Tenosynovitis: Inflammation of the tendon sheath

Thoracic outlet syndrome: Trauma to the brachial plexus, subclavian artery and vein by compression

Diagnostic Tests

A. **Lower back and upper extremity soft tissue pain**
   Arthroscopic surgery
   Coordination testing
   Electromyelogram (EMG)/nerve conduction velocity (NCV)
   Injections—diagnostic and nerve blocks
   Isokinetic testing
   Laboratory studies
   Maneuvers (to reproduce symptoms)
      Finkelstein's—stretching thumb abductor/extensor muscles
      Phalen's—nerve compression
      Straight leg raising—stretching sciatic nerve
      Tinel's—nerve tapping
      Valsalva—increasing interabdominal pressure
   Manual muscle test
   Measuring leg length and extremity circumference
   Medical history
   Neurologic examination of spine and extremities
   Orthopaedic examination of spine and extremities
   Performance measures: heel/toe raising, heel/toe walking, one leg standing
   Radiologic techniques
   X-ray
   Discrography
   Magnetic resonance imaging (MRI)
   Computerized axial tomography (CT or CAT scan)
   Myelogram
   Bone scan
      Arthrogram
      Angiogram
   Range of motion
   Reflex testing
   Sensory testing
   Thermogram
   Tomogram
   Vascular examination—presence/absence of hair, pulses, ulcerations, and swelling

B. **Psychologic tests**
   Beck depression inventory
   Chronic pain battery
   Illness behavior questionnaire
   McGill pain questionnaire
   Milton behavioral health inventory (MBHI)
   Minnesota multiphasic personality inventory (MMPI)
   Pain drawing
   Pain rating scale
   Personality orientation inventory (POI)
   Psychosocial pain inventory (PSPI)

Medications

Generic Name	Brand Name	Action	Indication	Potential Side Effects	Usual Adult Dose & Availability
Aspirin (salicylates)	Anacin, Bayer, Bufferin, Norgesic Forte with orphenadrine*, Empirin with codeine*	Analgesic, antiinflammatory, antiplatelet, antipyretic, antiprostaglandin	Relief of minor aches & pains, headache, arthritis pain, neuralgia, myalgia, chronic pain	Mild: vertigo, tinnitus Moderate: gastrointestinal (GI) distress, drowsiness, headache, confusion, dimming of vision, talkativeness Severe: pulmonary edema, cardiovascular decomposition, seizure, hepatotoxicity	325–650 mg every 4–6 hr Max = 6 or 8/24 hr Over the counter; *by prescription
Acetaminophen	Anacin-3 Fioricet* Tylenol (with codeine*) Vicodin (with hydrocodone)* Zydone*	Analgesic, antiinflammatory (weak), antipyretic	Relief of minor aches and pains, headache, aspirin allergy, chronic pain	Mild: rash, drug fever Early severe: GI distress, abdominal pain relayed severe: hypoglycemia, myocardial arrythmia, hepatoxicity renal disease, coma, death	325–650 mg every 4–6 hr Max = 6 or 8/24 hr Over the counter; *by prescription

NONSTEROIDAL ANTI-INFLAMMATORY DRUGS (NSAIDS)

Generic Name	Brand Name	Action	Indication	Potential Side Effects	Usual Adult Dose & Availability
	The following applies to all medications listed below	Analgesic, antiinflammatory (nonsteroidal), antipyretic; antiprostaglandin	Acute musculoskeletal disorders; rheumatoid arthritis, sciatic pain; chronic pain; degenerative joint diseases; severe exacerbation of chronic pain (Toradol)	GI distress, severe headaches, vertigo, confusion, depression	Over the counter; *by prescription **intramuscular administration
Ibuprofen	Advil, Midol, Nuprin, Motrin IB Motrin*				200 mg every 4–6 hr 400–800 mg every 4–8 hr
Diflunisal	Dolobid*				500 mg every 8–12 hrs
Meclofenamate	Meclomen*				50–100 mg every 6–8 hr Max = 400 mg/24 h
Naproxen	Anaprox* Naprosyn*				250 mg every 6–8 hr Max = 1250 mg/24 hr
Piroxicam Sulindac	Feldene* Clinoril*				20 mg every 24 hr 150 mg every 12 hr Max = 400 mg/24 hr
Tolmetin	Tolectin*				400 mg every 6–8 hr Max = 2000 mg/24 hr

Generic	Brand	Action / Use	Side Effects	Dosage
Indomethacin	Indocin*			25–50 mg every 8–12 hr; Max = 200 mg/24 hr
Ketorolac Tromethamine	Toradol**	Short-term treatment of acute exacerbations of mild-to-moderate musculoskeletal pain	GI distress	60 mg
Narcotic analgesics: Propoxyphene (narcotic or opiate analgesic)	Darvocet Darvon Talwin Nx	Mild, centrally acting narcotic analgesic (may have additional ingredient of aspirin or acetaminophen)	respiratory depression, physical dependence, constipation, sedation, dysphoria and hallucination (more likely with Talwin)	50–65 mg every 4 hr Max = 400–600 mg/24 hr By prescription

TRICYCLIC ANTIDEPRESSANTS

The following applies to all medications listed below

Generic	Brand	Action / Use	Side Effects	Dosage
		Blocks reuptake of serotonin & norepinephrine (neurotransmitters)		
		Depression, adjunctive therapy in chronic pain	Sedation, dizziness, blurred vision, postural hypotension, weakness, fatigue, confusion, cardiac arrythmias, increased sensitivity to heat stress	Dosages below are maintenance levels By prescription
Amitriptyline	Elavil			75–150 mg/day
Imipramine	Tofranil			75–150 mg/day

MUSCLE RELAXANTS

The following applies to all medications listed below

Generic Name	Brand Name	Action	Indication	Potential Side Effects	Usual Adult Dose & Availability
		Muscle relaxation, prevents flexor and extensor spasms	Decrease musculoskeletal pain, short-term treatment of exacerbations	Sedation (unlikely with Norflex), insomnia, dizziness, weakness, ataxia, confusion, respiratory depression, seizure, sudden withdrawal from chronic use may cause anxiety, tachycardia, & hallucination	See below By prescription
Carisoprodol	Soma				350 mg every 6 hr
Chloroxazone	Parafon Forte				500 mg every 6–8 hr
Cyclobenzaprine	Flexeril				10 mg every 8 hr Max = 30 mg/24 h
Orphenadrine	Norflex				100 mg every 8–12 hr

OTHER DRUGS

Generic Name	Brand Name	Action	Indication	Potential Side Effects	Usual Adult Dose & Availability
Hydromorphone	Dilaudid	Narcotic analgesic	Relief of moderate-to-severe pain from soft tissue trauma, short-term treatment of exacerbation	Sedation, physical dependence, GI distress, respiratory depression	2 mg every 4–6 hr By prescription
Oxycodone	Percodan Percocet	Narcotic analgesic	Relief of moderate-to-severe pain, short-term treatment of exacerbation	Sedation, physical dependence, GI distress, respiratory depression	One tablet every 6 hr By prescription

| Amitriptyline | Elavil | Antidepressant | Chronic pain, relieve depression* | Gi distress, cardiovascular disturbances, sedation, weakness, fatigue, dizziness | 10 mg 2–3 mg times per day *50–100 mg every 24 hr 24 hr (maintenance) By prescription |
| Steroids | Medrol Prednisone | Anti-inflammatory, acute exacerbation of chronic pain with inflammatory component | Acute inflammation | Weakness, atrophy, GI distress, vertigo, headache, potential for multisystem side effects | Decreasing doses over 7-day therapy; 20 mg the 1st day decreasing to 4 mg by the 7th day By prescription |

[a]References: (25–30.)

9

Organic Mental Disorders

JOYCE FRAKER AND JACQUELINE McKILLOP

Leah advances warily down the hallway. A staff person greets Leah, and cautiously, Leah approaches.

"You're going to think I'm dumb, honey. I can't find the bathroom," Leah confesses.

The staff person escorts Leah to the restroom, pointing out landmarks to follow. This instruction has been repeated several times a day over the 3 weeks since Leah was admitted to the state psychiatric hospital.

A short time later, Leah is back again, in tears.

"Honey, I'm so worried about my little dog. She'll be hungry if I don't get home to feed her. Have you seen my purse and keys? I can't find them. I'm getting so stupid."

The staff member gently reminds Leah once more that her dog will be fine, neighbors are caring for it, and again explains that she is in the hospital. Leah has been told three times today that her keys and purse will be kept safely until she is ready to leave the hospital.

Leah was petitioned into the hospital by a social worker from Adult Protective Services alerted by a Meals on Wheels delivery person about decline in Leah's personal appearance and a foul odor in Leah's home. Upon investigation, the social worker found dog excrement throughout the house, no running water, and the toilet full of human waste.

Since her admission, Leah has failed to learn any of the staff members' names. She cannot remember coming to the hospital and does not recognize it as a hospital. She does not remember when meals are served or where the bathroom, dining room, and her bedroom are located. You're so sweet to help me," Leah thanks the staff member with a tearful smile.

"It's a horrible thing to lose your mind."

INTRODUCTION

The *Diagnostic and Statistical Manual of Mental Disorders* (DSM-III-R) differentiates between organic mental syndromes and organic mental disorders. Organic mental syndrome refers to a cluster of psychologic or behavioral signs or symptoms that tend to occur together. No reference is made to etiology for the diagnosis of organic mental syndromes.

Organic mental disorder refers to a specific organic mental syndrome in which the cause is known or presumed. Therefore, a basic understanding of organic mental syndromes is necessary. The DSM-III-R lists six categories of organic mental syndrome as seen in Table 9.1. The first category, delirium and dementia includes conditions more commonly seen by occupational therapists.

Delirium

The abnormalities and symptoms that tend to be present with delirium include dif-

Table 9.1
Six Categories of Organic Mental Syndrome[a]

1. *Delirium and dementia:* Impairment of cognitive functioning is relatively global.

    Delirium: Poor attention span with at least two of the following: reduced level of consciousness, sensory misperceptions, disturbance of sleep-wake cycle, change in level of psychomotor activity, disorientation, memory impairment. Relatively rapid onset, fluctuation of symptoms.

    Dementia: Impairment in recent and remote memory. There are also problems in at least one of the following: abstract thinking, judgment, higher cortical functioning (such as aphasia, apraxia, agnosia) or personality change. Onset is gradual, with a deteriorating course.

2. *Amnestic syndrome and organic hallucinosis:* Impairment of relatively select areas of cognition.

3. *Organic delusional syndrome, organic mood syndrome, and organic anxiety syndrome:* These syndromes have features that are similar to schizophrenia, mood, and anxiety disorders.

4. *Organic personality syndrome:* Persistent personality disturbance is the main feature.

5. *Intoxication and withdrawal:* In this category, the disorder is associated with the ingestion of or the withdrawal from a psychoactive substance.

6. *Organic mental syndrome not otherwise specified:* This residual category includes any other organic mental syndrome not classifiable as one of the above syndromes.

[a]Reprinted by permission: American Psychiatric Association: Diagnostic and Statistical Manual of Mental Disorders, 3rd ed., revised, Washington, D.C.: American Psychiatric Association, 1987:100.

ficulty sustaining and shifting attention, impaired concept formation, rambling or irrelevant speech, reduced levels of arousal, sensory misperceptions, disturbances of sleep-wake cycle, disturbance of level of psychomotor activity, disorientation, and memory impairment. Emotional disturbances are commonly seen, especially fear or depression. Neurologic signs are uncommon in delirium, though tremors are frequently present (1).

Delirium may occur at any age, but children and those over 60 years of age are most susceptible. The causes of delirium include systemic infections, metabolic disorders, postoperative states, psychoactive substance use, and hypertensive encephalopathy (related to seizures and head trauma) (1).

With delirium, as with all organic mental syndromes, an underlying organic cause is assumed. However, delirium tends to be transient, and the severity of symptoms, which are most marked at night, may fluctuate over the course of a day (2).

Dementia

The most significant characteristic of dementia is impairment in recent and remote memory. Dementia also has disturbances in cognitive integration, including orientation, recognition, categorization, problem solving, and learning (generalization, integration, and synthesis). There may also be disturbances of higher cortical functioning or a personality change (1).

Dementia is most often found in the elderly and primary degenerative dementia of the Alzheimer type is the most common dementia. It is important to note that dementia is not part of the normal aging process. Dementia results from an organic disturbance, and the need for investigating the organic cause is implicit in the diagnosis of dementia.

Some of the causes, in addition to Alzheimer's disease, include vascular disease (multiinfarct dementia), central nervous system infections, toxic metabolic disturbances, normal-pressure hydrocephalus, neurologic diseases, and postanoxic or posthypoglycemic states (1). The course of dementia varies according to the underlying etiology. Primary degenerative dementia of the Alzheimer type progresses slowly, and the affected person may live for many years in a state of gradual decline. When the underlying cause can be treated, as in hyperthyroidism or subdural hematoma, the dementia can be halted or even reversed.

The diagnosis of dementia is made only when the cognitive impairment is severe enough to interfere with performance in activities of daily living, work, and social activities.

In differentiating between delirium and dementia there are two points to consider. First, the person with delirium has a reduced level of arousal, whereas the person with dementia is alert. Second, with delirium the symptoms fluctuate, while in dementia the symptoms remain stable over the course of a day.

ORGANIC MENTAL DISORDERS

There are three categories of organic mental disorders, as seen in table 9.2. The first group, dementias arising in the senium and presenium (primary degenerative dementia of the Alzheimer type and multiinfarct dementia) are related to pathologic changes of the brain. The second category, psychoactive substance–induced organic mental disorders, are related to the ingestion of a substance. The last category includes organic mental disorders associated with axis III physical disorders or conditions, or those whose etiology is unknown (1).

This chapter discusses the first type, dementias arising in the senium and presenium. These disorders, especially dementia of the Alzheimer type, are more commonly seen by occupational therapists, who are concerned about losses in occupational performance areas. The course of primary degenerative dementia of the Alzheimer type is generally progressive and deteriorating. The resulting

loss of function is irreversible. The second disorder in this category, multiinfarct dementia, also causes permanent dysfunction, but its course may not be as debilitating when the condition is stabilized with medical treatment.

Psychoactive substance–induced organic mental disorders are caused by the direct effects of psychoactive substances on the nervous system. The course varies, depending upon the type and amount of the psychoactive substance ingested, but the symptoms disappear at some point after cessation of the use of the toxic substance. The exceptions include (*a*) alcohol amnestic disorder (Korsakoff's syndrome), which can result in a major impairment of memory, and (*b*) several of the hallucinogen-induced organic mental disorders, which may result in long-lasting episodes that are difficult to distinguish from a nonorganic psychotic disorder or a mood disorder (1).

Although we will not discuss psychoactive substance–induced organic mental disorders in depth, the occupational therapist should know that they are usually caused by substances taken nonmedically to alter mood or behavior. However, these disorders are distinguished from psychoactive substance use disorders, or the behavior associated with taking psychoactive substances that affect the central nervous system (1). For the occupational therapist working in substance abuse programs, there are Recommended Readings for psychoactive substance use disorders at the end of the chapter.

Organic mental disorders, which are associated with physical disorders or whose etiology are unknown, are not discussed in this chapter. This category allows the clinician to classify the involvement of a physical illness that contributes to any of the above disorders. This chapter does not address the many physical causes associated with organic brain disorder.

Dementias Arising in the Senium and Presenium

There is a popular misconception that the term *senile* refers to impaired cognitive

Table 9.2.
Three Categories of Organic Mental Disorders[a]

Type I: Dementias arising in the senium and presenium
  A. Primary degenerative dementia of the Alzheimer type
     The onset of dementia is insidious with a progressive, deteriorating course.
  B. Multi-infarct dementia
     Dementia is due to cerebrovascular disease. There is step-wise deterioration in cognitive functioning.

Type II: Psychoactive substance–induced organic mental disorder
  A. Alcohol-induced organic mental disorders
     There are seven disorders attributed to the ingestion of alcohol.
  B. Amphetamine- or similarly acting sympathomimetic–induced organic mental disorders
     This category includes four disorders attributed to the ingestion of amphetamine or a similarly acting sympathomimetic.
  C. Caffeine-induced organic mental disorder
     The one disorder in this category, caffeine intoxification, results from recent use of caffeine-containing substances.
  D. Cannabis-induced organic mental disorder
     There are two disorders attributed to the use of cannabis.
  E. Cocaine-induced organic mental disorder
     There are four disorders attributed to the use of cocaine.
  F. Hallucinogen-induced organic mental disorders
     There are four disorders attributed to the use of hallucinogens.
  G. Inhalant-induced organic mental disorders
     Inhalant intoxification is the one disorder and is attributed to recent use of an inhalant.
  H. Nicotine-induced organic mental disorders
     Nicotine withdrawal is the one disorder in this category.
  I. Opioid-induced organic mental disorders
     There are two disorders which are attributed to the use of opioids.
  J. Phelcyclidine (PCP)- or similarly acting arylcyclohexylamine–induced organic mental disorders.
     The five disorders result from recent use of phencyclidine (PCP) or a similarly acting arylcyclohexylamine.
  K. Sedative-, hypnotic-, or anxiolytic-induced organic mental disorders
     The four disorders in this category result from the recent use of a sedative, hypnotic, or anxiolytic.

Type III: Organic mental disorders associated with axis III physical disorders or conditions, or whose etiology is unknown
     This category allows identification of organic mental disorders on axis I when associated with physical disorders entered on axis III. For example, this category is used when dementia is associated with a brain tumor.

---

[a]Reprinted with permission: American Psychiatric Association, Diagnostic and Statistical Manual of Mental Disorders, 3rd ed., revised. Washington, D.C.: American Psychiatric Association, 1987.

functioning. Senium and senile are terms that refer to persons over age 65. Impaired cognitive functioning is not part of the normal aging process, and most people who are 65 years of age or older do not experience this loss. Presenium, or presenile, refers to persons 65 years of age and under. The age of onset does not seem to affect the nature or severity of symptoms. Naturally, the course of the disease may be shorter, from onset to death, in senile dementia because the affected person is older at onset.

PRIMARY DEGENERATIVE DEMENTIA OF THE ALZHEIMER TYPE

Nearly all cases of dementias arising in the senium and presenium are primary degenerative dementia of the Alzheimer type. Alzheimer's disease is considered a physical disorder, according to the DSM-III-R. The definitive diagnosis can be made only through autopsy. The diagnosis of primary degenerative dementia of the Alzheimer type can be made when there is dementia that is insidious and progressive and other causes of dementia have been ruled out. For simplification, in further discussion we will refer to this dementia as Alzheimer's disease (AD), which in other texts is synonymous with primary degenerative dementia of the Alzheimer type.

MULTIINFARCT DEMENTIA

In the past, the diagnosis of psychosis with cerebral arteriosclerosis was made when dementia was associated with vascular disease. Now it appears that the dementia results from repeated infarcts in the brain rather than cerebral arteriosclerosis, so it is called multiinfarct dementia (1). In multiinfarct dementia the course of the dementia is more uneven than in Alzheimer's disease. There is a stepwise deterioration in cognitive functioning that correlates with the incidence of insults to the brain. Early in the course there is patchy deterioration in which some functioning may remain intact, as opposed to the global impairment found in Alzheimer's disease. The most characteristic cognitive deficits include disturbances in memory, concept formation, and problem solving, as well as poor self-control and personality change. Multiinfarct dementia also results in focal neurologic signs and symptoms, such as weakness in the limbs and gait abnormalities (1).

Vascular disease is always assumed to be present, and early treatment may prevent further progression of the dementia. It should be noted that a single stroke may result in memory impairment, but dementia results from multiple strokes at different times (1).

Table 9.3, Comparison of Features Associated with Dementias, summarizes the differences and similarities between dementias and delirium. Alzheimer's disease and multiinfarct dementia differ primarily in onset and progression of symptoms. Features common to both delirium and dementia include memory loss, cognitive impairment, emotional incontinence, vegetative symptoms, and paranoia/hallucinations (3).

Normal age-related decline may result in some mild memory loss. Other symptoms associated with dementia do not occur in the normal aging process. Memory loss, the hallmark of dementia, does not occur in depression or chronic schizophrenia. Memory loss is clearly a significant symptom that indicates a need for medical investigation.

ALZHEIMER'S DISEASE

In the past decade, studies on Alzheimer's disease have proliferated. Although many questions remain unanswered, the impact of the disease on occupational performance can be predicted to some degree, but other individual variables may affect performance as well.

Many psychosocial variables influence the severity of dementia. The individual's personality may undergo an alteration or accentuation of premorbid traits (1). For example, a person who was characteristically neat and organized may become untidy and careless about self-care and home management. Or the meticulous personality may become accentuated, resulting in obsessive-compulsive or paranoid behavior. The person's emotional state is important to consider, as stress, anxiety, and depression tend to reduce functional performance (2). The very fact that persons can sense their cognitive deficits, especially in the area of recent memory, creates stress. In the early stages, an intelligent person may be able to compensate for deficits in memory, thus reducing the impact of disease on functioning. Other people may use less adaptive

Table 9.3.
Comparison of Features Associated with Dementias[a]

	Slow Onset	Reduced Level of Consciousness	Progression of Symptoms	Memory Loss	Cognitive Impairment	Emotional Incontinence[b]	Vegetative Symptoms[c]	Paranoia Hallucinations
Normal age-related decline	Yes	No	None	Mild	No	No	No	No
Alzheimer's disease	Yes	No	Slow	Yes	Yes	Yes	Yes	Yes
Multi-infarct dementia	No	No	Stepwise	Yes	Yes	Yes	Varies	Varies
Depression	No	No	Rapid	No	No	No	Yes	No
Delirium	No	Yes	Fluctuates	Yes	Yes	Yes	Yes	Yes
Chronic schizophrenia	Yes	No	May be episodic	No	Yes	Yes	Varies	Yes

[a] Reprinted with permission: Glickstein JK. Therapeutic interventions in Alzheimer's disease. Rockville, MD: Aspen, 1988.
[b] Inappropriate or sudden crying or laughing for no apparent reason.
[c] Vegetative symptoms include: changes in the sleep-wake cycle, loss of appetite, and excessive eating.

coping mechanisms such as denial or fabrication.

General health may also affect occupational performance. Conditions such as heart disease, diabetes, and chronic pain are possible causes of declining functioning or behavioral change, and they should especially be considered with the elderly person. Isolation and sensory deprivation will also contribute to the decline of cognitive functioning.

Etiology

The precise cause of Alzheimer's disease is unknown. The hallmarks of dementia (memory loss, acquired deficit in cognition, and the persistence of symptoms) imply an organic disease (3). A senile dementia, which may have many causes, is considered to be Alzheimer's disease when specific behavioral, structural, and neurophysiologic changes occur. Pathologies specific to Alzheimer's disease have been identified in autopsy specimens, including degeneration of specific nerve cells, neuritic plaques, neurofibrillary tangles, and changes in forebrain cholinergic systems (3). Also identified is gross atrophy of the brain, particularly in the parietal, temporal, and frontal lobes (4). There are changes which can be identified in vivo. Computerized tomographic (CT) studies have shown dilation of the third and fourth ventricles and progressive cortical atrophy. There are significant relationships between these findings and progressive cognitive impairment. A strong positive relationship between the severity of electrophysiologic changes and the degree of dementia has been found. In positron emission tomographic (PET) techniques, used to evaluate whole-brain glucose utilization, a significant relationship between decline in glucose utilization and progressive cognitive loss has been found in early investigations (4).

Six different models are the focus of current research on the cause of the neuropathologies particular to Alzheimer's disease: the genetic model, the infectious agent model, the abnormal protein model, the toxin model, the immunologic model, and the neurochemical model (3).

The models are driven by epidemiologic studies that have identified possible risk factors, and they are the bases for research into the etiology of AD.

GENETIC MODEL

There is a greater incidence of AD among parents, siblings, and offspring in proband families than among the general population (5). Three groups of AD patients have been distinguished. In the first group autosomal dominant inheritance can be established between members who develop presenile dementia. The second group contains those who develop presenile dementia without a strong genetic component. In the third group, members develop dementia in the senium, and only weak evidence of heredity can be shown (6). Research is indicating an abnormality in chromosome 21 in Alzheimer's disease (7). A defective gene that codes for amyloid precursor proteins has been detected in pathogenesis similar to that of Alzheimer's disease (8).

INFECTIOUS MODEL

With the discovery of viruses that transmit encephalopathy, such as scrapie (9) and Creutzfeldt-Jakob disease (10), attention has been given to finding a virus that causes Alzheimer's disease. Research aimed at detecting evidence of human herpesvirus, herpes simplex, neuroborreliosis, and lentiviruses in persons with AD has not shown an association between these viruses and Alzheimer's disease (11–14).

ABNORMAL PROTEIN

The hallmark pathologies of AD, neurofibrillary tangles, amyloid placques, and amyloid around and within cerebral blood vessels, indicate abnormal deposits of protein within the brain. While a deficiency in RNA is suspected, there is no precise explanation for abnormal protein accumulation (3).

TOXIN MODEL

Toxins known to produce dementias are alcohol, poisons (ingested or inhaled), and heavy metals (3). In Alzheimer's disease, great attention has been paid to aluminum neurotoxicity. Initial attention was given to aluminum as a toxin over 50 years ago (15). Accumulations of aluminum have been detected in neurofibrillary tangles of neurons of Alzheimer's disease and other neuropathologies. Although research has been unable to assign a causative role to aluminum in the production of neurofibrillary tangles, it suggests that environmental factors may play a role in this pathology (16).

The metabolism of cadmium and zinc by the liver is also altered in AD (17).

IMMUNOLOGIC MODEL

Aging brings both an increased incidence of AD and deterioration of the immune system (3). A recent study has shown a significant reduction in lymphocyte count in patients with AD. The reduction in lymphocytes was correlated with the degree of dementia (18).

NEUROCHEMICAL MODEL

Investigations into brain biochemistry have shown changes and disturbances of the neurotransmitters and neurotransmitter systems. Damage in the acetylcholinergic system has been found to be especially important in the etiology of AD (19).

Incidence

In the United States, more than 1 million individuals over age 65 have cognitive loss severe enough to justify the diagnosis of dementia. This is approximately 5% of those over the age of 65, 20% of those at age 80, and 30% of those aged 90 (3, 4).

Of those with dementia, the percentage with Alzheimer's disease runs between 54 and 65% (2, 3). Surveys indicate that AD is the major cause of institutionalization in nursing homes in the United States. Thousands of AD victims are institutionalized in state facilities and veterans' hospitals. Perhaps most of those afflicted are maintained in their homes with continuous care and supervision from family and home health aides (4). Indeed, only 1% of persons between the ages of 65 and 75 years are in nursing homes (3).

Signs and Symptoms

The signs and symptoms of AD begin insidiously and become progressively more pronounced and debilitating. The disease has been described as following stages or phases of increasing cognitive disability. Terms used for the stages or phases are not uniform. The DSM-III-R refers to three stages: an early stage marked by memory impairment while socially appropriate behavior remains intact; a middle stage during which cognitive deficits are remarkable and disturbances in personality and behavior are prominent; and the late stage in which the person may be uncommunicative, inattentive, and incapable of self-care (1).

Glickstein uses a four-stage scale of general features, symptoms, and speech and language abilities (3). She suggests the stages be used by therapists in providing concrete behavioral landmarks for AD clients and their families during treatment sessions.

Reisberg, Ferris and Crook developed the global deterioration scale (GDS) for age-associated cognitive and Alzheimer's disease (4). This highly detailed scale defines seven stages according to clinical characteristics and psychometric concomitants. The GDS ranges from stage 1 in which there is no cognitive decline, a normal clinical phase, to stage 7, very severe cognitive decline or the clinical phase of late dementia.

The signs and symptoms described here are broken into three phases, using Reisberg's descriptive terms of "forgetfulness" phase, "confusional" phase, and "dementia" phase (4).

Initially, individuals may seek assistance in an early, or "forgetfulness" phase of AD. The symptoms or subjective feelings about which they complain focus on memory loss. They have trouble remembering where objects have been placed and difficulty recalling names of familiar objects and places. Despite these complaints, the individuals and their intimates do not feel a sense of helplessness. In the forgetfulness phase, they may be able to maintain psychosocial skills and satisfactory job performance. They may have slight feelings of shame. At this point, there are no observable signs of the disease.

As the disease progresses into the second, or "confusional" phase, they experience growing problems with memory and difficulty with cognition. Relevant others report a greater inability to remember names, recover "lost" objects, recall past events, and manage finances. Incidences of becoming hopelessly lost while traveling to a location that should have been easy to find are reported. They have become less sociable (4) and may be more passive or hostile toward others (3). They cannot function as well on the job (4), and those who remain employed depend increasingly on others as memory loss and cognitive deficits become more pronounced (3).

Clinical signs become evident during the "confusional" phase. They have sleep disturbances. Deficits in concentration and attention span are elicited by attempts to perform serial subtractions. Deficits also appear in long-term memory. They cannot recall the current president, a personal address, the current year, or the present location (4). Short-term memory is affected. When given three objects, they cannot recall them after 5 minutes (3).

Disorders of higher cortical function become apparent. They may have aphasia, apraxia, or agnosia. "Constructional difficulty" also develops. When given a specific design to replicate, they cannot assemble blocks or sticks correctly.

The third, or "dementia" phase begins when they can no longer survive without constant supervision and support (4). They wander without regard for their whereabouts or personal safety. They may become increasingly agitated and combative or excessively passive and socially withdrawn.

The ability to maintain nourishment by feeding and eating and to maintain cleanliness deteriorates and ultimately disappears. They cannot manipulate utensils and make no attempt to eat. They become unaware of the urge to urinate or defecate and are incontinent of bladder and bowel. Gait becomes unsteady. They lose the urge and talent to bathe themselves and must be coerced to allow another person to assist with the bath. A fear of water may develop, complicating baths. They may refuse to get into bath water or may become combative when bathed.

All memories and cognition are lost. They do not know their own names nor that of a spouse. They do not recall any personal life history. The ability to count from one to five disappears. Eventually they lose the ability to speak and merely grunt in response to stimuli.

During this phase, they may develop psychiatric symptoms of overt paranoia, delusions, and visual or other hallucinatory experiences, which makes caring for the afflicted individual extremely difficult and forces families to consider institutionalization (4).

Progression—Prognosis

Alzheimer's disease is insidious in onset and progresses slowly, with gradual worsening of memory and other cognitive functions (3).

The forgetfulness stage may last from 2 to 4 years. What appear to be minor deficits in memory that may be dismissed at first become more irritating and disconcerting. The severity of symptoms and how readily they become apparent depends on psychosocial factors. These factors include the individual's ability to cope with stress, the support of family/employer, and environment demands. How well the individual copes with and compensates for cognitive losses is influenced by premorbid personality, intelligence, and level of education (2). The greater the individual's fund of knowledge, resources, and coping strategies, the greater is that person's ability to compensate for cognitive losses.

The confusional phase lasts an average of 4 years. Losses in cognitive function can no longer be ignored or dismissed. It is at this point that families seek help for the affected individual, who becomes unable to maintain employment and increasingly dependent on others for assistance with activities of daily living and psychosocial skills.

The length of the dementia phase is unknown. Some have remained in this final stage of the disease well beyond 2 years. Others have died within 6 months (3).

The disease process is irreversible. At this time there are no known medications that can halt or reverse the progression of the disease (3).

Diagnosis and Medications

The *definite* diagnosis of Alzheimer's disease is made when the individual has demonstrated signs and symptoms of dementia while living, and histopathologic evidence is found on autopsy.

The *probable* diagnosis of Alzheimer's disease is given when an individual has dementia that cannot be attributed to systemic disorders or other brain diseases. Arriving at the probable diagnosis of Alzheimer's disease involves testing to eliminate other possible causes of dementia (3). A comprehensive physical examination and laboratory tests (blood chemistry, venereal disease, and thyroid studies) are performed to rule out systemic disease. Neurologic evaluation, mental status examination, and neuropsychologic testing of cognitive function are conducted to eliminate the possibility of psychiatric disorders. Lumbar puncture to evaluate spinal fluid, electroencephalogram (EEG), computed axial tomographic scan (CAT), positron emission tomographic scan (PET), nuclear magnetic resonance (also called magnetic resonance imaging), and cerebral blood flow studies are used to rule out other organic brain disorders (3).

Medication is given to persons with AD for two purposes: to improve memory and cognition and to control troublesome symptoms such as sleep disturbances, agitation, combative behaviors, paranoia, and hallucinations.

Current research in the development of medications to improve memory and cognition is based on the theory that AD is the result of deterioration of cholinergic neurotransmitters. Drugs that boost cholinergic neurotransmission have been studied. Physostigmine has been tested in double-blind studies and found to be of doubtful efficacy (20), producing nonsignificant intergroup differences (21). It has been suggested that physostigmine may be of value when given concomitantly with clonidine, an agent that augments norandrenergic neurotransmitters. As both drugs may have serious adverse effects, researchers suggest that pilot studies be conducted to ensure that these medications can be safely given together to AD patients (22).

Preliminary studies of the cholinesterase inhibitor tetrahydroaminoacridine (THA) have shown that while THA is not a cure or definitive treatment, it has a palliative effect (23). The safety of THA administration is a concern, with reports of side effects, especially frequent indications of hepatotoxicity (24).

Table 9.4.
Occupational Performance Profile—Early or Forgetful Phase

		Performance Areas		
		Work Activities		Care of Others
	Vocation	Education	Home Management	
SENSORIMOTOR — **SENSORY INTEGRATION** Intact **NEUROMUSCU-LAR** Intact **MOTOR** Intact				
PERFORMANCE COMPONENTS — COGNITIVE — **COGNITIVE** Memory loss begins to affect work activities and activities of daily living	Difficulty recalling names and faces, forgetting where objects have been placed, difficulty with calculations result in decreased job and educational performance; may use adaptive skills to effectively deal with memory loss		Budgeting and managing finances becomes difficult	
PSYCHOSOCIAL — **PSYCHOLOGIC** Psychologic components include shame, depression, irritability **SOCIAL** **SELF-MANAGEMENT**				

EXTERNAL FACTORS WHICH INFLUENCE PERFORMANCE; CULTURE, ECONOMY, ENVIRONMENT

Grid adapted from Uniform Terminology (2nd ed.) Developed by the occupational therapy faculty at Eastern Michigan University.

Client initials:
Diagnosis:
Age:

Play or Leisure Activities		Activities of Daily Living				
Exploration	Performance	Self-Care	Social ization	Functional Communication	Functional Mobility	Sexual Expression
				Anomia and expressive aphasia		
				Depression and irritability may strain family and social relationships		

Medications, especially those given to control problematic behaviors, must be prescribed cautiously to the geriatric client. The neuroleptics, psychoactive drugs given to control behavioral problems and psychotic symptoms, can cause considerable adverse reactions (25). Physiologic changes associated with aging necessitate smaller doses for geriatric patients than those given younger patients. Absorption delayed by other medications, increased fat-muscle ratio leading to increased apparent volume of lipid-soluble drugs, reduced hepatic metabolism, and age-related decrease in renal blood flow may make a drug toxic to the elderly when given in standard doses (26). Indeed, the sedative hypnotics, especially long-acting benzodiazepines, may cause cognitive impairment in the elderly (27). In one study, patients were given low doses of a benzodiazepine, lorazepam. In addition to mild sedation, patients showed "attentional" impairments, making omission errors on a continuous performance task. No decrease in memory was found (28).

Medications that are reported to improve agitated behaviors in limited trials are very low dose haloperidol, very low dose thioridazine (29) and carbamazepine (30).

Because medications have not been shown to be of remarkable value in the management of the symptoms of AD, treatment relies heavily on environmental and psychotherapeutic interventions (4). Environmental interventions include maintaining a calm and relaxed atmosphere, improving lighting, and using signs to identify specific living areas. Assessing and maximizing the individual's remaining social and functional skills is recommended (31).

Impact of AD on Occupational Performance

Cognitive integration and cognitive components are most seriously affected by Alzheimer's disease. As the disease progresses, there is an increase in the number of performance areas affected as well as the severity of the dysfunction. We will address the impact of the condition on occupational performance for each of the three identified phases of Alzheimer's disease. (See Tables 9.4, 9.5 & 9.6 for summaries in chart form.)

EARLY OR FORGETFUL PHASE

Early in the disease process the individual develops difficulty in short-term and recent memory. In the orientation component, there is intermittent or consistent confusion about time and place. Concept formation tends to be concrete and problem solving begins to be difficult (3). Integration and synthesis of learning are also affected.

These cognitive losses begin to affect several occupational performance areas. The individual who cannot adapt to the memory loss and other cognitive deficits has difficulty with job performance. The inability to recall names and faces, the tendency to forget where objects have been placed, poor orientation to time and place, the inability to learn new procedures and to resolve problems in a timely manner may result in a change of work assignment or the loss of a job.

In the performance area of home management, affected individuals begin to need assistance with shopping and money management. Functional communication is also affected. They may experience anomia (the inability to find a name for something) or expressive aphasia (the inability to say what one wants to say) (5). There may also be perseveration (the uncontrollable repetition of a word or phrase) and some inability to speak in a coherent manner (3).

The awareness of increasing cognitive loss often leads to problems in psychosocial skills and components. Depression may manifest early in the disease process, as well as irritability and hostile behavior (32). An altered self-concept results in feelings of shame. Coping skills and time management begin to disintegrate, and socialization may be affected. There is a strain on family relationships, and the affected individual may begin to curtail social and leisure activity. Feelings of inadequacy may impair the fulfillment of sexual expression (33).

CONFUSIONAL PHASE

The confusional phase is marked by increasing deficits in recent memory, as well as short-term, long-term, and remote memory. Individuals cannot recall their address, familiar telephone numbers, or the names of close family members. Orientation to person, place, and time is impaired, with concepts of time most seriously affected (3). There is difficulty concentrating and lessened ability to make sense of incoming stimuli (4).

At this phase, occupational performance becomes so dysfunctional that these individuals require the aid of a care-giver. They can no longer perform on the job, and home management skills are seriously impaired. They may lose valuables and can no longer manage finances, as number concepts are very poor or nonexistent (3, 4). They may create hazards, such as turning on a stove and forgetting to turn it off. Habits become rigid and a self-care routine, if interrupted, may be difficult or impossible to complete. Dressing problems include difficulty selecting proper clothing and difficulty dressing in a sequential fashion. Bathing problems include fear of bathing, refusal to bathe, or inadequate performance (3).

Functional communication continues to deteriorate. Speech content may be confused or irrelevant, with increased difficulty choosing words and addition of irrelevant words at the end of a sentence. Circumlocution appears, in which the individual avoids the issue by speaking in a roundabout way, and never getting to the point. There is increased anomia and paraphasia (substituting inappropriate words in a sentence). Agnosia, which is difficulty seeing or reading, also impacts on functional communication (3). Functional mobility becomes impaired, as the individual begins to wander and habitually gets lost.

In the second phase of Alzheimer's disease, psychosocial skills and components also continue to decline. Self-concept further deteriorates, and there is a sense of helplessness and feelings of impotence (4). Social conduct is affected. There may be excessive passivity or impulsive verbalizations. Time management is seriously affected, and disturbances of the sleep-wake cycle create difficulties for the care-giver. Individuals may display frequent repetitive behaviors, making termination of activity difficult. In addition, there may be hallucinations, paranoia, and emotional lability (3).

Dysfunction in psychosocial skills and components also affect occupational performance. Depression can cause loss of appetite, and intimacy becomes increasingly impaired (33). Personality changes found in organic mental disorder include overtly antisocial behavior and sexual excesses and indiscretions (34). Problems related to these behaviors may surface during the second phase and worsen as the disease progresses.

DEMENTIA PHASE

In the dementia phase, Alzheimer's disease begins to take its toll not only on the cognitive and psychosocial components, but also on the sensorimotor components of functioning. At this point, the affected individuals need complete supervision and eventually total care.

The cognitive components of memory and orientation are severely impaired. These individuals cannot identify close relatives, though they may be able to distinguish between strangers and people who are familiar. Eventually they may lose this awareness as well as the ability to recall their own name. There is confusion in fa-

Table 9.5.
Occupational Performance Profile—Confusional Phase

		Performance Areas			
		Work Activities			
		Vocation	Education	Home Management	Care of Others
SENSORIMOTOR	**SENSORY INTEGRATION** Intact				
	NEUROMUSCULAR Intact				
	MOTOR Intact				
PERFORMANCE COMPONENTS — **COGNITIVE**	**COGNITIVE** Increased memory loss, lessened ability to process and make sense of incoming stimuli	Difficulty concentrating or processing information results in job change, need for assistance on the job, or loss of a job	Decreased ability to process (new) information	Loses objects & cannot find them; may lose valuables; increased difficulty managing finances	Neglects care of others due to memory loss & poor organization
PSYCHOSOCIAL	**PSYCHOLOGIC** Sense of helplessness, flattening of affect				
	SOCIAL				
	SELF-MANAGEMENT				

EXTERNAL FACTORS WHICH INFLUENCE PERFORMANCE; CULTURE, ECONOMY, ENVIRONMENT

[a]Grid adapted from Uniform Terminology (2nd ed.) Developed by the occupational therapy faculty at Eastern Michigan University.

Client initials:
Diagnosis:
Age:

Play or Leisure Activities		Activities of Daily Living				
Exploration	Performance	Self-Care	Social ization	Functional Communication	Functional Mobility	Sexual Expression
Lifelong leisure activities become difficult due to memory loss	Routines are rigid, performance is slow; change in routine or environment seriously impacts performance	Difficulty recalling names of friends and family	Does not remember own or other phone numbers; may have impulsive verbalizations	Does not remember address; gets lost		May become sexually indiscreet; intimacy impaired due to poor cognition and feelings of impotence
Sense of helplessness may result in withdrawal from activities	Depression may cause loss of appetite or may not know when to stop eating	May withdraw from social activities				

Table 9.6.
Occupational Performance Profile—Dementia Phase

| | | Performance Areas | | |
| | | | Work Activities | |
	Vocation	Education	Home Management	Care of Others
SENSORIMOTOR — **SENSORY INTEGRATION** Perceptions are distorted; poor postural control, gross motor coordination				
COGNITIVE — **COGNITIVE** Memory very poor; severely disoriented; communication severely impaired	No longer can function			
PSYCHOSOCIAL — **PSYCHOSOCIAL** Psychotic symptoms may manifest; these may be a result of cognitive and sensory impairments as opposed to a true psychosis				

(left vertical label: PERFORMANCE COMPONENTS)

EXTERNAL FACTORS WHICH INFLUENCE PERFORMANCE; CULTURE, ECONOMY, ENVIRONMENT

Grid adapted from Uniform Terminology (2nd ed.) Developed by the occupational therapy faculty at Eastern Michigan University.

miliar surroundings, and no awareness of season or year. The ability to process information is severely limited, and they may not be able to follow through with an action such as picking up a spoon and putting it into the mouth (3).

These cognitive losses result in the inability to perform work activities and severe limitations in leisure and daily living activities. These individuals cannot bathe alone, may be incontinent, and may need assistance with feeding. Functional communication continues to deteriorate. Comprehension of language is impaired, and they tend to lapse into unintelligible mumbling. At the very end of this stage, speech is limited to a few words or there is no intelligible vocabulary (3).

Sensory integration is impaired. Distortions in sensory perceptions may lead

Client initials:
Diagnosis:
Age:

Play or Leisure Activities		Activities of Daily Living				
Exploration	Performance	Self-Care	Socialization	Functional Communication	Functional Mobility	Sexual Expression
		Wandering pain, unable to locate internal cues; difficulty swallowing			Unsteady gait or loss of ambulation; eventual loss of motor abilities	
		Loss of ability to feed or bathe self; incontinent	Forgets spouse and own name	Speech may be unintelligible or lost; impaired comprehension of speech		No longer can function
		Paranoia may lead to aggression and resistance to care-givers				

to paranoia and aggression. They may experience wandering pain, being unable to locate internal cues of physiologic distress (33). Motor skills are affected, they become unsteady and eventually lose ambulation and voluntary movement. Speech becomes slurred due to motor dysfunction (dysarthria). There is visual agnosia (difficulty interpreting visual stimuli in the absence of significant visual impairment)

(3). Eating problems become a primary concern. Whereas early in the dementia phase they may have an overeating problem, at the end of this phase they cannot swallow food. The end-stage of Alzheimer's disease involves physical complications.

Death certificates on which senile and presenile dementia were mentioned were studied to determine which conditions might be associated with reduced survival in AD patients. The conditions that reached statistical significance are infections, trauma, nutritional deficiency, chronic ulcer of the skin, foreign body in the pharanx, losses in vision and hearing, and epilepsy (35). The length of survival for AD patients after the onset is highly variable. The severity of the disease, the combination of wandering and falling, and behavioral problems have been associated with shorter survival (36).

CASE STUDY

This case history chronicles the loss of cognitive function and concomitant loss of activities of daily living skills by R.P. over 4 years. Note the impact that the individual's premorbid personality has on his ability to cope with and compensate for loss of memory, cognition, and performance skills.

Background

R.P. is one of three brothers born to a very poor family. There are reports that his mother was abusive towards him. He achieved an eighth grade education. As an adult, R.P. worked a number of jobs, including underwater welding. He eventually found and maintained a job as a welder in an automobile factory and is now retired.

R.P. had few outside interests or social connections during his adulthood. He earned a reputation for having a short temper, yelling, swearing, kicking, and hitting things when frustrated.

He married at age 26 and was abusive toward his wife. On several occasions, the police were called to intervene in incidences of domestic violence. R.P.'s wife divorced him after 20 years of marriage. Following the divorce, R.P. drank heavily for a decade, until age 56.

"Forgetfulness" Phase (Table 9.4)

At age 65 and again 1 year later, R.P. was hospitalized for apparent problems with mentation and behavior, which the family labeled "attacks." During this time, R.P. also suffered a myocardial infarction and was hospitalized. He was not a cooperative patient and refused to take prescribed medication.

R.P. experienced a period of confusion and weakness and "passed out" at 67 years of age. He was hospitalized for 1 week and discharged with no definitive diagnosis. While hospitalized, he struck two nurses.

"Confusional" Phase (Table 9.5)

At age 68, R.P. was hospitalized again for difficulty with cognition and behavior for a period of 1 week. R.P. had become agitated and violent, striking others for no apparent reason. His family and girlfriend reported that R.P. had been increasingly unpredictable and showed poor judgment. R.P. had recently been known to roam local streets and become lost. He would give money to strangers. He was unable to complete sentences. His girlfriend reported that his memory was poor and that he was becoming very forgetful. R.P. required constant supervision and care, which was difficult to provide, as he was having violent outbursts several times a month. It was determined that R.P. was suffering from probable Alzheimer's disease. Upon discharge from the hospital, he was placed in a nursing home, as his girlfriend felt that she could no longer maintain him in her home.

R.P. remained in the nursing home for 3 weeks. During his brief stay, he presented many problematic behaviors. He made several attempts to climb out a second-floor window. When staff tried to deter him, R.P. became violent and struck them. On one occasion, the sheriff's department was called to assist in subduing him. When moved to a first-floor room to prevent a potential fall from a second-floor window, R.P. began wandering out of the facility. He refused to return to the facility, pushing and striking staff, swearing at them and yelling, "I hope you die, you bitch!" He was confined to a traychair or restrained in bed with wrist and leg limiters for management of violent and agitated behavior. Restraint escalated his agitation. He began tipping over his traychair. On one occasion, R.P. tipped over violently, struck his head on the floor, and lost consciousness. He was seen in the emergency room of a local hospital for skull x-ray and evaluation for closed head injury. No fracture or injury was found. Upon return to the nursing home, R.P. began receiving tranquilizers and antianxiety agents. None were effective.

He was then transferred to a state psychiatric hospital as an involuntary patient. He was evaluated by a psychiatrist, who described him as "taciturn." A mental status examination showed R.P. to be disoriented to person, place, and time. He demonstrated agnosia, being unable to identify a pen and a set of keys. He could not complete sentences, give rational answers to questions, or give any reliable information about himself, including his last name. He was given a diagnosis of primary progressive dementia, Alzheimer's type.

Initial evaluations by the occupational therapist found remarkable dysfunction in activities of daily living and leisure activities. R.P. required physical assistance in grooming and dressing. He appeared not to recognize grooming and dressing articles and could not use them appropriately. He required an escort to the dining room and bathroom, as he could not locate them when given verbal directions. When food was placed directly in front of him on a table and an eating utensil was placed in his hand, he could initiate and maintain feeding, chewing, and swallowing until his meal was finished. When escorted to a toilet, R.P. could remove his clothing and use the toilet appropriately, but he needed occasional assistance adjusting his clothes after toileting. During the night, R.P. was regularly incontinent, defecating and urinating on the floor next to his bed.

R.P. often misinterpreted staff's intentions when they offered help or guidance. He often appeared baffled or angered by assistance rendered by staff and often struck the staff helping him. When greeted, he would smile and offer a spontaneous "Hi!" Other attempts at communication were not successful. He often looked perplexed when asked questions. He might begin to speak, but would stop abruptly, as if he could not think of how to say the words he wanted. Often he would shrug his shoulders and quip, "Well, I'll be damned."

R.P. could ambulate without difficulty, but his ambulation was not directed. He would wander aimlessly. If he chanced upon a door, all of which were kept locked on his hospital unit, he would kick and bang it until staff intervened.

He appeared to have no leisure interests. When the therapist would attempt to engage him in activities, he often appeared unable to recognize or appreciate the task being performed. With repeated directions and demonstrations, R.P. was able to attend to one-step tasks for 1 to 2 minutes.

"Dementia" Phase (Table 9.6)

One month later, at the time of this writing, R.P. shows deterioration, with increasingly frequent and more intense agitated episodes toward staff and his peers. When escorted into an activity, he seems panicked and hyperventilates. He immediately begins looking for an escape from the room. He appears less able to process information. He often looks puzzled when others speak to him, frightened when others approach him. He regularly fails to respond to his name.

R.P. now assaults others who offer no provocation except that they happen to be seated in his path. He assaults staff daily as they provide assistance in dressing, feeding, hygiene, and grooming. R.P.'s toilet hygiene has deteriorated. When escorted to the toilet, he no longer independently removes his clothing before urinating. Unless a staff member pulls down his pants, he wets himself and his clothes. He seems not to notice his wet clothing and becomes angry when encouraged to change into clean, dry clothing. At mealtimes, he must be escorted to the dining area and reminded to seat himself. He sometimes requires physical prompts to sit down. He can no longer use utensils correctly or refuses to use utensils placed in his hand. He requires spoon-feeding. Recently, he picked up a peeled banana as if it were a spoon and tried to scoop up pieces of food.

Communication skills have also deteriorated. R.P. is unable to exchange greetings. He regularly grunts in response to auditory, tactile, and visual stimuli. Replacing smiles and other facial expressions is a flat affect, devoid of emotion.

R.P. spends an increasing proportion of his waking hours sitting in one chair with his eyes closed. He has developed difficulty in locating the origins of noises and peoples' voices. When approached by others, he fails to initiate eye contact. When the therapist deliberately gets in his line of vision, he avoids eye contact.

R.P. is still ambulatory. He continues to wander about the unit aimlessly, but less frequently. He has been observed on occasion kneeling down and crawling on the floor, apparently trying to pick up designs in the floor tile and the lines between the tiles.

REFERENCES

1. Diagnostic and statistical manual of mental disorders, 3rd ed, revised. Washington, D.C.: American Psychiatric Association, 1987.
2. Kaplan H, Sadock B. Modern synopsis of comprehensive textbook of psychiatry, 4th ed. Baltimore: Williams & Wilkins, 1985.
3. Glickstein J. Therapeutic interventions in Alzheimer's disease. Rockville: Aspen Publishers, 1988.
4. Reisberg B, ed. Alzheimer's disease. New York: Free Press, 1983.
5. Constantinidis J. Heredity and dementia. Gerontology 1986;32(suppl 1):73–79.
6. Davies P. The genetics of Alzheimer's disease: a review and a discussion of the implications. Neurobiol Aging 1986;7(6):459–466.
7. Davous P., Roudier M, Nicole A, Amouyel P, Stehelond D, Delabar JM, Lamour Y, Gegonne A, Rearrangement of chromosome 21 in Alzheimer's disease. Ann Genet 1986;29(4):226–228.
8. Schellenberg GD, Bird TD, Wijsman EM, Moore DK. Martin GM. The genetics of Alzheimer's disease. Biomed Pharmacother 1989;43(7):463–468.
9. Fraser H, Bruce ME, McBride PA, Scott JR. The molecular pathology of scrapie and biological basis of lesion targeting. Prog Clin Biol Res 1989;317:637–644.

10. Kimberlin RH. Introduction to scrapie and perspectives on current scrapie research. Prog Clin Biol Res 1989;317:559–566.

11. Dealty AM, Haase AT, Fewster PH, Lewis E, Ball MJ. Human herpes virus infections and Alzheimer's disease. Neuropathol Appl Neurobiol 1990;16(3):213–223.

12. Walker DG, O'Kusky JR, McGeer PL. In situ hybridation analysis for herpes simplex virus nucleic acids in Alzheimer's disease. Alzheimer Dis Assoc Disord 1989;3(3):123–131.

13. Andorn A, Suarez M, Pavia C, Weinstein A, Shank D, Davis K, Burderfer W, Pappolla MA, Omar R, Saran B, Concurrent neuroborreliosis and Alzheimer's disease: analysis of the evidence. Hum Pathol 1989;20(8):753–757.

14. Friedland RP, May C, Dahlberg J. The viral hypothesis of Alzheimer's disease. Absence of antibodies to lenteviruses. Arch Neurol 1990;47(2):177–178.

15. Hewitt CD, Savory J, Wills MR. Aspects of aluminum toxicity. Clin Lab Med 1990;10(2):403–422.

16. Perl DP, Pendlebury WW. Aluminum neurotoxicity—potential role in the pathogenesis of neurofibrillary tangle formation. Can J Neurol Sci 1986;13(4 suppl):441–445.

17. Lui E, Fisman M, Wong C, Diaz F. Metals and the liver in Alzheimer's disease. An investigation of hepatic zinc, copper, cadmium, and metallothionein. J Am Geriatr Soc 1990;38(6):633–639.

18. Tollefson GD, Godes M, Warren JB, Haus E, Luxenberg M, Garvey M. Lymphopenia in primary degenerative dementia. J Psychiatr Res 1989;23(3–4):191–199.

19. Gottfries, CG. Alzheimer's disease. Gerontology 1986;32(suppl 1):98–101.

20. Jenike MA, Albert M, Baer L, Gunther J. Oral physostigmine as treatment for primary degenerative dementia: a double-bind placebo-controlled inpatient trial. J Geriatr Psychiatry Neurol 1990;3(1):13–16.

21. Jenike MA, Albert MS, Heller H, Gunther J, Goff D. Oral physostigmine treatment for patients with presenile and senile dementia of the Alzheimer's type: a double-blind placebo controlled trial. J Clin Psychiatry 1990;51(1):3–7.

22. Davidson M, Bierer LM, Kaminsky R, Ryan TM, Davis KL. Combined administration of physostigmine and clonidine to patients with dementia of the Alzheimer's type: a pilot safety study. Alzheimer Dis Assoc Disord 1989;3(4):224–227.

23. Boller F, Forette F. Alzheimer's disease and THA: a review of the cholinergic theory and of preliminary results. Biomed Pharmacother 1989;43(7):487–491.

24. Kumar V, Becker RE. Clinical pharmacology of tetrahydroaminoacridine: a possible therapeutic agent in Alzheimer's disease. Int J Clin Pharmacol Ther Toxicol 1989;27(10):478–485.

25. Wragg RE, Jeste DV. Neuroleptics and alternative treatments: management of behavioral symptoms and psychosis in Alzheimer's disease and related conditions. Psychiatr Clin North Am 1988;11(1):195–213.

26. Salzman C. A primer on geriatric psychopharmacology. Am J Psychiatry 1980;139:67–74.

27. Larson EB, Kukull WA, Buchner D, Reifler BV. Adverse drug reactions associated with global cognitive impairment in elderly persons. Am Intern Med 1987;107(2):169–173.

28. Tariot PN, Newhouse PA, Thompson KE, Lawlor BA, Muella EF, Sunderland T, Weingartner H, Cohen RM, Low-dose oral lorazepam administration in Alzheimer subjects and age-matched controls. Psychopharmacology (Berlin) 1989;99(1):129–133.

29. Risse SC, Lampe TH, Cubberly L. Very low-dose neuroleptic treatment in two patients with agitation associated with Alzheimer's disease. J Clin Psychiatry 1987;48(5):207–208.

30. Gleason RP, Schneider LS. Carbamazepine treatment of agitation in Alzheimer's outpatients refractory to neuroleptics. J Clin Psychiatry 1990;51(3):115–118.

31. Taira E, ed. Therapeutic interventions for the person with dementia. New York: Haworth Press, 1986.

32. Kalicki A, Confronting Alzheimer's disease. Owings, MD: Rynd Communications, 1987.

33. Ninos M, Makohon R. Functional assessment of the patient. Geriatric Nurs 1985;6:139–142.

34. Mancall E. Essentials of the neurological examination, 2nd ed. Philadelphia: FA Davis, 1982.

35. Chandra V, Bharucha NE, Shoenberg BS. Conditions associated with Alzheimer's disease at death: case control study, Neurology 1986;36(2):209–211.

36. Walsh JS, Welch HG, Larson EB. Survival of outpatients with Alzheimer-type dementia. Ann Intern Med 1990;113(6):429–434.

RECOMMENDED READINGS

Bennett G, Vourakis C, Woolf D, eds. Substance abuse: pharmacological, developmental, and clinical perspectives. New York: John Wiley, 1983. This book offers easy to read information on the autonomic and central nervous system as well as central nervous system depressants and stimulants. It includes information on substance abuse problems throughout the life span and clinical practice in substance abuse treatment.

Gold M. The facts about drugs and alcohol, 3rd ed. New York: Bantam Books, 1988. This book discusses addiction, adolescent drug abuse, cocaine, marijuana, alcohol, prescription drugs, drug testing, and assessing treatment programs.

Milkman H, Shaffer H, eds. The addictions: multi-disciplinary perspectives and treatments. Lexington, MA: Lexington Books, 1985. This book discusses several theories of addiction and reviews various treatment perspectives.

Nicholi AM Jr, ed. The new Harvard guide to psychiatry. Cambridge, Mass: Belknap Press of Harvard University Press, 1988. The chapter on substance use disorders gives a description of the disorders as well as adverse effects, tolerance, and withdrawal.

Glossary

Agnosia: Inability to recognize the import of sensory impressions despite being able to recognize the elemental sensation of a stimulus. Language deficits must be absent for this diagnosis; the varieties correspond to several senses and are distinguished as auditory (acoustic), gustatory, olfactory, tactile, and visual. Visual agnosia, for example, is the inability to recognize familiar objects by sight. Specific sensory agnosias can occur when the connections are interrupted between the primary cortical receptor region for a stimulus and the memory of that abstraction (parietal lobe damage). An example is the incapacity to identify a familiar faces despite seeing the face.

Alzheimer's disease: A primary degenerative dementia (PDD) of the Alzheimer type characterized by loss of cognitive and intellectual abilities that is severe enough to impair social or occupational performance. The full clinical picture consists of impairment of memory, abstract thinking, and judgment, with some degree of personality change.

Anomia: Loss of the ability to name objects or recognize/recall names; may be both receptive and expressive.

Aphasia: Defect or loss of the power of expression by speech, writing, or signs or of comprehension of spoken or written languages, caused by disease or injury of the brain centers.

Broca's aphasia: Expressive aphasia, in which the patient understands written and spoken words and knows what he wants to say, but cannot utter the words. Also called apraxia of speech, motor aphasia, and nonfluent aphasia. Wernicke's aphasia: Receptive aphasia, in which a patient cannot understand written, spoken, or tactile speech symbols.

Apraxia: A disorder of skilled purposeful movement that is neither caused by deficits in primary motor skills nor comprehension problems. It can affect the praxic components of ideation and concept formation, as well as programming and planning of movement. Apraxia can include loss of the ability to use objects correctly. Disturbances of motor execution, on the contrary, are usually related to primary motor skills.

Cholinergic: Stimulated, activated, or transmitted by choline (acetycholine), a neurotransmitter: a term applied to those nerve fibers that liberate acetylcholine at the synapse when a nerve impulse passes, such as at the parasympathetic nerve endings

Circumlocution: An indirect or lengthy way of expressing something; speaking in a roundabout way, never getting to the point during conversation.

Cognition: A conscious thought process that refers to awareness and knowledge of objects, perceptions, thoughts, and memories. In addition to knowledge, it includes the abilities to understand, reason, make decisions, and apply judgment.

Confabulation (fabrication, fabulation): Unconscious filling in of gaps in memory with fabricated facts and experiences, commonly seen in organic amnestic syndromes. It differs from lying in that the individual has no intention to deceive and believes the fabricated memories to be real.

Constructional apraxia: A failure to produce or replicate a specific design or object from parts in two or three dimensions, either drawings or block designs. The failure may manifest spontaneously, upon command, or by copying.

Delirium: A mental disturbance of relatively short duration usually reflecting a toxic state and marked by illusions, hallucinations, delusions, excitement, restlessness, and incoherence. Almost any acute illness accompanied by very high fever can bring on delirium. Other causes are metabolic, neurologic trauma, congestive heart failure, thyrotoxicosis, physical and mental exhaustion, and drug and alcohol intoxication and withdrawal.

Dementia: An organic mental disorder characterized by a general loss of intellectual abilities involving impairment of memory, judgment, and abstract thinking, as well as changes in personality. It does not include a loss of intellectual functioning caused by clouding of consciousness (as occurs in delirium) nor that caused by depression or other functional mental disorders. Common causes are Alzheimer's disease, cerebrovascular disease (multiinfarct), central nervous infection, brain trauma or tumors, pernicious anemia, folic acid deficiency, Wernike-Korsakoff syndrome, hydrocephalus, and neurologic diseases such as Huntington's chorea, multiple sclerosis, and Parkinson's disease.

Dysarthria: Imperfect articulation of speech caused by disturbances of muscular control resulting from central or peripheral nervous system damage.

Fabrication: The telling of imaginary events or tales as if they were true; the recitation of imaginary experiences to fill gaps in the memory, especially seen in organic psychoses.

Focal: Chief center of a morbid process.

Hallucination: False sensory perceptions not associated with real external stimuli; there may or may not be a delusional interpretation of the hallucinatory experience. Hallucinations indicate a psychotic disturbance only when associated with impairment in reality testing.

Infarction: A localized area of ischemic necrosis produced by occlusion of the arterial supply or the venous drainage of the heart.

In vivo: Within the living body.

Korsakoff's syndrome: The amnestic component of the Wernike-Korsakoff syndrome associated with chronic alcoholism and vitamin B_1 (thiamin) deficiency. It is characterized by retrograde and anterograde amnesia, sometimes with disorientation, confabulation, and lack of insight into the memory deficit.

Lability: The quality of being unstable or fluctuating. In psychiatry, emotional instability; a tendency to show alternating states of gaiety and somberness.

Neurofibrillary tangles: Neurofibrils are the delicate threads running in every direction through the cytoplasm of a nerve cell, extending into the axon and dendrites. These bundles of fibrous proteins are not normally present in large quantities in the human brain (3). In Alzheimier's disease, these threads proliferate and become tangled and disorganized, generally with an accumulation in the hippocampus, amygdala, and pyramidal cells of the neocortex.

Paraphasia: Partial aphasia in which the person employs wrong words, or uses words in wrong and senseless combinations.

Perseveration: Continuation of an activity after cessation of the causative stimulus.

Plaques: Senile plaques are microscopic lesions in the brain, representing tissue deterioration, composed of fragmented axon terminals and dendrites surrounding a core of amyloid. Neuritic plaques: Glycoproteins that collect in scaly patches, replacing degenerating nerve terminals (3). These plaques are present in the cerebral cortex, hippocampus, amygdala, corpus striatum, and thalamus.

Presenium: Pertaining to a condition occurring in early or middle life (e.g., presenile) usually before the age of 65.

Proband (propositus): The original person with a mental or physical disorder who serves as the basis for a hereditary or genetic study; one from whom a genetic line of descent is traced.

Psychotropic: Exerting an effect on the mind; capable of modifying mental activity; a drug that affects the mental state. There are several classes of psychotropic drugs. Antidepressants are used for the relief of symptoms of major depression; lithium for the treatment of manic episodes of manic-depressive illness; neuroleptics (major tranquilizers) for management of the manifestations of psychotic disorders (schizophrenia); and antianxiety agents (minor tranquilizers) for relief of symptoms of anxiety and tension (phobias, anxiety neurosis).

Senium: Pertaining to old age (i.e., senile). Pertaining to a condition occurring in the later years of life, usually after the age of 65.

10

Spinal Cord Injury

LAURA VINCENT MILLER

. . . of the many forms of disability which can beset mankind, a severe injury or disease of the spinal cord undoubtedly constitutes one of the most devastating calamities in human life.

Sir Ludwig Guttmann

Pioneer in twentieth century management of spinal cord injury

The future lies in our own hands, and if a challenge should enter our life, it is important to remember we have tremendous strength, courage, and ability to overcome any obstacle.

Douglas Heir, Esq.

Attorney-at-Law

The full impact of the preceding statements (1, 2) may not strike the reader unless the whole story is known. The latter author, Doug Heir, sustained a spinal cord injury at age 18. He dove into a pool to save a boy who appeared to be drowning. The boy was only playing—but Doug's injury rendered him quadriplegic. Now, at age 29, Doug is many things, among them: an author, U.S. delegate to the Soviet Union, cover athlete for Wheaties cereal, associate legal editor of the *National Trial Lawyer*, and a gold medalist in the 1989 Seoul, Korea, Olympics. An impressive list of accomplishments for someone who sustained "one of

the most devastating calamities in human life!"

The goal of the health-care team should include empowering clients to take charge of their futures. To accomplish this end, the health professional must understand the complexities of the diagnosis. This chapter explores the ramifications of spinal cord injuries, beginning with a brief overview of the central nervous system (CNS) and surrounding structures.

OVERVIEW OF CNS AND RELATED STRUCTURES

The brain and spinal cord make up the CNS. The spinal cord receives sensory (afferent) information from the peripheral nervous system and transmits this information to higher structures (i.e., the thalamus, cerebellum, cerebral cortex) in the CNS. Descending motor (efferent) information, originating from the cortex, is also transmitted by the spinal cord back to the peripheral nervous system.

The consistency of the spinal cord has been compared to that of a ripe banana, and it is fortunate that the spinal cord and cerebral cortex are protected by bony structures. While the skull protects the brain, the vertebral column protects the spinal cord. The vertebral column is com-posed of 33 vertebrae, with 7 cervical vertebrae in the neck region (C1–C7), 12 thoracic vertebrae in the chest region (T1–T12), 5 lumbar vertebrae in the midback region (L1–L5), 5 sacral vertebrae (S1–S5) which are actually fused in the lower back and pelvic region, and 4 fused coccygeal vertebrae that make up the coccyx, or tailbone (Fig. 10.1).

There are 31 pairs of spinal nerves, which exit from the spinal cord and branch to form the peripheral nervous system. The nerves exit through the openings formed between each two vertebrae. The spinal nerves are named according to the

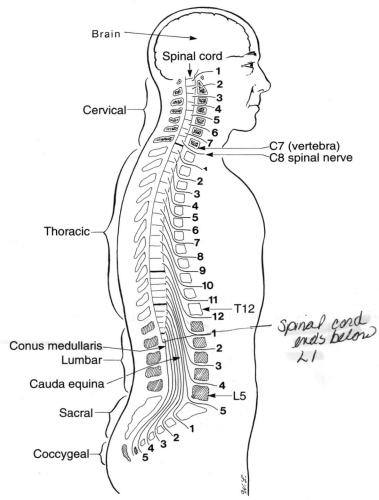

Fig. 10.1. The spinal cord, spinal nerves, and vertebral column. (Courtesy, Rehabilitation Institute of Michigan. Used with permission.)

vertebrae above or below which they exit. Note that spinal nerves C1 through C7 exit above the corresponding vertebrae, while the remaining spinal nerves (C8–S5) exit below the corresponding vertebrae. Thus, while there are seven cervical vertebrae, there are eight cervical spinal nerves. The actual spinal cord ends just below the L1 vertebra. However, some spinal nerves continue, to exit beyond the point where the spinal cord ends. Due to their visual resemblance, this bundle of nerves is referred to as the cauda equina, which is Latin for "horse's tail" (3). The meningeal covering of the spinal cord, which contains the cerebrospinal fluid (CSF) that bathes the structures of the CNS, also extends past the end of the spinal cord to the L4 vertebral level. The CSF-filled meningeal space between L2 and L4, referred to as the lumbar cistern, is the site where spinal taps are performed, since the spinal cord is not present, but CSF is accessible.

Sensory and Motor Tracts

The terms *tract, pathway, lemniscus,* and *fasciculus* all refer to bundles of nerve fibers that have a similar function and travel through the spinal cord in a particular area. It is important to know the names, locations, and functions of these tracts to understand the possible outcomes of a spinal cord injury at a given level. The location of major tracts within a cross-section of the spinal cord can be seen in Figure 10.2.

Two basic types of nerve tissue make up the spinal cord. Gray matter is located centrally and resembles a butterfly in cross-sections of the cord. Gray matter is composed of cell bodies and synapses. White matter encompasses most of the periphery of the cord. The white matter contains the ascending and descending pathways. A more detailed description of the functions of the various sensory and motor pathways that travel through the white matter of the spinal cord is provided in Table 10.1. It may be helpful to remember that many pathways are named according to their origin and the location of their final synapse (e.g., spinocerebellar, corticospinal).

Specific motor and sensory information is carried by each pair of spinal nerves. Very generally, the cervical nerves (C1–

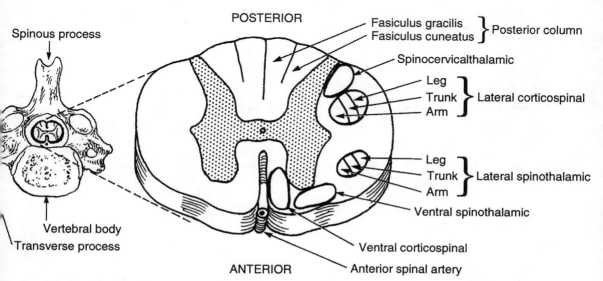

Fig. 10.2. Cross-section of cervical spinal cord, shown in relation to surrounding vertebral structures. Selected ascending and descending pathways are illustrated. (Adapted from materials provided courtesy of Rehabilitation Institute of Michigan. Used with permission.)

C8) carry afferent and efferent impulses for the head, neck, diaphragm, arms, and hands. The thoracic spinal nerves (T1–T12) serve the chest and upper abdominal musculature. The lumbar spinal nerves (L1–L5) carry information to and from the legs and a portion of the foot, while the sacral spinal nerves (S1–S5) carry impulses for the remaining foot musculature, bowel, bladder, and muscles involved in sexual functioning. A more detailed outline of muscles innervated by each level of the spinal cord, as well as a dermatomal segmentation (sensory map) of the body are presented in Table 10.2 and Figure 10.3.

Reflex Arc

Most nerve impulses move up the spinal cord to the brain and back through the cord to the peripheral nerves. However, some impulses merely enter the cord through the dorsal nerve root, synapse, and exit via the ventral nerve root. This causes certain muscle functions or responses without direction from the brain. A simple example of this "looping" can be seen in the knee-jerk reflex. If the knee is tapped with a reflex hammer, the knee will extend without any influence from the brain. The stimulation by the hammer causes afferent impulses to enter the cord, synapse, and exit, causing a contraction of the muscle fibers (Fig. 10.4). This activity is called a *reflex arc*. In persons with an intact spinal cord, afferent nerve impulses also travel to the brain almost instantaneously. This allows an awareness, or "feeling," of the initial stimulation (knee tap) and subsequent response (knee jerk).

This concept is important to an understanding of spinal cord injuries (SCI). It explains why some persons with SCI continue to have reflexes but do not have voluntary control of their muscles. It also explains why others have no reflexes at all below the level of their injury. This is discussed in much greater detail in the section on classification of injuries.

ETIOLOGY AND INCIDENCE

Many sources of statistics attempt to account for the number of persons who have sustained spinal cord injuries. Unfortunately, only recently has the United States made strides in collecting comprehensive data on a national level. In 1985, the Centers for Disease Control began promoting surveillance mechanisms at state and national levels for the collection and reporting of these data. Nonetheless, current data sources do provide a picture of

Table 10.1.
Noninclusive Listing of Ascending and Descending Pathways

Ascending afferent (sensory) pathways	Function
Spinocerebellar	Nonconscious proprioception
Lateral spinothalamic	Pain, temperature
Ventral spinothalamic	Touch, pressure
Fasiculus gracilis/fasiculus cuneatus[a]	Two-point tactile discrimination, vibration, conscious proprioception, stereognosis
Spinocervicothalamic	Touch, proprioception, stereognosis, vibration
Descending efferent (motor) pathways	**Function**
Lateral corticospinal	Movement to extremities
Ventral corticospinal	Movement for neck and trunk
Vestibulospinal	Equilibrium
Reticulospinal	Autonomic functions: motor respiratory functions

[a]Called the "posterior column."

Table 10.2.
Spinal Cord Innervations/Function

Spinal Cord Level	Primary Muscle Groups	Primary Movements
C1–C3	• Infrahyoid muscles • Head/neck extensions • Rectus capitus • (anterior & lateral) • Sternocleidomastoid • Longus colli • Longus capitus • Scaleni	• Depression of the hyoid • Neck extension, flexion, rotation, and lateral flexion
	Additional Primary Muscle Groups	Additional Primary Movements
C4	• Trapezius • Upper cervical paraspinals • Diaphragm	• Shoulder elevation, scapular adduction and depression • Independent breathing
C5	• Rhomboids • Deltoids • Rotator cuff muscles (partially– some nerve supply is at C6 level) • Biceps • Brachialis (partially) • Brachioradialis (partially)	• Scapular downward rotation • Weak shoulder external rotation, flexion, and extension • Shoulder abduction and rotation • Weak approximation of humeral head in glenoid fossa • Elbow flexion
C6	• Rotator cuff muscles (complete innervation) • Serratus anterior (partially) • Pectoralis (clavicular segments) • Total innervation of elbow flexors • Supinators • Extensor carpi radialis • Flexor carpi radialis	• Full shoulder rotation, adduction, flexion, extension • Scapular abduction • Horizontal shoulder adduction • Strong elbow flexion and supination • Wrist extension (weak) • Tenodesis action of hand • Very weak wrist flexion
C7	• Latissmus dorsi • Pectoralis major (sternal portion) • Triceps • Pronator teres • Flexor carpi radialis • Flexor digitorium superficialis • Extensor digitorum (partially) • Extensor pollicis longus and brevis	• Elbow extension • Forearm pronation • Wrist flexion • Finger flexion (trace) • Finger extension (weak) • Thumb extension (weak)
C8	• Flexor carpi ulnaris • Extensor carpi ulnaris • Flexor digitorum profundus and superficialis • Flexor pollicis longus and brevis • Abductor pollicis longus • Adductor pollicis • Opponens pollicis • Lumbricals (partially)	• Complete wrist extension, adduction, and abduction • Finger flexion (stronger) • Thumb flexion, abduction, adduction, opposition • Weak flexion at MCP with IP extension

Table 10.2.   (Continued)
Spinal Cord Innervations/Function

Spinal Cord Level	Primary Muscle Groups	Primary Movements
T1	• Dorsal interossei • Palmar interossei • Abductor pollicis brevis • Lumbricals (complete innervation) • Erector spinae muscles (partially) • Intercostal muscles (partially)	• Finger abduction • Finger adduction • Thumb abduction (strong) • MCP flexion with IP extension (strong) • Thoracic spine extension • Increased respiratory function with presence of intercostals
T4–8	• Erector spinae muscles (partially) • Intercostal muscles (partially) • Abdominal muscles (beginning at T7)	• Stronger thoracic spine extension • Stronger respiratory function • Thoracic flexion • Weak trunk flexion
T9–12	• Lower erector spinae muscles • Lower intercostal muscles • Abdominal muscles • Quadratus lumborum (partially)	• Strong thoracic spine extension • Trunk flexion, extension, rotation and stability • Pelvic control and stability
L1–3	• Quadratus lumborum (full innervation) • Iliopsoas • Erector spinae (lumbar segment)	• Pelvic elevation • Hip flexion • Lumbar extension
L4–5	• Lumbar erector spinae • Hip adductors • Hip rotators • Quadriceps • Hamstrings (partially) • Tibialis anterior	• Lumbar extension and stability • Hip adduction • Hip rotation • Knee extension • Knee flexion (weak) • Ankle dorsiflexion (weak)
S1–2	• Hip extensors • Hip abductors • Hamstrings (complete innervation) • Plantar flexors • Invertors of ankle • Evertors of ankle	• Hip extension • Hip abduction and stability • Knee flexion • Ankle plantar flexion • Ankle inversion and stability • Ankle eversion and stability
S2–5	• Bladder • Lower bowel • Genital innervations	• Genitourinary functions • Bowel functions

the etiology and incidence of SCI in this country.

The leading causes of SCI in the United States are motor vehicle accidents, followed by falls and gunshot wounds (Fig. 10.5). Sports-related injuries account for most of the remaining SCIs, with diving being by far the most common (and preventable) cause (Table 10.3).

Analyzing the etiology of spinal cord injuries makes for well-targeted preven-

tion programs. Public awareness is certainly heightened on the effects of using substances while operating a vehicle. Tougher penalties for driving under the influence of altering substances have been enacted, and many states have adopted seat belt and child restraint legislation. Grant monies have even been awarded to hospital-based programs that evaluate the home environments of senior citizens. Their recommendations may reduce the

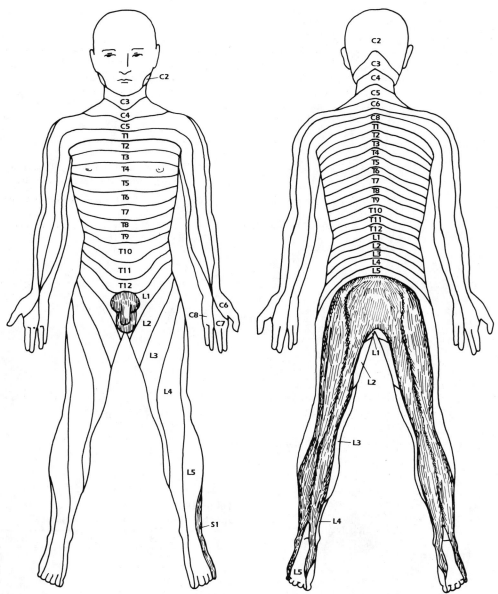

Fig. 10.3. Dermatome map. (From Hammond M, Umlauf R, Matteson B, Fulginiti SP. *Yes, you can! A guide to self care for persons with spinal cord injury*. Washington, D.C.: Paralyzed Veterans of America, 1989. Used with permission.)

risk of falls—a major cause of SCI in the elderly. An innovative program sponsored by the Southeastern Michigan Spinal Cord Injury System tells high-risk youths about the consequences of interpersonal violence and presents strategies to avoid those tragic outcomes. This program is brought to elementary and high schools, where weapons are, unfortunately, too prevalent.

Incidence rates for SCI in the United States are estimated to be between 28 and 50 per million population per year (5). This translates to between 6,700 and 12,000 new cases of SCI every year. But who is the "average" person with SCI? The sta-

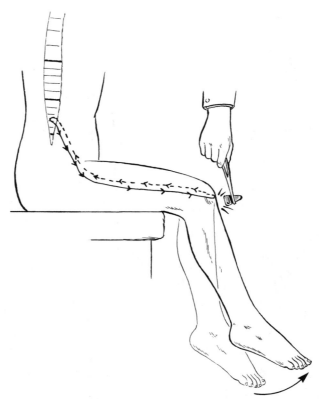

Fig. 10.4. Knee-jerk reflex.

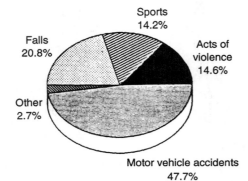

Fig. 10.5. Etiologic distribution of spinal cord injury. (Adapted from Stover SL, Fine PR, eds. Spinal cord injury: the facts and figures, 1986. The National Spinal Cord Injury Statistical Center, University of Alabama at Birmingham: Birmingham, Alabama. Used with permission.)

Table 10.3.
Sports-related Spinal Cord Injuries[a]

Sport	Percentage
Diving	66.0
Football	6.1
Snow Skiing	3.8
Surfing	3.1
Trampoline	2.6
Other Winter Sports	2.3
Wrestling	2.3
Gymnastics	2.2
Horseback Riding	2.0
Other	9.6

[a]From Stover SL, Fine PR, eds. Spinal cord injury: the facts and figures, 1986. The National Spinal Cord Injury Statistical Center, University of Alabama at Birmingham: Birmingham, Alabama. Used with permission.

tistics indicate an 18-year-old white male involved in an auto accident, but this can vary widely, both geographically and seasonally. Seasonal sports cause fluctuations in etiology statistics, and some urban hospitals are reporting that over 40% of their SCI cases are secondary to gunshot wounds.

Although much of the literature focuses on trauma, there are many non-traumatic causes of spinal cord damage. Developmental conditions, such as spina bifida, scoliosis, and spinal cord agenesis, may yield the same clinical signs as traumatic SCI. There are also many acquired conditions, such as bacterial or viral infections, benign or malignant growths, embolisms, thromboses, hemorrhages—even radiation or vaccinations—which could lead to damage of spinal cord tissue.

CLASSIFICATION OF INJURY

There are two major classifications of spinal cord injuries: complete and incomplete. A complete spinal cord injury occurs when there is a total transection of the cord. In this case, all ascending and descending pathways are interrupted, and there is a total loss of motor and sensory function below the level of injury. The injury may additionally be referred to as an upper motor neuron (UMN) injury if the reflex arcs are intact below the level of injury, but are no longer mediated by the brain. Upper motor neuron lesions are characterized by (a) a loss of voluntary function below the level of the injury, (b) spastic paralysis, (c) no muscle atrophy, and (d) hyperactive reflexes (Fig. 10.6).

Complete injuries below the level of the conus medullaris (Fig. 10.1) are referred to as lower motor neuron (LMN) injuries, because the injury has affected the spinal nerves after they exit from the cord. In fact, injuries involving spinal nerves after they exit the cord at any level are referred to as LMN injuries. In LMN injuries, the reflex arc cannot occur, since impulses cannot enter the cord to syn-

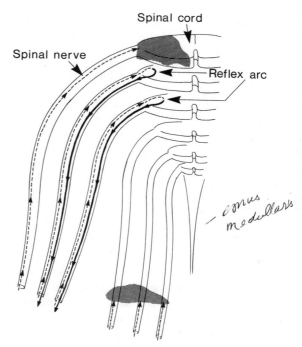

Fig. 10.6. A diagrammatic representation of the reflex arc. The shaded lesion above denotes an upper motor neuron (UMN) lesion, with the exception of the spinal nerve entering at the level of the lesion. The shaded lesion below represents a lower motor neuron lesion. (Courtesy, Rehabilitation Institute of Michigan. Used with permission.)

apse. As a result, LMN injuries are characterized by (a) a loss of voluntary function below the level of the injury, (b) flaccid paralysis, (c) muscle atrophy, and (d) absence of reflexes.

UMN and LMN injuries may be complete or incomplete. There may also be a mixture of UMN and LMN signs with an incomplete lesion in the lower thoracic/upper lumbar region. The following section discusses incomplete injuries in greater detail. See Appendix 10.2 for some common diagnostic procedures.

INCOMPLETE INJURIES

If damage to the spinal cord does not cause a total transection, there will still be some degree of voluntary movement and/or sensation present below the level of injury. This is known as an incomplete injury. Incomplete injuries may be further categorized according to the area of the spinal cord which was damaged, and the clinical signs present.

Anterior Cord Syndrome. This syndrome results from damage to the anterior spinal artery, or indirect damage to anterior spinal cord tissue (Fig. 10.7). Clinical signs include

Loss of motor function below the level of injury;

Loss of thermal, pain, and tactile sensation below the level of injury;

Light touch and proprioceptive awareness are generally unaffected.

Brown-Séquard's Syndrome. This syndrome occurs when only one side of the spinal cord is damaged (Fig. 10.8). A hemisection of this nature is frequently the result of a stab or gunshot wound. The clinical signs that would indicate Brown-Séquard's syndrome generally include

Ipsilateral loss of motor function below the level of injury;

Ipsilateral reduction of deep touch and proprioceptive awareness (there is a reduction rather than loss as many of these nerve fibers cross);

Contralateral loss of pain, temperature, and touch.

Clinically, a major challenge presented by Brown-Séquard's syndrome is that the extremities with the greatest strength have the poorest sensation.

Central Cervical Cord Syndrome. In this lesion, the neural fibers serving the upper extremities are more impaired than those of the lower extremities (Fig. 10.9). This occurs because the fibers that innervate the upper extremities travel more centrally in the cord and, as the name of the syndrome implies, the central struc-

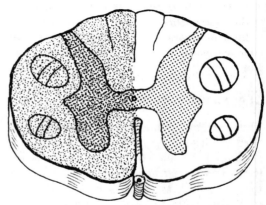

Fig. 10.8. Cross-section of the cord, illustrating the damage that results in Brown-Séquard's syndrome. (Courtesy, Rehabilitation Institute of Michigan. Used with permission).

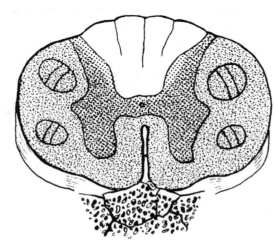

Fig. 10.7. A cross-section of the spinal cord illustrating the damage that causes anterior cord syndrome. The anterior artery is involved, resulting in damage to most areas, with the exception of the posterior columns. (Courtesy, Rehabilitation Institute of Michigan. Used with permission.)

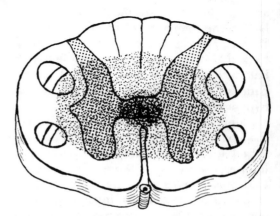

Fig. 10.9. Cross-section of the cord, illustrating the damage resulting in central cervical cord syndrome. (Courtesy, Rehabilitation Institute of Michigan. Used with permission.)

tures are the ones that are damaged (Fig. 10.2). Injury to the central portion of the spinal cord is often seen, along with structural changes in the vertebrae. Most commonly, hyperextension of the neck, combined with a narrowing of the spinal canal, results in this type of injury. Because arthritic changes can lead to spinal canal narrowing, this syndrome is more prevalent in aging populations. The signs of central cord syndrome often include

> Motor and sensory functions in the lower extremities less involved than in the upper extremities.
> A potential for flaccid paralysis of the upper extremities, as the anterior horn cells in the cervical spinal cord may be damaged. Since these are synapse sites for the motor pathways, a LMN injury may result.

Cauda Equina Injuries. Cauda equina injuries do not involve damage to the spinal cord itself but, rather, to the spinal nerves that extend below the end of the spinal cord (Fig. 10.1). Injuries to the nerve roots and spinal nerves composing the cauda equina are generally incomplete. Since this type of injury actually involves structures of the peripheral nervous system (exiting spinal nerves), there is some chance for nerve regeneration and recovery of function if the roots are not too severely damaged or divided. These injuries are usually the result of direct trauma from fracture dislocations of the lower thoracic or upper lumbar vertebrae. Clinical signs of cauda equina injuries include

> Loss of motor function and sensation below the level of injury.
> Absence of a reflex arc, since the transmission of impulses through the spinal nerves to their synapse point is interrupted. Motor paralysis is of the LMN type, with flaccidity and muscle atrophy seen below the level of injury.

In both complete and incomplete injuries, the terms "quadriplegia" and "paraplegia" may be used to further describe the impact of the injury. Quadriplegia refers to lost or limited function of all extremities as a result of damage to cervical cord segments. Paraplegia, which refers to lost or limited function in the lower extremities, occurs after lesions to thoracic, lumbar, and/or sacral cord segments.

POSTTRAUMATIC PROGRESSION

Immediately following a traumatic spinal cord injury, there is a time of altered reflex activity, commonly referred to as spinal shock. As a result of injury, spinal cord segments below the level of the lesion are deprived of excitatory input from higher CNS centers. What is observed clinically during this phase is a flaccid paralysis of muscles below the level of injury and an absence of reflexes (6). The bladder is also flaccid, requiring catheterization, and there is no voluntary control of the bowel. Depending on the level of the injury, the person with an SCI may also require the aid of a ventilator because of lost or temporarily interrupted innervation to the diaphragm, intercostals, and abdominal muscles.

Spinal shock generally lasts from 1 week to 3 months after injury. Once spinal shock subsides, the areas of the spinal cord *above* the level of the lesion operate as they did premorbidly. *Below* the level of the lesion, reflexes will resume if the reflex arc is intact. This is an important concept to understand. Unlike a plant, which may die entirely if its stem is cut in half, the spinal cord is still alive and functional above and below the level of injury. The problem is one of communication; the brain cannot receive sensory information beyond the lesion site and also cannot voluntarily control motor function below that point.

After spinal shock subsides, there is often an increase in spasticity, especially in the flexor muscle groups. The reflex arc "fires" and the brain is unable to interfere. Following this phase, there may be a period of 6 to 12 months postinjury when it is not uncommon to see an increase in spasticity of the extensor groups. Usually, after a year postinjury, the wide fluctuations in tone will cease.

COMPLICATIONS

There is an array of complications that can greatly affect the prognosis of a person sustaining an SCI. Some of the more common medical complications are addressed in this section.

Autonomic Dysreflexia (Hyperreflexia)

As implied by its name, autonomic dysreflexia, or hyperreflexia, involves an exaggerated response of the autonomic nervous system (ANS). You may recall that a function of the ANS is the integration of body functions in the "fight-or-flight" response—heart rate, blood vessel constriction/dilation, regulation of glands, and smooth muscle. The condition usually occurs in persons with spinal cord injuries above the T6 level. Signs to look for include a sudden, pounding headache, diaphoresis, flushing, "goosebumps," and tachycardia followed by bradycardia. All of this is caused by an irritation of nerves below the level of injury. Common sources of irritation include an overfull bladder or bowel, urinary tract infections, or decubitus ulcers. Even irritations such as ingrown toenails can trigger the response. All these irritations would be bothersome to a person with an intact spinal cord—you would feel uncomfortable and act to remedy the situation. But the person with a spinal cord injury lacks this "feeling," and autonomic dysreflexia is the body's way of warning that something is wrong below the level of the injury.

The most important aspect of managing autonomic dysreflexia is to find the cause and alleviate it. This may require emptying the bladder, checking for blockages or "kinks" in the urinary drainage tubing, checking for bowel impaction, or evaluating for other factors. If the person assumes an upright position, it helps to decrease blood pressure. Most persons with quadriplegia will experience an episode of autonomic dysreflexia at least once, but if the signs of autonomic dysreflexia appear frequently, medication may be indicated. Although autonomic dysreflexia may appear suddenly, it must be managed promptly. As blood pressure tends to elevate dramatically, there is risk of stroke or death if the situation is ignored or mismanaged.

Postural Hypotension

In contrast to autonomic dysreflexia, blood pressure is decreased in postural hypotension. This condition, often seen in persons who have sustained cervical or thoracic spinal cord injuries, may also be referred to as orthostatic hypotension (7). Blood tends to pool distally in the lower extremities as a result of reduced muscle tone in the trunk and legs. The symptoms of postural hypotension frequently occur when a person attempts to sit up after prolonged periods of bed rest. Symptoms include lightheadedness, dizziness, pallor, sudden weakness, and unresponsiveness. Preventive measures include the use of antiembolism hosiery and abdominal binders, which externally assist circulation. Additionally, assuming an upright position slowly can often help avoid these symptoms. If symptoms do occur, a semireclined or reclined position should be maintained until the symptoms subside.

Respiratory Complications

Persons with spinal cord injuries at or below the level of T12 generally have a normal respiratory status. Injuries above that level, however, compromise the respiratory system to some degree. The abdominal musculature is innervated by segments T7 through T12; the intercostal muscles are served by segments T1 through T12; and the diaphragm is innervated by C4. Persons with complete injuries above C4 are usually dependent on a respirator. Some may be candidates for a phrenic nerve stimulator if the nerve shows the ability to conduct an impulse. Generally, persons with C4 complete injuries and below are off respirators, but respiratory complications may persist. Breathing may be shallow, and the ability to cough productively may be weak. Various deep-breathing and assisted-coughing techniques may be taught, along with other procedures to keep the lungs clear.

Deep Vein Thromboses

Deep vein thromboses (DVT) can be a serious complication in many types of medical conditions. They are a potential complication in SCI for three main reasons: reduced circulation due to decreased tone, frequency of direct trauma to legs causing vascular damage (e.g., repeated trauma during transfer or bed mobility activities), and prolonged bed rest. Edema is often seen in SCI for the same reasons.

Clinical signs of DVT may include swelling in the lower extremities, localized redness, and a low-grade fever. However, a DVT may be relatively asymptomatic on bedside evaluation. Vigilant medical screenings for DVT should be performed in all cases of SCI. An undetected and unmanaged DVT may result in an embolism and resultant death.

Thermal Regulation

You have already seen that damage to the spinal cord can disrupt the ANS, possibly resulting in autonomic dysreflexia. Thermal regulation is another function of the ANS that can be disturbed after SCI. Maintaining the appropriate body temperature is often a problem for persons whose injuries are above T6. During the first year postinjury, the body tends to assume the temperature of the external environment. This condition is called *poikilothermia* (8). In time, some adjustment usually occurs. Discomfort is often experienced in cold weather, as blood vessels below the level of injury do not constrict sufficiently to conserve the body's heat. Conversely, excessive sweating may occur above the level of injury in warmer weather, but not below, which hampers the body's efforts to prevent hyperthermia. Because of this, extreme temperatures should be avoided, and attention should be given to the extent and type of clothing worn in all conditions.

Spasticity

In persons who have UMN lesions, increased tone appears in muscles below the level of injury after spinal shock subsides. Virtually all persons with cervical cord injuries experience spasms; 75% of those with thoracic lesions, less than 58% of those with lumbar injuries, and less than 25% of persons with cauda equina injuries report spasms (9). An increase in spasticity can be triggered by a variety of factors including infections, positioning, pressure sores, urinary tract infections, and heightened emotional states. Spasms are not necessarily disadvantageous. Being able to trigger their spasms can aid some persons in maintaining muscle bulk, circulation, bowel and bladder management, transfers, and other self-care activities. Excessive spasticity, however, may result in contractures, pain, and a reduced ability to participate in activities. At this point, medical or surgical options may be recommended.

Heterotopic Ossification (Ectopic Bone)

Heterotopic ossification (HO) refers to the abnormal formation of bone deposits on muscles, joints, and tendons. It occurs most often in the hip and knee, less frequently in the shoulder and elbow. It has been estimated that 20% of all persons with SCI have some degree of ectopic bone growth (10).

Clinical signs of heterotopic ossification (HO) may include heat, pain, swelling, and a noted decrease in active or passive range-of-motion. These signs should always alert the clinician, as they may indicate other serious complications, such as DVT. Many facilities specializing in the care of per-

sons with SCI routinely provide prophylactic medications that have shown promise in halting this abnormal calcification.
In extreme cases, where range of motion
is permanently and severely limited by
HO, surgery may be indicated.

Urinary System Complications

Urinary tract infections (UTI) are a common and dangerous complication of SCI.
Prior to modern medical management,
many persons with SCI who survived the
initial trauma died within a few years
postinjury, with one of the most common
causes being kidney failure due to chronic
UTI. Persons with SCI are more prone to
UTI—or bladder infections—for several
reasons.

The bladder is composed of smooth
muscle, innervated by sacral segments of
the spinal cord. As such, it is affected by
a loss of sensory and motor function, as
are other parts of the body, depending on
the level and extent of injury. The nature
of bladder function will depend on

whether the injury caused LMN or UMN
deficits. To understand this more clearly,
refer to Figure 10.10. Injury at point *A*
yields an UMN bladder, also referred to
as a *reflex* or *spastic* bladder. In this case,
the bladder can contract and void reflexively. Although this action is involuntary,
some persons with SCI can trigger the
reflex through various stimuli, much as
the knee-jerk reflex is triggered by tapping with a reflex hammer. That is because impulses can still enter the cord
below the level of injury, synapse, and
exit.

Persons with an UMN bladder may use
various types of catheters and additional
techniques to ensure that the bladder does
not become distended or retain urine.
They generally cannot rely on sensation
to alert them that the bladder has ex-
ceeded its normal capacity; rather, they
must rely on an established voiding
schedule.

An LMN bladder may also be referred
to as a *nonreflex* or *flaccid* bladder. This
type of bladder function is usually seen

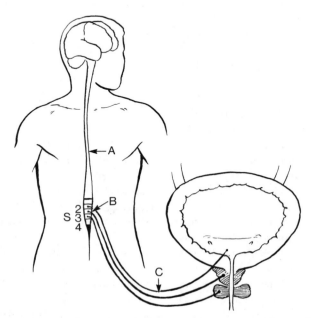

Fig. 10.10. Bladder and corresponding spinal segment innervations. Injuries at point *A* would result in
a UMN, or spastic bladder. Injuries at points *B* or *C*
would result in LMN, or flaccid, bladder function.
(Courtesy, Rehabilitation Institute of Michigan. Used
with permission.)

during the spinal shock phase and may remain if the injury has affected the cauda equina area. An injury at point B or C (Fig. 10.10) can result in an LMN bladder. With this type of injury, a reflexive emptying of the bladder cannot occur, as the reflex arc is destroyed. Since the bladder is flaccid and does not spontaneously empty, urine will accumulate continuously. Persons with an LMN bladder must catheterize according to a schedule and/or must apply external pressure to the abdomen with their fists, which forces urine from the bladder. This application of external pressure is called *Credé's technique*.

With either type of bladder (UMN or LMN), voiding must occur routinely and completely. Chronic overstretching of the bladder will reduce its ability to void adequately. Residual urine is a breeding ground for infections that can spread to all structures in the urinary system, including the ureters and kidneys. Chronic infections can lead to renal calculi (kidney stones) and, unfortunately, result in kidney failure and, potentially, death. Warning signs of a urinary tract infection include urine that appears cloudy or has excessive particles, dark or foul-smelling urine, an elevated fever, chills, or an increase in spasticity. The best treatment of UTI is prevention—adhering to an effective voiding schedule, using clean or sterile techniques, maintaining a proper diet and adequate fluid intake, and prompt attention to warning signs.

Complications Associated with the Bowel

Normally, elimination occurs when stool is present in the rectum. Nerves in the rectal musculature are stimulated, triggering a reflexive peristalsis and a relaxation of the rectal sphincters. A bowel movement may be prevented at this step of the process if the brain "overrides" this reflex, sending down an impulse to tighten the sphincter muscles until an appropriate time. We have all experienced the sensation of urgency caused by a full rectum, but perhaps we have not fully appreciated our brain's ability to allow us to forestall the inevitable until a socially acceptable time.

Unfortunately, a SCI can interfere with bowel function in much the same way as it impedes the bladder. The bowel can become spastic (also referred to as a reflex or UMN bowel) or flaccid (also called a nonreflex or LMN bowel).

A reflex bowel can be caused by a lesion at point A (Fig. 10.11). In this case, stool can be eliminated reflexively if nerves located in the rectum are stimulated. This stimulation may be done manually through digital stimulation, or in conjunction with the use of suppositories. Establishing and following a regular schedule for bowel management can often prevent incontinence.

The bowel is usually flaccid during the phase of spinal shock and may remain in that state if the injury involves the areas illustrated at points B and C (Fig. 10.10). As with the flaccid bladder, the flaccid bowel cannot be stimulated to empty reflexively. Stool may often remain in the rectum after attempts at evacuation, and it may be necessary to remove it manually to prevent impaction.

Constipation or impaction may result if elimination does not occur regularly. Aside from the standard discomfort associated with this, autonomic dysreflexia may be triggered in persons with lesions above the T6 level.

Diarrhea is another complication that can be particularly frustrating for the person with a SCI who is trying to establish a set schedule for bowel management. While this condition is also frustrating for the general population, they have the benefit of intact sensation to provide a warning. The best prevention for diarrhea is to make sure to appropriately use (not overuse) laxatives if they are prescribed, eat a proper diet, and follow a scheduled

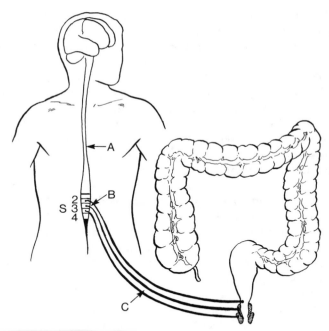

Fig. 10.11. The bowel and corresponding spinal segment innervations. Injuries at point *A* would result in a UMN, or spastic, bowel. Injuries at points *B* or *C* would result in LMN, or flaccid, bowel function. (Courtesy, Rehabilitation Institute of Michigan. Used with permission.)

bowel program that reduces the chance of impaction, which can result in diarrhea.

Dermal Complications

Your skin is the largest organ of your body, and it performs essential functions in maintaining your health. Skin assists in thermal regulation, insulating you in cold weather and sweating to prevent hyperthermia during hot conditions. Aside from literally keeping you together, skin acts as a barrier to the external environment. At the cellular level, skin provides the site for O_2/CO_2 exchange via the capillary system. Keeping skin intact is essential and requires conscious effort by a person with SCI, as sensations that would normally provide warning of potential skin damage—pain, extremes in temperature—are not perceived below the level of injury.

Damage to the skin as a result of pressure sores, or decubitus ulcers, are a major reason for hospital readmissions in SCI populations. The major cause, as the name implies, is continued pressure due to lack of movement. Circulation is impaired because of the pressure, and capillary exchange is impeded. This can result, rather quickly, in tissue necrosis. The severity of pressure sores can be classified in four stages.

Stage I. Clinical signs are reddened or darkened skin. Damage is limited to more superficial (epidermal and dermal) layers. At this stage, tissue breakdown can be halted merely by removing pressure until the skin returns to its normal color.

Stage II. The skin now appears reddened and open. A blister or scab formation is present. The scab is not a sign of healing; rather, the tissue beneath it is necrotic. This involves the epidermal and dermal layers, as well as deeper adipose tissue. Wound dressings may be involved at this stage, and it is imperative that pressure be kept off the site.

Stage III. The skin breakdown is deeper, and the wound is now draining. Muscle may be visible through the open wound. An ulcer is developing in the necrotic tissue. In addition to wound dressings, surgical intervention may be indicated if more conservative treatment is unsuccessful.

Stage IV. All structures, from the superficial levels to the bone, are destroyed. Infection and bone decay occur. Surgical intervention is likely, and the person with a pressure sore at this stage often must spend weeks after a skin graft with pressure totally removed from the involved site (11).

Pressure sores are preventable with diligent attention and preventive strategies. There are a variety of pressure relief methods that a person with SCI should use or instruct another person to assist with. Also, visual skin inspections should be performed at least twice daily, taking particular note of areas most prone to breakdown. These would include areas where bony prominences (e.g., the sacrum, ischium, calcanaeous, and scapula) can add to pressure. Proper nutrition should also be heeded, as healthy skin is less apt to break down and is more responsive to healing in early stages of pressure sore development.

Other dermal complications, such as burns or frostbite, are prevented by attentiveness and common sense. Even commonly encountered things, such as space heaters or exposed pipes under a sink, can cause severe burns to persons with SCI, without their immediate knowledge. Therefore, it is important to be aware and to rely on other, intact senses, to avoid injury.

See Appendix 10.3 for a list of common medications used to treat the complications described in this section.

PROGNOSIS

Providing a prognosis implies that one can forecast or predict the outcome and chances for recovery from a particular disease or traumatic injury. That is very difficult to do for spinal cord injuries. While there are aspects of SCI that are highly predictable (e.g., specific muscle functions impaired with a total lesion at C5), other aspects are much more vague.

Part of the ambiguity lies in the definitions of the term "recovery." One definition is to "get back," or regain. That definition tends to be the patient's focus. Another definition for "recover" stresses compensation, which tends to be the thrust for the health-care professional working with SCI. While we will discuss the physiologic prognosis of SCI, the clinician should always be aware of, and acknowledge the validity of, the patient's perspective of recovery. To "get back" and to "compensate for" are dramatically different. When discussing prognosis with a person who has survived a SCI, the clinician should always be truthful, but also be acutely aware of the impact of what the patient is hearing. Perhaps the most crucial indicators of a patient's functional outcome are personal characteristics such as motivation, use of support systems, and coping mechanisms. The clinician must be skilled at fostering these strengths while at the same time providing accurate information to the patient.

Physiologically, while there is extensive, ongoing research, there is currently no way to induce functional axonal regeneration within a damaged human spinal cord. Recent research headlines have reported that the use of steroids—specifically methylprednisolone—may improve neurologic outcomes of SCI persons if administered within the first 8 hours after injury (12). However, it remains to be seen whether these neurologic gains actually result in significant functional improvements for persons with SCI. Additional research efforts are being aimed at a variety of strategies, including pharmacologic and enzyme therapy, fetal tissue transplants, and the highly sophisticated altering of the cellular environment to encourage actual regeneration. As was stated earlier, the spinal cord is alive above and below the level of injury; one goal of current research is to encourage functional reconnection of the disrupted pathways.

A different picture is presented with cauda equina injuries or injuries involving the nerve root. You may recall that with these types of injuries, there is the potential for regeneration if the nerve roots are not severely damaged or divided. The degree of regeneration to expect is very difficult to predict, and prediction must be done on an individual basis after extensive medical testing.

Aside from research on actual spinal cord regeneration, there is also significant work being done with high-tech devices to compensate for paralysis. Functional electrical stimulation (FES) is one example. Persons with UMN injuries have experienced increases in their functional abilities (improved upper extremity function, standing ability, ambulation) with the external application of electrodes that stimulate muscle contraction. Although some may feel that FES apparatus is cumbersome, unsightly, time-consuming, and difficult to apply, refinements are ongoing. Many persons with SCI feel that, although not ideal, the technology provides an appealing alternative to outcomes from traditional methods of rehabilitation.

Overall, while actual regeneration of the cord does not appear to be on the immediate scientific horizon, there are promising advances in all phases of SCI management. Everyone has the right to hope for what is not yet reality, without being labeled as having "unrealistic expectations." Assisting someone to be hopeful, while simultaneously working to maximize today's function, is to truly master the art of the therapeutic relationship.

IMPACT ON OCCUPATIONAL PERFORMANCE

Occupational performance relates to a person's ability to engage in activities that are essential and meaningful to them. Occupational performance includes work activities, play or leisure activities, and activities of daily living. It should be apparent that a spinal cord injury can have a catastrophic effect on a person's ability to function in these areas, because a SCI can affect performance components that underlie the ability to participate in these activities. Occupational performance components relevant to SCI include sensory integration, and neuromuscular, motor, and psychosocial components. (See Table 10.4 for a quick summary of the occupational performance components affected by SCI.) The importance of understanding the theory of occupational performance cannot be overstated. We cannot begin to holistically treat a person with SCI until we can visualize the impact that this diagnosis has on the various aspects of life that are important for that person. The following sections explore occupational performance areas and components to present a comprehensive view of the impact of SCI.

Activities of Daily Living

Grooming, Oral Hygiene, Eating, Bathing, Dressing. For a person with quadriplegia, grooming, oral hygiene, and eating may be extremely laborious. The use of extensive adaptive devices or reliance on a caregiver may be required, because of deficits in sensory and neuromuscular performance components. Persons with paraplegia are generally independent in these tasks, but they must often "think ahead," making sure that items are available and sufficient time is allocated.

Bathing and dressing present major challenges for persons with quadriplegia. With higher-level injuries (C1–C4), total assistance is required. At lower levels of injury, with extensive adaptive equipment and assistance from others in some task components, the person with quadriplegia can be a more active participant. It is extremely important for the person's own goals to be acknowledged. A recent study revealed that a person with a complete C6 injury required from 20 to 60 minutes to dress independently (13). Yet none of the 10 patients in the study re-

Table 10.4.
Occupational Performance Components

Sensory Motor Component	Cognitive Integration & Cognitive Components	Psychosocial Skills & Psychologic Components
1. **Sensory integration**	1. Level of arousal	1. **Psychologic**
a. **Sensory awareness**	2. Orientation	a. **Roles**
b. **Sensory processing**	3. Recognition	b. Values
1. **Tactile**	4. Attention span	c. **Interests**
2. **Proprioceptive**	5. Memory	d. **Initiation of activity**
3. Vestibular	a. Short-term	e. **Termination of activity**
4. Visual	b. Long-term	f. **Self-concept**
5. Auditory	c. Remote	2. Social
6. Gustatory	d. Recent	a. Social conduct
7. Olfactory	6. Sequencing	b. Conversation
c. Perceptual skills	7. Categorization	c. Self-expression
1. **Stereognosis**	8. Concept formation	3. **Self-management**
2. **Kinesthesis**	9. Intellectual operations in space	a. **Coping skills**
3. **Body scheme**	10. Problem solving	b. **Time management**
4. Right-left discrimination	11. Generalization of learning	c. Self-control
5. Form constancy	12. Integration of learning	
6. Position in space	13. Synthesis of learning	
7. Visual-closure		
8. Figure ground		
9. Depth perception		
10. Topographic orientation		
2. **Neuromuscular**		
a. **Reflex**		
b. **Range of motion**		
c. **Muscle tone**	*Note*: All occupational performance areas are affected depending on degree on disability.	
d. **Strength**		
e. **Endurance**		
f. **Postural control**		
g. **Soft tissue integrity**		
3. **Motor**		
a. **Activity tolerance**		
b. **Gross motor coordination**		
c. **Crossing the midline**		
d. **Laterality**		
e. Bilateral integration		
f. Praxis		
g. **Fine motor coordination**		
h. Visual-motor integration		
i. Oral-motor control		

Table 10.4.   (Continued)
Occupational Performance Components

Occupational Performance Areas		
Activities of Daily Living	Work Activities	Play/Leisure Activities

1. Grooming
2. Oral hygiene
3. Bathing
4. Toilet hygiene
5. Dressing
6. Feeding and eating
7. Medication routine
8. Socialization
9. Functional communication
10. Functional mobility
11. Sexual expression
	1. Home management
	  a. Clothing care
	  b. Cleaning
	  c. Meal preparation and cleanup
	  d. Shopping
	  e. Money management
	  f. Household maintenance
	  g. Safety procedures
	2. Care of others
	3. Educational activities
	4. Vocational activities
	  a. Vocational exploration
	  b. Job acquisition
	  c. Work or job performance
	  d. Retirement planning
		1. Play or leisure exploration
		2. Play or leisure performance

ported dressing themselves routinely after discharge from the hospital. Assistance was sought from another person, due to feelings that the task was too time-consuming and exhausting. The question becomes, "Is this functional?" If a person is attempting reentry into the work force or return to school, is it "functional" to spend an entire hour, as well as all the physical energy, in just getting dressed? Or is it a greater sign of autonomy to delegate some tasks to a care-giver to allow participation in activities that are more meaningful?

Secondary conditions aside, persons with paraplegia are usually independent in bathing and dressing. Many even have the strength to transfer to the bottom of a tub without assistive devices.

Toileting. Managing altered bowel and bladder function is a challenge for virtually all SCI persons. There are two aspects to this challenge: the actual physiologic management and the various techniques and equipment used in the toileting process.

Medications may be required for physiologic management. Stool softeners are often used, as well as suppositories to assist in evacuation. A goal of effective bowel management is to eliminate reliance on medications. For persons with injuries at C7 or below, independence in toileting can usually be achieved with an array of equipment that may include: suppository inserters, digital stimulators (devices that trigger reflexes to relax the rectal sphincter in UMN injuries), catheterization devices, leg separators, mirrors, and adapted commode chairs that allow access to the perianal area for bowel-training procedures.

Aside from medications and equipment, additional strategies include maintaining a specific schedule for elimination, eating a healthy diet that promotes regularity, assuming positions that facilitate elimination, and the use of Crede's method. If toileting appears to be tiring, then it has been portrayed correctly! But many persons with SCI become adept at its management. It may be a very different picture, though, when a person attempts these procedures in a community environment (i.e., rest rooms at work, school).

The person with a higher-level cervical injury faces another scenario. Although the bowel- and bladder-management concepts are the same, neuromuscular deficits limit performance of the tasks, even with adaptive equipment. Generally, persons with injuries above the C6 level require a caregiver to perform functions such as suppository insertion, digital stimulation, catheterization, and general perianal care. The person with SCI must be the one to indicate who the care-giver is to be, particularly for tasks that are socially sensitive to them. Even though family members may be willing to assist, it is perfectly justifiable for the person to request someone else as a care-giver. Some persons may have no reservations about who assists them, while others may feel strongly that it would negatively affect established roles. Whatever the case, whenever feasible, the preferences of the person should be the decisive factor in selecting care-givers for various tasks.

Socialization and Functional Communication. In pure spinal cord injuries, there are no cognitive deficits that would preclude a person from socializing in an appropriate contextual manner. What is challenging, though, are a variety of barriers that may inhibit socialization. Architectural/environmental barriers, transportation barriers, reduced endurance, and increased reliance on others may discourage or actually prevent someone from traveling to the places where they socialized prior to their injury. Psychologic barriers may also prevent reintegration into a premorbid social support system, and these "barriers" are as real to overcome as physical ones.

In all but the highest of injuries, verbal communication is quite functional. Persons with injuries at C7 or below are generally independent with a variety of forms of communication (e.g., writing, keyboard use, phone use), without the use of adaptive equipment. Above this level, however, adaptive devices are needed.

Functional Mobility. Persons with complete injuries at the T3 level and above must usually rely on wheelchairs for household and community mobility. Persons with injuries at C6 or above may require additional assistance in wheelchair

management or may use an electric wheelchair with adapted controls. Acquisition of an electric wheelchair may depend not only on need but also on financial resources. Persons with complete injuries at T4 and below can often ambulate short distances with ambulation devices (walkers, Lofstrand crutches) and orthotic devices. Persons with sacral injuries can often ambulate community distances without orthoses or devices.

Frequently, it is not so much the ability or inability of the SCI person but the inaccessibility of the environment that limits functional mobility. While the home environment can be modified through creative thought, planning, and finances, the community environment is much harder to change. Many states have laws related to accessibility, but enforcement and compliance are less than ideal. Many physically challenged persons are fighting discriminatory situations (e.g., inaccessible public transportation, restaurants, offices, classrooms) in court. As they become more visible and numerous, increased legislation will be introduced to ensure their rights. A lighter side to inaccessibility was recalled recently by Ed Roberts, founder of the first Center for Independent Living. He reminisced that early protestors in the disability-rights movement were released from police custody . . . due to inaccessible paddy wagons and jail cells (13)! But, in the vast majority of situations, an inaccessible environment is frustrating, demeaning, and personally violating. The health-care team can do its part by helping physically, emotionally, or cognitively challenged persons to be aware of their rights, as well as by providing them with information on advocacy groups.

An extension of the functional mobility category includes driving. Occasionally, a strong C5-injured person may be able to drive with specially adapted low-effort steering, braking, and acceleration hand controls. Generally, though, persons with C5 level injuries and above cannot drive. Persons with C6 injuries and below can generally drive independently using conventional hand controls and adaptive devices. A van with an electric lift may be recommended for someone who has difficulty maneuvering a wheelchair in and out of a car or van. Again, finances, more than need, may dictate the type of transportation used.

Sexual Expression. As with bowel and bladder function, most persons with SCI experience alterations in their ability to perform sexually, as compared with their premorbid status. The nerves that innervate the genital area (both motor and sensory components) originate at the sacral spinal cord levels, so there are relatively few cases where sexual function is not affected.

For the most part, a variety of sexual activities can be participated in despite SCI, although the level of sensation and motor response will vary, depending on the extent and level of injury. Medications, surgical implants, and sexual enhancement devices may be recommended by specialists, but this is highly individualized.

Advances in the field of fertility have improved the chances for a spinal cord–injured male to father a child. Although fertility rates for men with SCI are estimated at less than 10% (15), techniques such as electrostimulation to induce ejaculation in paraplegics have proven successful in many cases (16). Men may be well-advised to delay a decision about surgical penile implants until at least 1 year postinjury. This allows time to evaluate the full impact of the spinal cord injury on sexual function and to determine the extent, if any, of sensory or motor return in an incomplete injury. The reproductive capabilities of women are generally unaltered by a SCI, and women and their partners should be made aware that the potential for pregnancy exists.

Addressing sexual function should be an integral part of each person's treatment plan, but a distinction should be made between purely physiologic sexual performance—arousal, orgasm, ejaculation—and sexuality, which is the totality of a person's attractiveness, personality, and self-perception as a sexual being. Sexuality does not have to rely on physiology. While performance may be hampered as a result of a SCI, one's sexuality can be quite healthy and intact. The health-care provider must make accurate information available and identify sources of more detailed information or expertise. It is entirely at the discretion of the person with a SCI to explore—or not explore—options available to them.

Work Activities

Home Maintenance. Tasks such as household maintenance, meal preparation, shopping, cleaning, clothing care, and safety procedures are included in the general category of home maintenance. Usually, persons with a C6-level injury or above require assistance with all of these activities and need some attendant care. Persons with injuries at C7 or lower can live independently (without attendant care) in accessible environments. Heavier home-maintenance tasks may be performed by others, but most routine activities can be accomplished with adaptive techniques/equipment.

Care of Others. A SCI can certainly make caring for others difficult, particularly if the injured person had been the primary care-giver for a child, spouse, or parent. While a major goal of persons with SCI is mastering self-care, a concurrent goal may be the introduction of activities (e.g., diapering, bathing a child) that can allow them to assume some premorbid roles. Often, many of these previous responsibilities must be delegated to others. In these cases, it is ideal if the person with SCI retains the responsibility for the verbal direction of care.

Education. Persons with SCI can generally resume educational activities, even while still inpatients in rehabilitation facilities. Many specialty hospitals retain the services of teachers from local school districts, and educational instruction is often scheduled along with other therapies for elementary, secondary, and high school students, which allows smoother reintegration after discharge.

College students would most likely be able to resume their studies. Depending on the level of injury, however, persons may reevaluate their course of study to prepare for a more feasible career.

Adaptive writing devices, page turners, tape recorders, and computers have made returning to the classroom less intimidating. Laws have also improved the accessibility of public buildings such as schools. It is challenging for the student to manage bowel and bladder schedules, adjustment of clothing, eating devices, and so forth, but with planning and the assistance of others if needed, many individuals have successfully returned to the classroom.

Vocation. It is appropriate for a person with any level of SCI to begin to formulate vocational options, even as an inpatient, with the members of the healthcare team. As individual situations are so variable—premorbid occupation, level of injury, educational level, other vocational interests, family support, cognitive abilities, motivation, financial resources—it is impossible to say definitively whether a person with a certain level of SCI can or cannot be gainfully employed. However, significant legislation mandates that work sites be accessible within reason. Additionally, many employers recognize the importance of a trained employee and will make additional accommodations to return a valued person to the workplace.

As we move from an industrial to an informational society, the jobs that will be increasingly available (and better compensated) are those that do not require the amount of menial labor as in the past. Job requirements for this "new society" will include analytical thought, problem solving, and creativity—all of which are certainly intact after a spinal cord injury!

Leisure Activities

For most people, leisure pursuits are an integral part of a meaningful life. While a SCI can alter the *way* in which one participates in leisure activities, it does not have to change the *intensity* of participation.

Sports, both individual and team, are excellent leisure pursuits that are growing in popularity for persons with SCI. Virtually any sport can be undertaken, from basketball to tennis to archery. True, adaptive equipment and modified regulations help make some sports more feasible and competitive for persons with SCI, but most athletes use "adaptive" equipment. How long would a catcher last in a hardball league without a mitt and a mask! The point is, adaptive equipment need not detract from the legitimacy of the contest. It is heartening to see that, even internationally, the wheelchair athlete is recognized for excellence, with designated events in the Olympic Games. Persons with SCI who want to participate have numerous avenues open to them.

Aside from sports, opportunities for social activities from square dancing to traveling abound. Travel agencies and tour groups have recognized the market created by the wheelchair traveler and have responded. Most hospitals with specialized SCI rehabilitation units have well-established programs that help persons get involved with special interest groups, which is an invaluable service. Often, during the acute phase of SCI, persons cannot envision themselves participating again in the things they enjoy. The healthcare professional must be available for these persons and encourage any renewed interest in their favorite pastimes.

There are a number of resources related to leisure activities and other issues discussed in this chapter. The reader is encouraged to consult the References and Suggested Readings at the end of this chapter for more information. Additionally, Table 10.5 gives an overview of spe-

Table 10.5.
Expected Functional Outcomes of Various Levels of Complete Injury (noninclusive)[a]

Last Spinal Cord Level Intact (spared)	Expected Functional Outcomes
C1–C3	• Requires 24-hour availability of caregiver • Generally ventilator-dependent • Requires maximal assistance of another for pressure relief, or requires an adapted switch and power reclining chair • May propel power chair independently with adapted switches (pneumatic, chin, head, mouthstick); requires maximal assistance for set-up • Maximal assistance needed for transfers, positioning, bed mobility, dressing, feeding, hygiene, grooming and bowel/bladder care • Dependent with driving
C4	• Requires 24-hour availability of caregiver • Generally off ventilator; continued difficulty with productive coughing and deep breathing • Pressure relief, wheelchair propulsion, transfers, bed mobility, dressing, hygiene, bowel/bladder care and driving comparable to C1–C3 level • Adaptive feeding and grooming devices are available, but are very time-consuming and exhaustive for a person at this level and generally do not result in task independence
C5	• May require 24-hour availability of caregiver • Decreased respiratory endurance, but off ventilator • A strong person with a C5 injury may be independent in pressure relief by leaning side to side; a weaker person may require maximal assistance • Independent on level surfaces with a power chair and occasionally wrist/forearm supports. A manual wheelchair with rim adaptations may be used by a strong person for short distances. • Moderate to maximal assistance is required for all transfers, and generally a sliding board is used. Moderate assistance is also required for bed mobility • A strong person with a C5 injury may assist with some dressing, hygiene and grooming activities with the aid of adapted equipment. Feeding is generally possible with the use of adapted utensils and set-up • Driving is generally not feasible at this level, but an exceptionally strong person may be able to drive with specially-adapted steering, braking, and acceleration hand controls
C6	• Amount of assistance needed from another person varies from moderate to very limited with just a few specific activities • Some decrease in respiratory capacity and productive cough • Has potential for independence in pressure relief • Independently uses a manual wheelchair on level surfaces, gradual inclines and down a curb backwards. May require an electric chair for long distances or rough terrain • Ability to transfer varies. Some strong persons with C6 injuries are able to transfer independently with the use of a sliding board to a car, chair, bed, commode, or tubseat • Has the potential for independent bed mobility and positioning with rails, power controls, and trapeze • With some adapted devices, usually independent with hygiene, shaving, and grooming. Potential for independence in bathing and bowel/bladder care with equipment. Generally independent with U.E. dressing, and potential for independence in L.E. dressing with adaptive devices. Independent with feeding, although a wrist-hand orthosis (W.H.O.) and set-up may be required • Generally able to drive independently using hand controls and adaptive devices

Table 10.5. **(Continued)**
Expected Functional Outcomes of Various Levels of Complete Injury (Noninclusive)[a]

Last Spinal Cord Level Intact (Spared)	Expected Functional Outcomes
C7–C8	• May be able to live independently without attendent care • Some decreased respiratory endurance • Independent in pressure relief • Independently uses manual wheelchair • Generally able to transfer without a sliding board. Very strong persons may be able to transfer to the floor and tub bottom independently • Generally independent with positioning, bed mobility, hygiene, feeding, shaving, hair care, dressing, bathing, cooking and light housekeeping (Independent with bowel/bladder care using adaptive equipment/techniques) • Drives independently with hand controls/steering adaptations • Can stand in parallel bars once assisted to upright, with the use of knee-ankle-foot orthoses (K.A.F.O.'s)
T1–T3	• Can live independently • Respiratory capacity and coughing abilities significantly improved • All transfers generally independent • Independent with all self-care. May require assistance with heavy household cleaning • Finger dexterity, strength, and coordination is functional • Drives independently with hand controls. Can get own wheelchair in and out of car • Able to stand with minimal assistance, K.A.F.O.'s and use of walker or parallel bars. Ambulation is generally not practical due to reduced balance and high energy expenditure
T4–T8	• Can live independently • Respiratory status stronger than T1–T3 level; only slightly decreased • Pressure relief, wheelchair use, positioning, bed mobility, and self-care all independent. May continue to require assistance with heavy cleaning • Driving: comparable to T1–T3 level • Generally able to ambulate short distances with the use of a walker or Loftstrand crutches and K.A.F.O.'s. Can stand independently with the use of a walker. May be able to manage curbs or stairs, but generally requires assistance. Ambulation requires high energy output
T9–T12	• Respiration is functional • Pressure relief, wheelchair use, transfers, positioning, bed mobility, self-care, homemaking (except heavy tasks) all independent • Able to drive with hand controls • Can generally ambulate short community distances with K.A.F.O.'s and Loftstrand crutches
L1–L3	• Same as T9–T12 level with the addition of improved ambulation distances. A wheelchair may still be required for long distances
L4–L5	• Same as above, with exceptions – Driving independent without adaptive devices – Generally able to ambulate with ankle-foot orthoses (A.F.O.'s) and canes – Wheelchairs generally not needed
S1–S2	•A person with an S2 spared injury has the potential to ambulate without devices or orthoses. A wheelchair is not required. Hip extensors/abductors, knee flexors and ankle plantar flexors are weak at the S1 level of injury. As with all other preceeding levels, bowel and bladder function is impaired; but managed independently at this level through adapted devices/techniques

[a](Developed from material compiled courtesy of the Rehabilitation Institute of Michigan. Used with permission.)

CASE STUDY

M.L. is a 19-year-old woman who sustained a spinal cord injury during a motor vehicle accident while on her honeymoon. Her husband was thrown from the vehicle but received only minor injuries. M.L. was transported by EMS to the local ER. She was diagnosed with a C5-6 vertebral subluxation and a C6 crush injury, resulting in a complete C6 spinal cord injury. She also sustained a left clavicular fracture. She received nasal O_2 for respiratory support. Once stabilized, she was transferred to the specialized trauma center near her home. A halo vest was applied, which stabilized her cervical spine. There was no indication for operative procedures at that time. After 22 days, her endurance improved so that she could tolerate sitting upright in a chair for up to 1 hour. She was transferred to the nearby rehabilitation facility's spinal cord injury unit. During her 12 weeks in the rehabilitation facility, the only complications she experienced were two episodes of autonomic hyperreflexia (ap-

parently secondary to hard stool in the lower rectum) and a mild UTI. Spasticity developed in her wrists, elbows, and lower extremities.

Prior to her injury, M.L. was a college student in a liberal arts curriculum. She and her new husband had recently signed a 1-year lease on an upstairs apartment close to the university. She had been totally independent in all of her ADL and home-management activities. Her leisure pursuits included recreational team sports (particularly softball) and more sedentary activities like reading and gourmet cooking. She was also quite involved with her family, particularly two sisters and her parents, who live close by.

Many occupational performance components are significantly affected by M.L.'s injury (Table 10.6). Her sensory-motor deficits are consistent with those anticipated for a C6 complete quadriplegia.

M.L. is challenged by the psychosocial/psychologic issues facing her as a result of her SCI. She feels that her role has changed significantly, especially in her relationship with her husband. He has been quite willing to assist her in those activities where she is physically limited; however, his assistance in some activities—particularly bowel management—has been difficult for her to accept. This has been a source of

Table 10.6.
Occupational Performance Deficit Profile (M.L.)

	Work Activities			
	Vocation	Education	Home Management	Care of Others
SENSORY INTEGRATION	X	X	X	X
NEURO-MUSCULAR	X	X	X	X
MOTOR	X	X	X	X
PSYCHOLOGIC	X	X	X	X
SOCIAL				
SELF-MANAGEMENT	X	X	X	X

EXTERNAL FACTORS WHICH INFLUENCE PERFORMANCE; CULTURE, ECONOMY, ENVIRONMENT

Grid adapted from Uniform Terminology (2nd ed.) Developed by the occupational therapy faculty at Eastern Michigan University.

frustration for her, and she has discussed with him the possibility of hiring an attendant on a limited basis to assist with specific activities. He resists this idea, stating that it is his desire and duty to care for her. He took a temporary leave of absence from the family-owned landscaping company where he is employed when she was discharged 2 weeks ago. There is no definitive timetable for his return. M.L. is also concerned about her ability to express herself sexually as well as her potential to have children in the future. She attended classroom sessions on these topics in the rehabilitation facility, but she did not seek any individual counseling. M.L. states that she probably wasn't ready to hear anything specific then, but she now wishes she had someone with whom she was comfortable asking questions.

M.L. has not begun to consider her work activities or return to school. Even before her accident, she had been undecided about a career path. She has expressed interest, however, in exploring her possible alternatives.

M.L. has stated that eventually she might like to get involved in team sports again. In the 2 weeks since her discharge, though, her main leisure pursuits have been reading and watching television.

REFERENCES

1. Guttmann L. Spinal cord injuries. Oxford, England: Blackwell Scientific, 1976.
2. Heir D. Personal communication, July 6, 1990.
3. Hanak M, Scott A. Spinal cord injury: an illustrated guide for health care professionals. New York: Springer Publishing, 1983.
4. Austin G. The spinal cord, 3rd ed. New York: Igaku-Shoin, 1983:28–42.
5. Kraus JF. Epidemiological aspects of acute SCI: a review of incidence, prevalence, causes and outcome. Central Nervous System Trauma Status Report. Bethesda, MD: National Institute of Neurological and Communicative Disorders and Stroke, National Institute of Health, 1985:313–322.
6. Yashon D. Spinal injury 2nd ed. East Norwalk, CT: Appleton-Century-Crofts, 1986:35–36.
7. Bloch RF, Basbaum M. Management of spinal cord injuries. Baltimore: Williams & Wilkins, 1983:153–154.
8. Hanak M, Scott A. Spinal cord injury: an illustrated guide for health care professionals. New York: Springer Publishing, 1983:30.

| Play or Leisure Activities | | Activities of Daily Living | | | | |
Exploration	Performance	Self-Care	Socialization	Functional Communication	Functional Mobility	Sexual Expression
	X	X		X	X	X
	X	X		X	X	X
	X	X		X	X	X
X	X	X	X			X
X	X	X	X			X

9. Burke DC, Murray DD. Handbook of spinal cord medicine. New York: Raven Press, 1975:67.
10. Hernandez AM, Fjorner JV, DeLaFuente T, Gonzalez C, Miro R. The paraarticular ossifications in our paraplegics and tetra-plegics: a survey of 704 patients. Paraplegia 1978;16:272–275.
11. Cassell BL. Treating pressure sores stage by stage. RN, 1986;49:36.
12. Bracken M, Holeord TR, Shepard MJ, Young W, Collins WE, Baskin DS, et al. A randomized, controlled trial of methylprednisolone or naloxone in the treatment of acute spinal cord injury. N Engl J Med 1990;322(20):1405–1411.
13. Weingarden S, Martin C. Independent dressing after spinal cord injury: a functional time evaluation. Arch Phys Med Rehabil 1989;70:518–519.
14. Price D. "Building Lives With No Barriers," Detroit News Washington Bureau, March 18, 1990, pp 17–23A.
15. Berczeller PH, Bezkor MF. Medical complications of quadriplegia. Chicago: Year Book Medical Publishers, 1986:165.
16. Perkash I, Martin D, Warner H, Speck V. Electroejaculation in spinal cord injury patients: simplified new equipment and technique. J Urol 1990;143:305–307.

Suggested Readings

General Texts Relating to SCI

Berczeller PH, Bezkor MF. Medical complications of quadriplegia. Chicago: Yearbook Medical Publishers, 1986.

Buchanan LE, Nawoczenski DA. Spinal cord injury: concepts and management. Baltimore: Williams & Wilkins, 1987.

Ozer MN. The management of persons with spinal cord injury. New York: Demos Publications, 1988.

Treischmann R. Spinal cord injuries: psychological, social and vocational rehabilitation, 2nd ed. New York: Demos Publications, 1988.

Whiteneck G, Lammertse D, Manley S, Menter R, Adler C, Wilmot C. et al. The management of high quadriplegia. New York: Demos Publications, 1989.

Yashon D. Spinal injury, 2nd ed. East Norwalk, CT: Appleton-Century-Crofts, 1986.

Patient/Family Resources

Corbet B. Options: spinal cord injury and the future. Denver: A.B. Hirschfield, 1980.

Hammond M, Umlauf RL, Matteson B, Fulginiti SP. Yes you can! A guide to self care for persons with spinal cord injury. Washington, D.C.: Paralyzed Veterans of America, 1989.

Phillips L, Ozer A, Axelson P, Chizeck H. Spinal cord injury: a guide for patient and family. New York: Raven Press, 1987.

General Neuroanatomy

Barr ML. The human nervous system: an anatomic viewpoint, 3rd ed. New York: Harper & Row, 1979.

Liebman M. Neuroanatomy made easy and understandable, 3rd ed. Rockville, MD: Aspen Publishers, 1986.

FES

Kralj A, Bajd T. Functional electrical stimulation: standing and walking after spinal cord injury. Boca Raton: CRC Press, 1989.

Glossary

Afferent: In the nervous system, a nerve that transmits impulses from the periphery toward the central nervous system (sensory).

Autonomic dysreflexia (hyperreflexia): An uninhibited and exaggerated reflex of the autonomic nervous system to stimulation. The response occurs in about 85% of all patients who have spinal cord injury above the level of the sixth thoracic vertebra. It is potentially dangerous because of attendant vasoconstriction and immediate elevation of blood pressure, which in turn can bring about hemorrhagic retinal damage or cerebrovascular accident. Less serious effects include severe headache, changes in heart rate, sweating and flushing above the level of the spinal cord injury, and pallor and "goose bumps" below that level.

Bradycardia: Slowness of the heartbeat, as evidenced by slowing of the pulse rate to less than 60 beats per minute.

Catheterization: Passage of a catheter into a body channel or cavity, especially introduction of a catheter via the urethra into the urinary bladder.

Cauda equina: ("Horse's tail") the collection of dorsal and ventral nerve roots descending from the lower spinal cord and occupying the vertebral canal below the cord at the L1 region.

Crede's method: A technique for manual expression of urine from the bladder, used in bladder training for individuals with paralysis. The hands are held flat against the abdomen, just below the umbilicus. A firm downward stroke toward the bladder is repeated 6 or 7 times, followed by pressure from both hands placed directly over the bladder to manually remove all urine.

Contralateral: Pertaining to, situated on, or affecting the opposite side.

Cryogenic: Producing low temperatures.

Decubitus ulcers: An ulcer due to local interference with the circulation, usually occurring over a bony prominence at the sacrum, hip (trochanter), heel, shoulder, or elbow. It begins as a reddened area and can quickly involve deeper structures and become an ulcer; also called bedsore and pressure sore. Persons most at risk for the development of decubitus ulcers are those who are emaciated, obese, or immobilized by traction or some other form of enforced immobility, and those who have diabetes mellitus or some type of circulatory disorder. Because urine and feces contribute to skin breakdown, incontinent patients are at high risk for pressure sores. Two major factors in their development are prolonged pressure on a part due to the weight of the body or an extremity, and a shearing force that exerts downward and forward pressure on tissues beneath the skin. The shearing action can occur when a patient slides downward while sitting in a bed or chair, or when bedclothes are forcibly pulled from under a patient.

Diaphoresis: Perspiration, especially profuse perspiration.

Efferent: In the nervous system, a nerve that conducts impulses away from the central nervous system toward the periphery (motor).

Ectopic bone: Bone that is situated elsewhere than in the normal place.

Fasciculus: Fascicle, a small bundle or cluster, especially of nerve or muscle fibers. Fasciculus, a tract or pathway in the nervous system.

Flaccid: Paralysis of muscles in which there is an absence of reflexes (in lower motor neuron disorders such as poliomyelitis).

Heterotopic ossification: The formation of bone in soft tissue and periarticular locations. Early clinical signs include warmth, swelling, pain, and decreased joint motion. Common joints for HO are the shoulder, elbow, hip, and knee.

Hyperreflexia: Exaggeration of reflexes during standard stretch of a muscle.

Ipsilateral: Pertaining to, situated on, or affecting the same side.

Lemniscus: A band or bundle of nerve fibers in the central nervous system; also called a tract or pathway.

Nonreflex neurogenic bladder or bowel: Also called autonomic bladder/bowel. A neurogenic bladder/bowel due to a lesion or injury in the sacral portion of the spinal cord that interrupts the reflex arc that controls the bladder/bowel. The lesion may be in the cauda equina, conus medullaris, sacral roots, or pelvic nerve. It is marked by loss of normal bladder/bowel sensations and reflex activity, inability to initiate urination/elimination normally, and stress incontinence.

Paraplegia: Paralysis of the legs and, in some cases, the lower part of the body due to central nervous system paralysis affecting all of the muscles of the parts involved.

Peristalsis: The wormlike movement by which the alimentary canal or other tubular organs with both longitudinal and circular muscle fibers propel their contents, consisting of a wave of contraction passing along the tube.

Poikilothermy: The state of having body temperature that varies with that of the environment (e.g., cold-blooded). The body tends to assume the temperature of the external environment for at least 1 year postinjury in a spinal cord injury.

Proprioception: Interpretation of stimuli originating in muscles, joints, and other internal tissues that give information about the position of one body part in relation to another. Perception is mediated by sensory nerve endings chiefly in muscles, tendons, and the labyrinth.

Quadriplegia: Paralysis of all four limbs (e.g., tetraplegia).

Reflex arc: A reflex is the total of any particular automatic response mediated by the nervous system, which is built in and does not need conscious thought to take effect. A reflex arc is usually a simple reflex such as a knee jerk, which involves only two nerves and one synapse. Other arcs may involve an interneuron. When the sensory nerve ending is stimulated, a nerve impulse travels along a sensory (afferent) neuron to the spinal cord. An association neuron or interneuron then transfers the impulse to a motor (efferent) neuron, which carries the impulse to a muscle, which then contracts and moves a body part.

Reflex neurogenic bladder or bowel: Also called autonomic or spastic bladder/bowel. A neurogenic bladder/bowel due to complete resection of the spinal cord above the sacral segments, marked by complete loss of micturition reflexes, violent voiding or eliminating, and an abnormal amount of residual urine/feces.

Scoliosis: Lateral curvature of the vertebral column. This deviation of the normally straight vertical line of the spine may or may not include rotation or deformity of the vertebrae.

Spasticity: Hypertension of muscles; the result of an upper motor neuron lesion.

Spina bifida: A defect of the vertebral column involving imperfect union of the paired vertebral arches at the midline; it may be so extensive as to allow herniation of the spinal cord and meninges, which may or may not be covered by intact skin.

Spinal shock: Result of an acute transverse lesion of the spinal cord that causes immediate flaccid paralysis and loss of all sensation and reflex activity (including autonomic functions) below the level of injury. On return of reflex activity, there is increased spasticity of muscles and exaggerated tendon reflexes.

Tachycardia: Abnormally rapid heart rate, usually over 100 beats per minute.

Thrombus: An aggregation of blood factors, primarily platelets and fibrin with entrapment of cellular elements, frequently causing vascular obstruction at the point of its formation and resultant medical problems such as stroke.

APPENDIX **10.2**

Common Test Procedures

Procedure	Purpose
Intravenous pyelogram (IVP)	Detects calculus formation or obstruction in kidneys, ureters, or bladder
Cystourethrogram	Determines (*a*) bladder capacity, (*b*) urine reflux, (*c*) urethral urine flow
Cystogram	Illustrates size of bladder and whether reflux is present
Cystometrogram (CMG)	Determines (*a*) bladder capacity, (*b*) degree of sensation intact, (*c*) degree of voluntary control over voiding
Sphincter electromyogram	Determines coordination of bladder contraction/sphincter relaxation during voiding
Urethral pressure profile (UPP)	Measures urethral pressure. To maintain continence, there must be a level of contraction in the urethral muscle fibers; for urination, the urethral muscle fibers must relax
Urinalysis	Laboratory studies of urine that determine (*a*) pH, (*b*) protein level, (*c*) glucose level, (*d*) the presence of blood or pus
Myelography	Determines structural changes in the spinal canal
Doppler testing	Determines adequacy of blood flow to extremities; may be used to diagnose deep vein thromboses
Computerized axial tomography	Provides serial pictures of sections of the spinal cord and surrounding structures
Roentgenogram	Illustrates the type and degree of vertebral displacement
Pulmonary function studies	Evaluate general condition of the lungs, as well as inhalation/exhalation volumes
Electromyography (EMG)	Records electrical activity brought about in a muscle by the stimulation of its innervating nerve; aids in diagnosing the type and extent of a lesion

Medications

Generic Name	Brand Name	Action	Indication	Potential Side Effects	Usual Adult Dose and Availability
Trimethoprim & sulfamethoxzole	Bactrim Septra	Antibacterial	Treatment of severe or complicated urinary tract infections	Early signs of serious reactions may include rash, sore throat, fever, cough, jaundice, arthralgia, shortness of breath, nausea, diarrhea, and/or headaches	Prescription
Phenoxybenzamine hydrochloride	Dibenzyline	Relaxes bladder sphincter/urethra; α-receptor blocking agent	Aids in complete bladder emptying; helps prevent autonomic hyperreflexia	Hypotension, nasal congestion, GI irritation, loose stool	Prescription
Bethanechol	Urecholine	Cholinergic, increases bladder tone	Induces spontaneous voiding; aids in bladder	Sweating, hypotension, headache, loose stool,	Prescription

Generic name	Brand name	Action	Use	Side effects	Availability
Oxybutynin chloride, phenobarbitol, hyoscyamine sulfate imipramine hydrochloride	Ditropan Donnatal Tofranil	Relaxes spastic bladder	contraction reducing urine residuals	nausea, flushing	Prescription
Docusate sodium	Colace	Laxative: stool softener	Helps prevent urinary accidents between intermittent catheterizations or nocturnally	Dry mouth, drowsiness, constipation, blurred vision	OTC
Casanthranol & docusate sodium	Peri-Colace	Mild stimulant laxative combined with stool softener	Augments bowel training program; aids passage of stool	Bitter taste, throat irritation, nausea	OTC
Bisacodyl	Dulcolax	Laxative: stimulates sensory nerve endings in the bowel to produce evacuation of stool	Augments bowel training program	Nausea, abdominal cramping, diarrhea, and rash are among rare side effects reported	OTC
Psyllium hydrophilic mucilloid	Metamucil	Laxative: bulk-forming natural fiber	Augments bowel training program; management of constipation	As with other laxatives	OTC
			Management of constipation	Contraindicated in person with intestinal obstruction or	OCT

Generic Name	Brand Name	Action	Indication	Potential Side Effects	Usual Adult Dose and Availability
				fecal impaction	
Magnesium hydroxide	Milk of magnesia	Laxative: increases intestinal mobility	Management of constipation, acid indigestion, heartburn, and sour stomach	Possible interaction with prescription drugs; should not be taken if abdominal pain, nausea, or vomiting persist	OTC
Diazepam	Valium	Appears to act on parts of limbic calming effects	Relief of skeletal muscle spasm due to upper motor neuron disorders	Common side effects include drowsiness, fatigue, and ataxia	Prescription
Sodium bicarbonate, potassium bitartrate	Ceo-Two	Rectal suppository that melts to form CO_2, which builds up pressure in the rectum and lower bowel, causing peristalsis or reflex evacuation	Augments bowel training program	As with other laxatives	OTC
Dantrolene sodium	Dantrium	Produces skeletal muscle	Treatment of debilitating spasticity	Potential for hepatotoxicity; common side	Prescription

Generic	Trade	Action	Use	Side effects	Availability
		relaxation		effects include drowsiness, weakness, dizziness, general malaise, fatigue, and diarrhea	
Baclofen	Lioresal	Muscle relaxant and antispastic	Helpful in alleviating signs and symptoms of spasticity	More common potential side effects include drowsiness, dizziness, weakness, and fatigue	Prescription
Prazosin hydrochloride	Minipress	Antihypertensive; causes a decrease in total peripheral resistance	Helpful in managing symptoms associated with autonomic hyperreflexia	May cause syncope with a LOC, lightheadedness, dizziness, tachycardia	Prescription
Hydralazine hydrochloride	Apresoline	Antihypertensive; appears to lower blood pressure via relaxation of vascular smooth muscle	Helpful in managing symptoms associated with autonomic hyperreflexia	Common side effects include headache, anorexia, nausea, vomiting, diarrhea, palpitations, tachycardia, and angina pectoris	Prescription
Etidronate disodium	Didronel	Prevents/retards	Indicated in the	No specific adverse	Prescription

Generic Name	Brand Name	Action	Indication	Potential Side Effects	Usual Adult Dose and Availability
		heterotopic ossification; modifies the crystal growth of calcium hydroxy-apatite; also slows the rate of bone turnover	prevention of heterotopic ossification due to spinal cord injury	effects; rare reports of angioedema/urticaria, rash, and/or pruritis	
Heparin sodium	Heparin	Inhibits blood clotting	Indicated in the prevention of deep vein thromboses	Possibility of hemorrhage at virtually any site in patients receiving heparin; potential also exists for local irritation,	Prescription

					Prescription
Methylpred-nisolone	Medrol	Corticosteroid: antiinflam-matory effect; in addition, modifies the body's immune responses to many stimuli	When initiated in the acute phase (within 8 hours posttrauma) it improves neurologic outcomes in SCI	chills, fever, vomiting, headache, and additional, rarer complications May cause a variety of adverse reactions, including but not limited to: fluid retention, muscle weakness, osteoporosis, peptic ulcers, convulsions, vertigo, headaches, CHF, HTN	

11

Adjustment Disorders

ELIZABETH FRANCIS-CONNOLLY

In the present age of psychiatry there is a strong basis for a biological frame of reference. Recognition of the brain as a complex biochemical organ, with multiple anatomical and biochemical networks playing a role in behavior, is a key concept within this orientation. Researchers and clinicians maintain interest in the question of whether psychiatric illnesses such as schizophrenia are organic diseases with underlying physical brain pathology (1). Unfortunately, the diagnostic criteria for adjustment disorder (Table 11.1), as compared with other DSM-III-R axis I categories such as schizophrenia and mood disorders, does not seem to fit this frame of reference as nicely.

Clinicians have long recognized the usefulness of this category, but very little systematic investigation has been undertaken, and the literature is restricted to only a handful of studies. In the past, the category of adjustment disorder was seen by some empirically oriented researchers studying adolescents as a catch-all category (2). One group noted that adjustment disorder is related to social and environmental influences that could be seen in other diagnoses and with non-ill people (3). Such situational factors remain vague as they are difficult to conceptualize and measure (4). Other researchers consider it to have face validity (5), confirming many clinicians' contention that, at the very least, it is useful in describing behavioral response to stress.

Adjustment disorder refers to short-term disturbances of nonpsychotic proportions that are provoked by an explicit stressor or stressors. This diagnosis is most commonly used with patients who exhibit a variety of emotional and behavioral symptoms in response to a stressful event or events but without enough symptoms to warrant a more severe diagnosis (such as a mood disorder or an anxiety disorder). Adjustment disorder carries a less negative connotation and has been used as a provisional or residual diagnosis reflecting reluctance and optimism. This benign diagnosis is often used with younger individuals and those first presenting in a mental health facility. The following case study of an adolescent with multiple diagnoses illustrates the difficulty in conceptualizing this category.

J.H. is a 14-year-old boy who was referred to the Department of Social Services via the courts. He is the eldest of three children whose parents appeared to have a solid marriage until recently. Father is an alcoholic who was dry for most of J.H.'s childhood, though 3 months previous, the father lost his job and started drinking again. The father's behavior is now quite unpredictable; he is moody with angry outbursts at his wife and children, and he is often absent from the home for long periods of time. The mother has responded by working at her job for longer hours and withdrawing to her room when at home. It has been made clear to J.H.

Table 11.1.
Diagnostic Criteria for Adjustment Disorder[a]

A. A reaction to an identifiable psychosocial stressor (or multiple stressors) that occurs within three months of onset of the stressor(s).
B. The maladaptive nature of the reaction is indicated by either of the following:
   1. Impairment in occupational performance (including school) Functioning or in usual social activities or relationships with others
   2. Symptoms in excess of a normal and expectable reaction to the stressor(s)
C. The disturbance is not merely one instance of a pattern of overreaction to stress or an exacerbation of one of the mental disorders previously described.
D. The maladaptive reaction has persisted for no longer than six months.
E. The disturbance does not meet the criteria for any specific mental disorder and does not represent Uncomplicated Bereavement.

[a]Reprinted with permission: American Psychiatric Association, Diagnostic and Statistical Manual of Mental Disorders, Third Edition, Revised. Washington, D.C.: APA 1987.

that he is expected to care for his two younger sisters after school and take on most of the daily housekeeping chores. J.H., though not an outstanding student, always maintained average grades and kept up with his homework. He enjoyed playing Nintendo with his friends and soccer. Within the past few months, his grades have noticeably declined, and he is loud and disruptive in classes. He was caught stealing in a local video store on two occasions, and the second time the store owners pressed charges.

The initial screening at the Department of Social Services showed that J.H. was angry, experienced difficulty controlling behavior, and was often sarcastic to the interviewer. He was unable to devise ways to help himself with his current situation, nor could he identify goals for himself. He felt his parents were not supportive of him and felt unable to cope with all of his new responsibilities. Current diagnosis for J.H. is adjustment disorder, rule out character disorder.

ETIOLOGY

The central cause of an adjustment disorder is the experiencing of one or more stressors. The severity of a reaction is not completely predictable from the intensity of the stressor(s) (2) and does not necessarily correlate with the severity of the adjustment disorder (6). However, the in-

dividual's overall reaction to these stressors is considered maladaptive and, with adolescents, can include a behavioral response typified by acting out. The response, in turn, has an impact upon the individual's ability to function in social or occupational arenas.

The term stressor is vague because stress is a part of life, and each individual's response to stress varies depending on a variety of factors, such as culture, age, personality, and available support systems (6). Woolston noted the importance of looking at the patient's age, gender, and coping mechanisms. He felt that women were more resilient in stressful situations than men (7). There may be a single stressor (e.g., the ending of a relationship) or multiple stressors (e.g., failing health and the loss of a job). Stress may be recurrent (e.g., experiences in dysfunctional families) or continual (e.g., chronic illness). Developmental life stages such as leaving home, getting married, having a child, and retiring may all be associated with an adjustment disorder (6). When faced with a stressful situation, some individuals will withdraw, some will respond with humor or dismay, and others will lash out with anger. In the following excerpt, each response is characteristic of that individual's long-standing pattern or mode of perceiving and relating to the world.

Destiny came down to an island centuries ago and summoned three of its inhabitants before him. "What would you do," asked Destiny, "if you were told that tomorrow this island will be completely inundated by an immense tidal wave?"

The first man, who was a cynic, said, "Why I would eat, drink, carouse, and make love all night long." The second man who was a mystic, said, "I would go to the sacred grove with my loved ones and make sacrifices to the gods and pray without ceasing." And the third man who loved reason, thought a while, confused and troubled, and said, "Why, I would assemble our wisest men and begin at once to study how to live under water!" (8)

All of these individual coping responses are attempts to integrate environmental information from a pending uncontrollable event into a meaningful cognitive procedure (action program) that attempts to regain or maintain control (9). Although the first two individuals would very likely perish when the tidal wave comes, they are showing coping behavior by at least maintaining illusory control over the situation via acceptable defense mechanisms (10). Control or the illusion of control can modify the impact of stressful events. If there is an imbalance between situational requirements (task demands) and available personal resources (intellectual or emotional capacity), there is decreased control over the outcome with changes in anxiety, arousal, and/or performance levels (11).

INCIDENCE AND PREVALENCE

Adjustment disorders seem to be relatively common, though the few studies available do not always support one another and there are sparse data on the incidence and prevalence of this disorder. A 1982 study found that approximately 5% of all inpatients of an urban psychiatric hospital were diagnosed with adjustment disorder; the estimate for outpatients was even higher (4). Another study, at the Western Psychiatric Institute and Clinic,

found an even higher incidence of adjustment disorders. This study looked at the diagnoses of all new patients over a 4-year period and found that 10% were diagnosed with adjustment disorder (12).

In looking at the male/female ratio, two studies contradict each other. The Western Psychiatric Institute and Clinic study found that adjustment disorders occur more frequently in females, 12.2% versus 9.5% of all male patients. A smaller study found that almost 70% of patients with adjustment disorders were males (3). When examined by age, 16.3% of all patients 18 years old or younger were diagnosed with adjustment disorder, 10% of all the 19- to 59-year-old patients, and only 3% of those 60 years and older (12). Two other studies found that 29% and 12.5%, respectively, of adolescent patients were diagnosed with adjustment disorders (13, 14). All three of these studies indicate a much higher incidence of adjustment disorder in adolescence. Clinicians may be more likely to use this diagnostic category with the younger patient population because adolescents do not have fully developed or adequate coping mechanisms and because adjustment disorder is a less damaging label.

SIGNS AND SYMPTOMS

The *Diagnostic and Statistical Manual of Mental Disorders*, 3rd ed., revised (DSM-III-R) defines adjustment disorder as a maladaptive response to one or more stressors that occur within three months after the stressful event (15). (See Table 11.1 for diagnostic criteria.) The signs and symptoms vary and are coded according to the predominant symptom. The following list describes the nine different categories of adjustment disorder and their associated essential features.

1. **Adjustment disorder with depressed mood** Essential features: depressed mood, feelings of hopelessness, helplessness, and tearfulness
2. **Adjustment disorder with anxious mood**

Essential features: worry, agitation, nervousness
3. **Adjustment disorder with mixed emotional features** Essential features: a combination of emotions, such as depression, anxiety, and other emotions, such as anger
4. **Adjustment disorder with disturbance of conduct** Essential features: behaviors that violate the rights of others or societal norms; examples include truancy, fighting, reckless driving
5. **Adjustment disorder with mixed disturbance of emotions and conduct** Essential features: this category is used when there are symptoms of both conduct disturbance and emotions, such as anger, depression, or anxiety
6. **Adjustment disorder with withdrawal** Essential features: social withdrawal but without a depressed or anxious mood
7. **Adjustment disorder with physical complaints** Essential features: physical manifestations, such as headache, fatigue, backache, or other physical complaints
8. **Adjustment disorder with work (or academic) inhibition** Essential features: significant difficulties functioning at work or school; for example, difficulty concentrating, writing reports, and taking tests. A depressed or anxious mood may also accompany the other symptoms
9. **Adjustment disorder not otherwise specified** This category is used when the patient's symptoms do not fit into one of the other categories or when the patient exhibits symptoms of more than one category

Overall, patients with a diagnosis of adjustment disorder appear healthy, as compared with patients with other diagnoses such as major depression, anxiety disorder, or schizophrenia. They tend to continue to dress neatly and appropriately, although they may have less interest in how they look. Their speech and thought processes are usually unchanged by the disorder. Patients with adjustment disorder exhibit fewer vegetative signs, have fewer problems with substance abuse, and exhibit fewer characterologic symptoms than patients with other specific diagnoses (3). Patients also score higher on axis V of the DSM-III-R, which looks at the patient's adaptive functioning over the past year in areas of work, family, and social relations. Therefore, one might expect to find that patients with an adjustment disorder have had consistent work histories or have done well academically prior to the current stressor in their lives. The area of the DSM-III-R in which patients with adjustment disorder do not score well is axis IV, the psychosocial stressor scale. These patients experience more stressors and/or higher levels of stress than those in the other diagnostic categories (3).

PROGNOSIS

It appears that the prognosis for adjustment disorder is very good (4, 6, 16). In one follow-up study, 71% of adults with adjustment disorder had completely recovered after 5 years (4). The same study showed less favorable results with the adolescent adjustment disorder population: only 44% were completely recovered after 5 years. The researchers theorized that the diagnosis of adjustment disorder was used more frequently with adolescents to avoid the stereotyping of the patients with a more severe diagnosis (4). Also, some adolescents with an initial diagnosis of adjustment disorder later develop a mood and/or substance abuse disorder (6). This study affirms the need to use adjustment disorder as a provisional diagnosis.

Though adjustment disorder seems to be transient, with the recovery period usually taking only 3 to 6 months, it is suggested that early intervention is a key factor in recovery (16). Early intervention helps to reduce the amount of stress experienced and helps the patient develop adaptive responses. Psychotherapy is usually adequate in providing support. However, an antianxiety agent may also be used to decrease anxious feelings that inhibit work or school performance (6, 16). Psychotherapy helps the patient explore the personal meaning of the stressor(s) and assists in the cognitive formulation of appropriate coping mechanisms. Development of individual and group skills in activities of daily living are also crucial and help increase feelings of competence. In the following paragraph, these techniques are used by an interdisciplinary team with J.H., who was mentioned earlier.

J.H. and his parents initially participated in an interdisciplinary counseling session to discuss evaluation results and

Table 11.2.
Occupational Performance Components Affected by an Adjustment Disorder[a]

Sensory Motor Component	Cognitive Integration & Cognitive Components	Psychosocial Skills & Psychologic Component

1. Sensory integration
  a. Sensory awareness
  b. Sensory processing
    1. Tactile
    2. Proprioceptive
    3. Vestibular
    4. Visual
    5. Auditory
    6. Gustatory
    7. Olfactory
  c. Perceptual skills
    1. Stereognosis
    2. Kinesthesia
    3. Body scheme
    4. Right-left discrimination
    5. Form constancy
    6. Position in space
    7. Visual-closure
    8. Figure ground
    9. Depth perception
    10. Topographic orientation
 	
2. Neuromuscular
  a. Reflex
  b. Range of motion
  c. Muscle tone
  d. Strength
  e. Endurance
  f. Postural control
  g. Soft tissue integrity
 	
3. Motor
  a. Activity tolerance
  b. Gross motor coordination
  c. Crossing the midline
  d. Laterality
  e. Bilateral integration
  f. Praxis
  g. Fine motor coordination
  h. Visual-motor integration
  i. Oral-motor control
	1. Level of arousal
	2. Orientation
	3. Recognition
	4. Attention span
	5. Memory
	  a. Short-term
	  b. Long-term
	  c. Remote
	  d. Recent
	6. Sequencing
	7. Categorization
	8. Concept formation
	9. Intellectual operations in space
	10. Problem solving
	11. Generalized of learning
	12. Integration of learning
	13. Synthesis of learning
		1. Psychologic
		  a. Roles
		  b. Values
		  c. Interests
		  d. Initiation of activity
		  e. Termination of activity
		  f. Self-concept
		2. Social
		  a. Social conduct
		  b. Conversation
		  c. Self-expression
		3. Self-management
		  a. Coping skills
		  b. Time management
		  c. Self-control

Table 11.2. (Continued)
Occupational Therapy Performance Areas

Activities of Daily Living	Work Activities	Play/Leisure Activities
1. Grooming	1. Home management	1. **Play or leisure explora-tion**
2. Oral hygiene	a. Clothing care	2. Play or leisure perfor-mance
3. Bathing	b. Cleaning	
4. Toilet hygiene	c. Meal preparation and cleanup	
5. Dressing	d. Shopping	
6. **Feeding and eating**	e. Money management	
7. Medication routine	f. Household mainte-nance	
8. **Socialization**	g. Safety procedures	
9. Functional communication	2. Care of others	
10. Functional mobility	3. Educational activities	
11. **Sexual expression**	4. Vocational activities	
	a. Vocational exploration	
	b. Job acquisition	
	c. **Work or job perfor-mance**	
	d. Retirement planning	

*a***Bold** items indicate components affected by an adjustment disorder.

recommendations. J.H.'s many strengths, his need for increased support and positive feedback at home, and his need for involvement with peers were discussed with him and his parents. He will continue to meet with his caseworker weekly, with his parents joining him monthly. Recommendations for his father to become reinvolved with Alcoholics Anonymous (AA) were also noted by the team. The goals for J.H. are to help him develop competence and confidence; improve work/study habits; increase frustration tolerance; encourage decision making and planning; and clarify personal values. In short, J.H. will learn coping skills.

IMPACT OF ADJUSTMENT DISORDERS ON OCCUPATIONAL PERFORMANCE

Performance Components

Sensorimotor skills are rarely affected by an adjustment disorder. If a deficit in sensorimotor skills is found, the deficit was most likely present before the onset of the adjustment disorder, and the therapist should look for other underlying reasons.

The cognitive skills most commonly affected are attention span and problem solving. Patients often comment that they have difficulty focusing on a task and feel anxious about their performance. As a result, they often avoid tasks or have a sense of decreased accomplishment when performing even ordinary daily activities. There is also a decreased ability to recognize problems and an inability to develop alternative plans to cope with stress. They often feel helpless and hopeless to make any changes ı their lives. This is seen commonly in adjustment disorder with depressed mood (9).

The performance component most profoundly affected by an adjustment disorder is the psychosocial skill area. A change or loss of roles is often experienced. In the case of a divorce, the person may lose the roles of wife, lover, and friend; with a job layoff, the worker role is lost. Interests and hobbies may be perceived with less pleasure and thus not pursued, resulting in another role loss. Patients find it difficult to initiate activity, especially any new, nonroutine activity (e.g., starting a report may be totally overwhelming). Patients often display a diminished self-concept and may express feelings of powerlessness and incompetence. Socially, they may be withdrawn, avoiding friends and social activities. Often, patients have difficulty expressing their feelings and needs. The coping skills of patients with an adjustment disorder vary, depending on the person's age and available support system.

Occupational Performance Areas

Changes in the activities of daily living may be less noticeable. Personal grooming may be difficult for those with an adjustment disorder, and they may take less interest in how they look. Nevertheless, they will usually bathe and dress adequately. Appetite may vary, resulting in

Table 11.3.
Occupational Performance Profile

		Performance Areas			
			Work Activities		
		Vocation	Education	Home Management	Care of Others
SENSORIMOTOR	**SENSORY INTEGRATION** Intact **NEURO-MUSCULAR** Intact **MOTOR** Intact				
COGNITIVE	**COGNITIVE**	Decreased problem solving	Decreased attention span, difficulty learning new material, resulting in poor grades		
	PSYCHOLOGIC				
PSYCHOSOCIAL	**SOCIAL**				
	SELF-MANAGEMENT		Decreased ability to cope with change in grade performance		

(Row labels at far left: OCCUPATIONAL PERFORMANCE COMPONENTS)

EXTERNAL FACTORS WHICH INFLUENCE PERFORMANCE; CULTURE, ECONOMY, ENVIRONMENT

Grid adapted from Uniform Terminology (2nd ed.) Developed by the occupational therapy faculty at Eastern Michigan University.

a significant weight change. Basic social skills usually remain intact, although the person may noticeably avoid friends or social activities. This is seen more commonly in a person who has an adjustment disorder with withdrawal. In an adjustment disorder with disturbance of conduct, there may be inappropriate social interactions, such as increased hostility and fighting. There may be an avoidance of sexual intimacy or, less commonly, some sexual acting out.

The therapist will often note a change of performance in work activities. For example, a college student who has suffered a death of a parent may have trouble at-

Client initials: S. P. (Case Study #2)
Diagnosis:
Age:

Play or Leisure Activities		Activities of Daily Living				
Exploration	Performance	Self-care	Socialization	Functional Communication	Functional Mobility	Sexual Expression
Decreased interest in leisure activities	Decreased interest in lacrosse, resulting in change in performance		Decreased interest in friends			
	Withdrawn from team members		Withdrawn, difficulty expressing self in concerns			
			Decreased self-control around potential limits, overdose of aspirin			

tending to lectures, be unable to concentrate on reading assignments, and feel more anxious about test taking, all culminating in poor grades. There may be less interest in leisure activities, and difficulty initiating tasks that were once pleasurable. Though there may be less interest in home management, significant change is usually not noted in this area.

CASE STUDIES

Case 1

V.L. is a 16-year-old female, whose parents separated about 4 months after her birth. She continued to live with her mother but spent the weekends with her father. Her parents' divorce proceedings took place when V.L. was age 7, with both parents fighting for custody. Her father remarried when she was 8 years old. Father and stepmother subsequently adopted two

Table 11.4.
Occupational Performance Profile

			Performance Areas		
			Work Activities		
		Vocation	Education	Home Management	Care of Others
SENSORIMOTOR	**SENSORY INTEGRATION** Intact				
	NEUROMUSCULAR Intact				
	MOTOR Intact				
COGNITIVE	**COGNITIVE**	Decreased attention span, decreased short-term memory			
PSYCHOSOCIAL	**PSYCHOLOGIC**	Decreased interest in work		Decreased interest in household tasks, passes some chores on to daughters though does complete tasks necessary for home management	Decreased initiation of activities with daughters, change in role as wife
	SOCIAL				Increased withdrawal from daughters
	SELF-MANAGEMENT	Decreased work effectiveness			

OCCUPATIONAL PERFORMANCE COMPONENTS

EXTERNAL FACTORS WHICH INFLUENCE PERFORMANCE; CULTURE, ECONOMY, ENVIRONMENT

Grid adapted from Uniform Terminology (2nd ed.) Developed by the occupational therapy faculty at Eastern Michigan University.

children, a girl now age 4 and most recently an infant son. About 4 years ago, when her father adopted the first child, her mother reported that V.L. started to have behavioral problems such as charging thousands of dollars on her mother's credit card and not responding to her parents' limit setting. At this point she started to get shuffled between her parents' respective homes. Two years ago, when she was 14 and entering the ninth grade, V.L. was sent to a boarding school. Both parents felt she needed more discipline than they could provide. V.L. reports feeling that her parents do not care about her and were too busy with their own work and lives.

A few months ago, V.L.'s maternal aunt died suddenly. V.L. was especially close to her aunt and felt she was the only person she could talk with. V.L. ap-

Client initials: S.P. (Case Study #2)
Diagnosis:
Age:

Play or Leisure Activities		Activities of Daily Living				
Exploration	Performance	Self-Care	Socialization	Functional Communica-tion	Functional Mobility	Sexual Expression
	Decreased interest in her hobbies		Doesn't want to be a "burden" to friends			Loss of sexual partner

peared to be quite upset, but she had difficulty communicating her sense of loss to anyone, preferring to be alone. She also had difficulty concentrating on her schoolwork, which resulted in some poor grades. She was frustrated by this change in her school performance, since she had always done quite well academically. V.L. had enjoyed playing lacrosse on the girls varsity team, as she found lacrosse to be a wonderful outlet for her frustrations and enjoyed the comraderie among the team members. After the death of her aunt, she lost interest in the team and found she was not playing well. Subsequently, she quit the team. Her friends found her to be quiet and preoccupied, preferring to be alone. Six weeks after her aunt's death, V.L. was hospitalized after taking an overdose of 40 aspirin. The attending psychiatrist diagnosed her as having an adjustment disorder with academic inhibition. V.L. was seen by the occupational therapist, who administered the occupational performance history interview (17) and the adolescent role assessment (18). The occupational therapist also placed V.L. in a task evaluation group to further assess her cognitive difficulties and an adolescent recreation group.

Case 2

S.P. is a 36-year-old, recently separated woman with two daughters, ages 12 and 10. She is an attorney, working in a small law firm for the past 6 years. S.P. reports that she is dedicated to her work and enjoys her colleagues there. Her interests include cooking, gardening, and reading, as well as spending time with her daughters.

S.P. is finding the separation from her husband very difficult. She described her marriage of 15 years as a good one with the normal ups and downs. Her husband's announcement that he wanted to leave the marriage came as a surprise to her. Since then she has experienced feelings of sadness, confusion, and helplessness. Although she finds it difficult to get herself up and to work in the mornings, she has not missed any days at work and continues to dress in a professional manner. She is often tearful and feels this is embarrassing, especially when she is at the law firm. She finds it difficult to concentrate on her work and feels she is slower at completing her normal work tasks.

She finds little enjoyment in her hobbies and only half-heartedly cooks and gardens to pass the time on weekends. S.P. knows she should be doing activities with her daughters but feels tired with all their questions surrounding the separation. She is pleased that the girls continue to do their household chores and surprised that they have offered to help out more since S.P. feels uninterested in the housework. She has tried to get together with friends but finds they are often busy with their own lives and does not want to be a burden to them.

S.P. contacted a psychologist to assist her in understanding her feelings and for support. The psychologist, upon meeting and interviewing S.P., diagnosed her as having an adjustment disorder with depressed mood and agreed to see S.P. weekly to work on her above-stated goals. The psychologist also referred S.P. to an occupational therapist to learn stress-management techniques and to join a women's group.

REFERENCES

1. Karno M, Norquist GS. Schizophrenia. In: Kaplan HI, Sadock BJ, eds. Comprehensive textbook of psychiatry. Baltimore: Williams & Wilkins, 1989:705–717.
2. Popkin MK. Adjustment disorder and impulse control disorder. In: Kaplan HI, Sadock BJ, eds. Comprehensive textbook of psychiatry. Baltimore: Williams & Wilkins, 1989:1141–1145.
3. Fabrega H, Mezzich JE, Mezzich AC. Adjustment disorder as a marginal or transitional illness category in DSM-III. Arch Gen Psychiatry 1987;44:6.
4. Andreasen NC, Hoenk PR. The predictive value of adjustment disorders: a follow-up study. Am J Psychiatry 1982;139:5.
5. Andreasen NC, Wasek P. Adjustment disorders in adolescence and adults. Arch Gen Psychiatry 1980;37:1166.
6. Kaplan HI, Sadock BJ. Synopsis of psychiatry, 5th ed. Baltimore: Williams & Wilkins 1988;408–411.
7. Woolston JL. Theoretical considerations of the adjustment disorders. J Am Acad Child Adolesc Psychiatry 1988;27:3.
8. Stuart ME. To bend without breaking. Nashville: Parthenon Press, 1978:38.
9. Kofta M, Sedek G. Learned helplessness: affective or cognitive disturbance. In: Spielberger C, Sarason I, Strelau J, eds. Stress and anxiety. New York: Hemisphere Publishing, 1989:81–96.
10. Lazarus RS, Launier R. Stress-related transactions between person and environment. In: Pervin LA, Lewis M, eds. Perspectives in interactional psychology. New York: Plenum Press, 1978:287–322.
11. Miller SM. Why having control reduces stress: if I can stop the roller coaster, I don't want to get off. In: Garber J, Seligman MEP, eds. Human helplessness: theory and applications. New York: Academic Press, 1980.
12. Mezzich JE, Fabrega H, Coggman GA, Haley R. DSM-III disorders in a large sample of psychiatric patients: frequency and specificity of diagnoses. Am J Psychiatry 1989;146:2.
13. Rey JM, Bashir MR, Schwarz M, Richards IN, Plapp JM, Stewart GW. Oppositional disorder: fact or fiction? J Am Acad Child Adolesc Psychiatry 1988;27:2.
14. Faulstich ME, Moore JR, Carey MP, Ruggiero L, Gresham F. Prevalence of DSM-III conduct

disorders and adjustment disorders for adolescent psychiatric inpatients. Adolescence 1986; 21:82.

15. American Psychiatric Association. Diagnostic and statistical manual of mental disorders; 3rd ed revised. Washington, D.C.: American Psychiatric Association, 1987.

16. Horowitz MJ. Stress-response syndromes: a review of post-traumatic and adjustment disorders. Hosp Community Psychiatry 1986;37:3.

17. Kielhofner G, Henry AD, Walens DA. Users guide to the occupational performance history interview. Rockville, MD: American Occupational Therapy Association, 1989.

18. Black MM. Adolescent role assessment. Am J Occup Ther 1976;30:73–79.

Glossary

Anxiety: A diffuse, highly unpleasant, often vague feeling of apprehension, accompanied by one or more bodily sensations (e.g., an empty feeling in the pit of the stomach, tightness in the chest, pounding heart, perspiration, headache, or the sudden urge to void). Restlessness and a desire to move around are also common. It is an alerting signal that warns of impending danger and enables the person to take measures to deal with a threat, either external or internal.

Stress: The sum of the biological reactions to any adverse stimulus, physical, mental, or emotional, internal or external, that tends to disturb the homeostasis of an organism. Inappropriate reactions may lead to disease states. The human body and mind normally can adapt to the stresses of a new situation; however, this ability has definite limits beyond which continued stress may cause a breakdown.

Stressor: Any factor that disturbs homeostasis, producing stress.

12

Coronary Artery Disease

BEN ATCHISON AND ROXANNE McTURNER-GILL

He awoke with distinct discomfort around his chest and hoped the pain would go away as it had before. However, this time it was different; the pain persisted. He had difficulty breathing and was sweating as if he had just run a mile. He felt very weak and nauseated. An alarm went off in his mind. He felt impending doom as he realized that he was having a heart attack.

Does this man have a chance of surviving his heart attack? What are the complications he might expect? How did he develop coronary artery disease that resulted in the heart attack? Will he be able to resume his usual life roles and activities if he does survive?

This chapter reviews cardiac anatomy and circulation, incidence and prevalence, etiology, pathophysiology and clinical manifestations of coronary artery disease (CAD) and medical-surgical management issues. At the end, two case studies illustrate the impact of CAD on occupational performance.

CARDIAC ANATOMY AND CIRCULATION

How do people develop coronary artery disease? What occurs in the cardiac anatomy and physiology to create pathologic changes? Understanding what goes wrong requires a basic comprehension of normal anatomy and physiology.

The heart is a muscle that works as a pump to provide oxygen and nourishment to the tissues in the body. It is hollow and is located slightly to the left of center in the chest. The major portion of the heart is a muscular wall called myocardium. The inner surface of the myocardium is raised into ridgelike surfaces that make up the papillary muscles. Lining the interior of the myocardium is smooth endothelial tissue called the endocardium. This smooth tissue allows the blood to pass through the heart chambers without cellular damage (1).

The interior of the heart is divided into upper and lower chambers called atria and ventricles. The ventricles, the lower chambers, are considerably larger and thicker than the atria, because they are required to perform heavier pumping action. These chambers of the heart are separated by two valves, called atrioventricular (AV) valves. The left one is called the mitral valve and the right is called the tricuspid. These valves prevent blood from flowing back into the atria from the ventricles when the heart is resting between beats. A review of these structures and cardiac circulation is provided in Figure 12.1.

The heart has its own system of arteries, called coronary arteries, that supply the heart with oxygen and nourishment. These major coronary arteries branch off the aorta, cross over the outside of the heart wall, and penetrate the muscle itself. The left main coronary artery divides into the left anterior descending (LAD) artery and the circumflex artery. The LAD

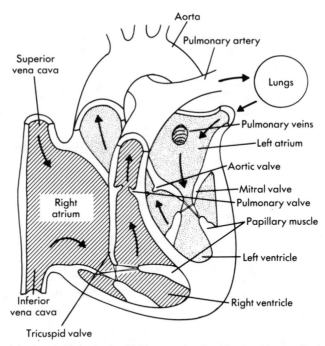

Figure 12.1. Anatomy of the heart. (From Andreoli KG, Fawkes VK, Zipes DR, Wallace AG, eds. Comprehensive cardiac care: a text for nurses, physicians and other health practitioners, St. Louis: CV Mosby, 1983, with permission.)

supplies the left ventricle, the interventricular septum, the right ventricle, the inferior areas of the apex, and both ventricles (1). The circumflex artery supplies blood to the inferior walls of the left ventricle and to the left atrium (2) (Fig. 12.2).

In the body, the smallest arteries empty into one end of a profuse network of tiny blood vessels called capillaries that deliver oxygen and other nutritional substances to individual cells. It is at the capillary level where oxygen and nourishment are exchanged for carbon dioxide. These capillaries supply the heart, head, arms, legs, and various organs such as the liver and stomach.

Like skeletal muscle, cardiac muscle requires innervation to contract. A specialized nervous conduction network of cells creates systematic depolarization creating an action potential that elicits myocardial contraction (3). The origin of the electrical impulse is the sinoatrial node (SA), or the "pacemaker" of the heart,

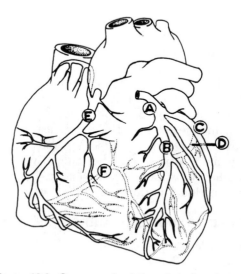

Figure 12.2. Coronary circulation. *A,* Left main coronary artery. *B,* Left anterior descending coronary artery. *C,* Left circumflex coronary artery. *D,* Posterior circumflex coronary artery. *E,* Right coronary artery. *F,* Posterior descending artery. From O'Sullivan S. Schmitz TJ, eds. Coronary artery disease. In: Physical rehabilitation: assessment 2nd ed., Philadelphia: FA Davis, 1988, with permission.)

which is located in the right atrium. This impulse spreads through both atria, which then contract simultaneously and stimulate the atrioventricular (AV) node. The impulse travels next to the bundle branches, then to the Purkinje fibers (4). Because the Purkinje fibers merge with the walls of the ventricle, the impulse spreads through the Purkinje system to the cells of the ventricles, and the ventricles contract together. This sequence occurs, on average, 72 times per minute (1).

Depolarization is the result of electrical cellular changes. Thus, it can be recorded graphically on an electrocardiogram (ECG, EKG) (5). To perform this test, surface electrodes are placed on the limbs and chest to monitor the sequence, timing, and magnitude of the impulse. Each graphic segment (P, QRS, and T waves) corresponds to the wave of depolarization as it travels through the heart chambers (6) (Fig. 12.3). The P wave indicates the electrical activity resulting from

depolarization in the atria, called atrial depolarization. The PR interval indicates the time that elapses from the beginning of the atrial contraction to the ventricular contraction. The QRS complex corresponds to the electrical activity known as ventricular depolarization, which occurs as electrical activity travels through the bundle branches and the ventricles. The T wave corresponds to ventricular repolarization, which is the reestablishment of an electrically polarized state in the ventricles.

The timing of depolarization can be determined by counting the blocks on the ECG graph paper. For example, if the PR interval is too wide or QRS is widened or longer than normal, a conduction abnormality would be suspected (7). See Figure 12.4 for examples of normal and abnormal ECGs.

The American Heart Association recommends that therapists using ECG during treatment be familiar with monitoring the equipment and be able to recognize

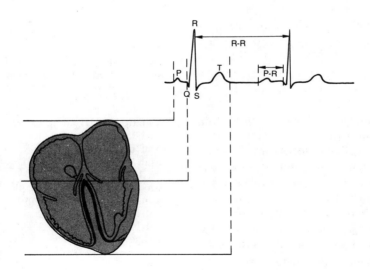

EKG COMPONENT	MYOCARDIAL EVENT
P wave	Atrial depolarization
QRS complex	Ventricular depolarization
T wave	Ventricular repolarization

Figure 12.3. Electrocardiographic (ECG) recording of myocardial activity. (From Rothstein JM, Roy SH, Wolf SL. The rehabilitation specialists handbook, Philadelphia: FA Davis, 1991, with permission.)

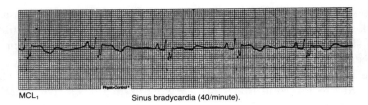

MCL₁   Sinus bradycardia (40/minute).

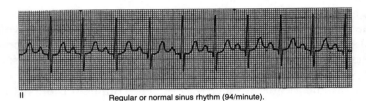

II   Regular or normal sinus rhythm (94/minute).

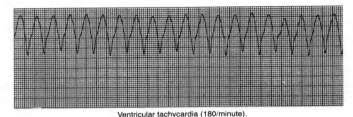

Ventricular tachycardia (180/minute).

Figure 12.4. Examples of normal and abnormal ECGs. Strips illustrate normal heart rate, bradycardia, and tachycardia. (From Rothstein JM, Roy SH, Wolf SL. The rehabilitation specialists handbook. Philadelphia: FA Davis, 1991, with permission.)

a minimum of twelve ECG dysrhythmias (Table 12.1).

ETIOLOGY

Coronary artery disease is the result of an arteriosclerotic process created by a thickening in the intimal, or inner, layer of the vessel. This progressive thickening is caused by an accumulation of fatty tissue. (A detailed description of this process is given later in this chapter.)

Risk factors are classified as controllable (smoking, obesity, blood lipid levels, inactivity) or noncontrollable (sex, age, family history of CAD).

Research has consistently found a relationship between the presence of certain risk factors and the development of arteriosclerosis (7). The most extensive work has been produced by an epidemiological study initiated in 1949 in Framingham, Massachusetts on 5209 men and

Table 12.1.
Dysrhythmias That Those Using EKG Equipment Must Be Able to Recognize[a]

Sinus tachycardia
Sinus bradycardia
Premature atrial complexes
Atrial tachycardia
Atrial flutter
Atrial fibrillation
Junctional rhythms
Atrioventricular blocks of all degrees
Premature ventricular complexes
Ventricular tachycardia
Ventricular fibrillation
Cardiac standstill or asystole

[a]Adapted from American Heart Association. Cardio-pulmonary resuscitation: advanced life support, JAMA Suppl Aug 1980.

women from 30 to 62 years of age. The Framingham study has identified major risk factors for the development of atherosclerosis (8, 9), including cigarette smoking, hypertension, elevated serum cholesterol or triglycerides, abnormal glucose tolerance (diabetes), sedentary lifestyle, family history of heart disease, age, and male sex. Recent reports on the Framingham study support the original data regarding risk factors, with increasingly convincing evidence that cigarette smoking and elevated lipids are strong predictive factors (23–25). The Framingham studies indicate that male cigarette smokers who smoke as few as 1 to 9 cigarettes per day have 1.6 times the risk of developing arteriosclerosis as a nonsmoker. The data are not much different for female smokers. Those who quit, however, reduce their risk of a coronary event by as much as 50% (9). There is a considerable degree of association between the risk factors. For example, low values of high-density lipoproteins (HDL) are associated with cigarette smoking, sedentary lifestyle, and diabetes. The presence of more than one risk factor enhances the chance of developing arteriosclerotic disease (8).

INCIDENCE AND PREVALENCE

According to the American Heart Association, heart disease is the number one cause of death, disability, and loss of income in the United States today. Approximately 66 million Americans have one or more forms of heart or blood vessel disease. Heart attacks caused one-half million deaths in 1986 and are the leading cause of death in this country. Some specific facts include the following (9):

- 4,940,000 people alive today have a history of heart attack, angina pectoris, or both.
- More than 300,000 people per year die of heart attack before they reach a hospital—studies indicate that 50% of heart attack victims wait more than 2 hours before seeking treatment.
- Based on the Framingham study, 5% of all heart attacks occur in people under the age of 40, and 45% occur in people under the age of 65.
- High blood pressure afflicts an estimated 60,130,000 Americans age 6 and older.

- Atherosclerosis was a leading contributor to many of the 671,900 deaths in 1986.
- The cost of cardiovascular disease in 1989 is estimated to be $88.2 billion.
- Mortality rates from coronary disease tend to equalize among the sexes at age 50 presumably due to higher risk in women postmenopause or the elimination of higher risk males at an earlier age.

PATHOPHYSIOLOGY OF CORONARY ARTERY DISEASE

Arteriosclerotic disease is a progressive destruction of the arterial structure and function. This destruction occurs in a series of changes caused by the development of plaques or lesions along the intimal layer of the vessel. These lesions are classified, in order of pathologic changes, into three types: fatty streak, fibrous plaque, and complicated plaque or lesion (1).

Fatty streaks are found throughout the inner lining of the arterial tree in individuals from infancy through late adulthood. They are composed mainly of cholesterol and appear soft and yellow. It is not clearly known whether these lesions progress to a raised fibrous lesion or are reversible.

Raised fibrous plaques are the typical lesions of arteriosclerosis. These lesions are yellowish gray lumps that thicken and begin to impinge on the lumen of the artery.

The complicated plaques are fibrous plaques that have progressed through one or more pathologic changes, including possible calcification, necrosis, internal hemorrhage, and thrombus formation. The changes in the intima may cause degeneration of the medial layer with the resultant loss of the artery's distension capability. This weakened condition may create an aneurysm, which may rupture and cause hemorrhage.

These three types of lesions may coexist at various sites in the arterial structure. Pathologic studies indicate that most lesions of the coronary arteries occur at proximal points in the two major coronary arteries at the bifurcation of the arteries (10).

As CAD progresses, structural changes in the artery result in a decreased coronary blood flow and a decrease in oxygen distribution to the myocardium. The functional inability of the vessel to carry oxygen creates an imbalance of myocardial oxygen demand and supply, called ischemia. When ischemia is prolonged, the tissues can undergo irreversible injury resulting in a myocardial infarction. Ischemia and infarction are accompanied by pain, elevated serum enzymes, and symptoms related to the affected organ or tissues, such as decreased renal function with renal ischemia or muscle cramps with peripheral ischemia (1). A transition from ischemia to infarction is not inevitable and depends on several factors, including the rate of onset and duration of ischemia, the ability of the tissue to compensate for the decreased blood flow, the oxygen requirements of the particular tissue, and the amount of oxygen in the blood (1).

When ischemia develops gradually, the tissue can tolerate it better because collateral circulation can develop, which allows alternate pathways for blood to flow. Tissues adapt to the decreased oxygen supply by increasing their oxygen extraction from available blood flow (1).

Coronary artery disease does not always result from the arteriosclerotic process. Medical conditions and disabilities that have associated and secondary cardiac involvement include alcoholism, cerebrovascular disease, drug abuse, diabetes, Friedreich's ataxia, obesity, progressive muscular dystrophy, rheumatoid arthritis, and systemic lupus erythematosus (6).

CLINICAL MANIFESTATIONS/SIGNS AND SYMPTOMS OF CAD

Coronary artery disease creates the potential for four clinical syndromes: angina, myocardial infarction, heart failure, and sudden cardiac death (10).

Angina pectoris is a reversible ischemic process that is caused by a temporary inability of the coronary arteries to supply sufficient oxygenated blood to cardiac muscle. The individual with angina experiences sudden anterior chest pain described as a pressure sensation. This sensation is described as a "vise-like" tightening around the chest, as if a large, tight rubber band is wrapped around the individual. Other symptoms can include a burning sensation in the throat or jaw, discomfort between the shoulder blades, and shortness of breath (1).

The frequency of attacks varies depending on the degree of coronary insufficiency, effectiveness of treatment, and the physical and emotional characteristics of the individual (1).

The second manifestation of CAD is myocardial infarction (MI). A portion of cardiac muscle is destroyed because of sustained myocardial ischemia resulting from acute occlusion of coronary vessels. Infarction may also result from hemorrhage or profound shock (1).

The pathology of MI is similar to that of angina and has comparable clinical symptoms and signs. Individuals who have MIs often have a history of angina, although the MI may be the first sign of cardiovascular problems. About 15% of individuals are asymptomatic and have what are referred to as "silent MIs" (11), i.e., episodes of ischemia, as documented by ECGs, that are not associated with the chest discomfort of angina. As a result, there is no "warning system," and the individual may experience severe ischemia without realizing the need to stop activity. Some patients with "silent MIs" may have symptoms of dyspnea rather than angina.

Complications of myocardial infarction include: arrhythmia, heart failure, thrombolytic complications, and irreversible damage to the heart structure.

Arrhythmia, an irregularity or loss of normal heart rhythm, occurs in 90% of individuals who are diagnosed with MIs. They are the leading cause of sudden death in persons with CAD, although the effect of arrhythmias on the morbidity rate varies from benign to life-threatening (12). Early intervention has decreased the overall morbidity rate of acutely diagnosed persons (13).

The types of arrhythmia vary with the area of the heart infarcted and the point on the conduction pathway where the tissue is damaged. Ninety-eight percent of arrhythmia disturbances can be detected by an ECG (1).

Heart failure, the second complication of an MI and the third clinical syndrome associated with CAD, occurs when the myocardium is unable to maintain adequate circulation of the blood for respiration and metabolism. Failure can occur in the right or left ventricle or both (1). There are several classifications of heart failure including backward, congestive, forward, high output, and low output (14). Backward heart failure occurs when reduced venous return to the heart results in venous stasis and congestion. Congestive heart failure occurs as a result of right heart failure and/or pulmonary congestion due to left heart failure. This leads to systemic congestion resulting in edema, an enlarged liver, and elevated venous pressure. Forward heart failure is a result of left ventricular failure following loss of ventricular contractility, post MI. High output heart failure results from conditions that increase the amount of circulation, as with a large arteriovenous fistula or anemia. Low output heart failure refers to the failure of the heart to maintain adequate cardiac output due to insufficient venous return, as with hemorrhage (14).

The third complication associated with MIs is thrombolytic, of two types: venous and mural thrombi. Both result from an interruption in the flow of blood. Venous, or deep vein thrombi (DVT), develop in the calf as a result of forced inactivity. Mural thrombi form in the ventricular wall and, like venous thrombi, have potential for embolism, or the development of a "traveling" clot (1).

Pulmonary embolism is the term used to indicate emboli that travel to the lung as a result of a venous thrombus. Although at one time a major complication and cause of death after MI, as a result of early rehabilitation efforts it now accounts for less than 1% of total deaths (1). Mural emboli may dwell in visceral arteries, resulting in infarction of the brain, kidney, spleen, or intestine. They may also lodge in the extremities creating sudden pain, numbness, and coldness in the affected part (1).

The fourth complication of a MI is heart structural damage. Possible structural damage includes ventricular aneurysm formation and rupture of papillary muscle, the ventricular wall, and/or the intraventricular septum. These complications may cause death or result in mild-to-severe heart failure. Surgical intervention may be required to repair the damage (1).

The fourth clinical syndrome associated with CAD is sudden cardiac death, commonly defined as an unexpected death in individuals without previous symptoms of heart disease. Cardiac death occurs as a result of sudden coronary artery occlusion that leads to ventricular fibrillation. There is a loss of ventricular contraction, leading to death in 4 minutes, if the occlusion is sustained (16). In 1984, one in three individuals who had an MI died as a result of sudden cardiac death (15). The only known prevention for sudden cardiac death is prompt initiation of cardiopulmonary resuscitation (1).

In summary, arteriosclerosis and the ischemia-infarction process are the basis for clinical manifestations of CAD. The clinical manifestations of CAD and major complications must be understood to effectively and safely manage persons with this disease.

PROGRESSION AND PROGNOSIS

Coronary artery disease is considered to be a progressive disease that can develop as early as the second decade of life. To assess the progression and prognosis of CAD, it is important to identify certain factors, relative to the severity of the disease at the time of initial assessment, which predict coronary events such as progression of symptoms, recurrent myocardial infarction, or cardiac death. In a 10-year study of 601 nonsurgical patients having coronary artery occlusion involving over 50% narrowing, a significant prognostic factor was the number of coronary arteries involved (13). Single vessel, double vessel and triple vessel disease were predicted to have 10-year survival rates of 63%, 45%, and 23%, respectively. Patients who had 50% or greater narrowing, specifically in the left main coronary artery, were predicted to have a 22% survival rate. Survival rates were also found to be related to ventricular function. Patients who experienced massive myocardial infarctions and left ventricular dysfunction had lower survival rates than those with small infarcts and normal ventricular function. Other factors included severity of angina pectoris and subsequent functional impairment, evidence of left ventricular hypertrophy, conduction deficits during depolarization, and continued presence of risk factors such as smoking, diabetes, and hypertension.

DIAGNOSTIC PROCEDURES

Coronary artery disease is diagnosed through a variety of clinical and laboratory studies. The symptoms of angina, which indicate an ischemic condition, are usually the initial reason for a person to seek medical attention. Ischemic symptoms are reversible events, but they may also indicate more serious cardiovascular pathology.

Diagnosis of angina is determined by the angina threshold (defined as the level of activity that initiates the sequelae of cardiac distress), ECG changes, substernal pain that lasts from 1 to 3 minutes, dyspnea, variable pulse rate, and ele-

vated blood pressure. The angina threshold is assessed through graded exercise testing, which is a measured exercise challenge designed to determine functional capacity during physical stress. Through a medical history, a physician is able to determine other factors that may precipitate angina, such as exposure to cold or eating. Persons with angina may also experience depressed left ventricular function, due to the ischemic episode, which is evident by changes in the ECG.

Diagnosis of a myocardial infarction, which is the result of prolonged, severe ischemia is assessed by physical examination, laboratory tests, and the ECG. The physician observes the person for hallmark signs of cardiac dysfunction including pain, nausea, sweating, and dyspnea. The heart rate may be abnormally slow (bradycardia) or fast (tachycardia).

Of the three diagnostic tools, serum enzyme studies are the most conclusive (1). Serum enzyme levels are useful in detecting myocardial infarctions and other heart diseases. They are also used in determining recovery status. Significant enzymes include creatine phosphokinase (CPK) and lactic dehydrogenase (LDH).

CPK levels increase after an MI during a 4-hour interval and peak at 36 hours. These levels continue to drop sharply and are back to normal in 2 to 4 days. Both CPK and LDH will elevate in an acute MI. CPK is more sensitive to myocardial ischemia than any other enzyme. Due to the rapid degeneration of CPK when stored, testing should be done on the same day.

LDH elevates in the first 12–18 hours, peaks in 2–3 days, and returns to normal with 7–10 days. Its elevation is also related to the extent of the injury. An increase of over 3000 units indicates a poor prognosis (19).

The occupational therapist should note serum enzyme levels when working with an individual, because any reelevation in these levels exceeding the normal time frame could indicate a new infarction or the extension of a previous one (1).

The occupational therapist selects a combination of low-level self-care activities in the initial evaluation. During these activities, the cardiovascular response is monitored by assessment of heart rate, blood pressure, ECG readings, signs and symptoms of cardiac dysfunction, and heart sounds. The primary purpose of this ongoing monitoring is to guide the therapist in treatment progression. One method of grading activity is to determine the energy expenditure of activities, measured by the amount of oxygen that is consumed, expressed as MET (basal *metabolic equivalent*) levels. One MET equals the amount of energy consumed when an individual is at rest in a semireclined position with extremities supported (semi-Fowler position) (6). This energy is equal to 3.5 ml of oxygen per minute per kilogram of weight (3.5/kg/min). As soon as one changes posture, sits up, ambulates, and performs activities, the metabolic demand and oxygen consumption increase (6).

While various MET lists provide guidance for the therapist in selecting safe levels of activity, caution is required. A person who can achieve four MET levels during one activity may not be able to resume all potential activities listed in the four MET level. Variables to consider include the person's pace, position, use of isometrics, environmental factors, muscles used, and emotional stress.

Resumption of activities must occur gradually, particularly in the initial, in-patient phase of recovery (phase I). Table 12.2 provides an example of a program of progressive activity with corresponding MET levels.

MEDICAL AND SURGICAL MANAGEMENT

The primary goal of medical management is to maintain myocardial integrity by controlling complications that might jeopardize the healing process. Prevention of myocardial ischemia and infarction, while improving the existing cardiac function, is

critical in long-term treatment. A major element in the medical management of CAD is the use of pharmacologic agents. Common therapies include the use of nitrates, β-blocking agents, antiarrhythmics, cardiac glycosides, calcium-channel blockers, and hypertensives (1). The specific drugs used, their effects and complications are described in Appendix 12.2.

Surgical intervention does not alter the process of arteriosclerosis (1). The primary purpose is to improve the quality of life, specifically to improve the person's tolerance for activity. Common surgical procedures include coronary artery bypass grafting (CABG), heart transplantation, and percutaneous transluminal coronary angioplasty (PTCA). These surgeries are recommended only in cases of severe, chronically disabling CAD, and their aim is revascularization of the myocardium.

PTCA involves the insertion of a "balloon"-tipped tube through a catheter into the coronary arteries to the point of the arteriosclerotic lesion. The balloon is then inflated to compress the lesion against the arterial wall (12) (Fig. 12.5).

A CABG procedure usually involves bypassing one or more obstructed arteries either by anastomosis, or surgical connection, of a vein graft from the aorta to the coronary artery at a point distal to the obstruction, or by patch grafting to widen the obstructed artery (12). This surgery often results in significant reduction of pain, increased tolerance for activity, and ECG ischemic changes. However, much controversy exists regarding the effectiveness of CABG conventional drug management in prolonging life, and it is currently a major issue in clinical research.

Heart transplantation is performed in end-stage coronary artery disease, when there is no expected recovery. The major complications are infection and rejection. Protective isolation is prescribed to minimize infection; an immunosuppressive regimen is used to prevent rejection. The first-year survival rate is 65%. Candidates for this surgery are usually under 50 to 60 years of age. They must be free of other

Table 12.2.
Suggested Interdisciplinary Stages for Patients with Cardiopulmonary History and/or Precautions[a]

Stage/MET Level	ADL and Mobility	Exercise	Recreation
Stage I (1.0–1.4 METS)	*Sitting:* Self-feeding, wash hands and face, bed mobility* Transfers Progressively increase sitting tolerance	*Supine:* (A) or (AA) exercise to all extremities (10–15 times per extremity) *Sitting:* (A) or (AA) exercise to *only* neck and LEs Include deep breathing exercise	Reading, radio, table games (noncompetitive), light handwork
Stage II (1.4–2.0 METs)	*Sitting:* Self-bathing, shaving, grooming, and dressing in hospital Unlimited sitting *Ambulation:* At slow pace, in room as tolerated	*Sitting:* (A) exercise to all extremities, progressively increasing the number of repetitions* NO ISOMETRICS	*Sitting:* Crafts, e.g., painting, knitting, sewing, mosaics, embroidery NO ISOMETRICS
Stage III (2.0–3.0 METs)	*Sitting:* Showering in warm water, homemaking tasks with brief standing periods to transfer light items, ironing *Standing:* May progress to grooming self *Ambulation:* May begin slow paced ambulation outside room on levels, for short distances	*Sitting:* W/C mobility limited distances *Standing:* (A) exercise to all extremities and trunk progressively increasing the number of repetitions* *May include:* 1. Balance exercises 2. Light mat activities without resistance *Ambulation:* Begin progressive ambulation program at 0% grade and comfortable pace	*Sitting:* Card playing, crafts, piano, machine sewing, typing*
Stage IV (3.0–3.5 METs)	*Standing:* Total washing, dressing, shaving, grooming, showering in warm water; kitchen/ homemaking activities while practicing energy conservation (e.g., light vacuuming, dusting and sweeping, washing light clothes) *Ambulation:* unlimited distance walking at 0% grade, in and/ or outside*	*Standing:* Continue all previous exercise, progressively increasing 1. Number of repetitions 2. Speed of repetitions *May include* additional exercises to increase workload up to 3.5 METs, balance and mat activities with mild resistance	Candlepin bowing Canoeing—slow rhythm, pace Golf putting *Light* gardening: weeding and planting Driving*

Table 12.2. **(Continued)**

Stage/MET Level	ADL and Mobility	Exercise	Recreation
		Ambulation: Unlimited on level surfaces in and/or outside* progressively increasing speed and/ or duration for periods up to 15–20 minutes or until target heart rate is reached* *Stairs:* May begin slow stair climbing to patient's tolerance up to two flights *Treadmill:* 1 mph at 1% grade, progressing to 1.5 mph at 2% grade* *Cycling:* Up to 5.0 mph without resistance	
Stage V (3.5–4.0 METs)	*Standing:* Washing dishes, washing clothes, ironing, hanging light clothes, and making beds	*Standing:* Continue exercises as in stage IV, progressively increasing 1. Number of repetitions 2. Speed of repetitions *May add* additional exercises to increase workload up to 4.0 METs *Ambulation:* As in stage IV, increasing speed up to 2.5 mph on level surfaces* *Stairs:* As in stage IV and progressively increasing, if increasing to patient's tolerance *Treadmill:* 1.5 mph at 2% grade, progressing to 1.5 mph at 4% grade up to 2.5 mph at 0% grade* *Cycling:* Up to 8 mph without resistance* May use up to 7–10 lbs* of weight for UE and LE exercise in sitting	Swimming (slowly) Light carpentry Golfing (using power cart) Light home repairs

Table 12.2. (Continued)

Stage/MET Level	ADL and Mobility	Exercise	Recreation
Stage VI (4.0–5.0 METs)	*Standing:* Showering in hot water, hanging and/or wringing clothes, mopping, stripping and making beds, raking	*Standing:* As in stage V *Ambulation:* As in stage V—increasing speed to 3.5 mph on level surfaces* *Stairs:* As in stage V *Treadmill:* 1.5 mph at 4–6% grade, progressing to 3.5 mph at 0% grade* *Cycling:* Up to 10 mph without resistance May use up to 10–15 lbs of weight in UE and LE exercises in sitting	Swimming (no advanced strokes) Slow dancing Ice or roller skating (slowly) Volleyball Badminton Table tennis (noncompetitive) Light calisthenics

[a]Spaulding Rehabilitation Hospital, Boston, MA, 1987, with permission.

cc

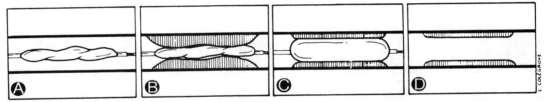

Figure 12.5. Percutaneous transluminal angioplasty. A, B, Deflated balloon-tipped catheter positioned within the atherosclerotic lesion. C, With controlled pressure, the balloon is rapidly inflated and deflated to compress the soft plaque into the vessel walls. D, Af-ter the balloon-tipped catheter is removed, the artery has improved patency. (From Brannon FJ, Geyer MJ, Foley MW. Cardiac rehabilitation. Philadelphia: FA Davis, 1988, with permission.)

chronic diseases, infection, and donor-specific antibodies. Emotional stability and a strong support system is required as well (18). A strong support system ideally includes the willingness and ability of family and significant others to provide the emotional and physical support required by the patient preceding and following the surgery.

IMPACT OF CORONARY ARTERY DISEASE ON OCCUPATIONAL PERFORMANCE COMPONENTS

The effects of CAD on occupational performance components is specific to each individual case. Age, the severity of the disease, complications of an infarct, and secondary diagnoses all are factors for consideration. It is highly possible that the person with an admitting diagnosis of myocardial infarction also has a history of a cerebral vascular accident, diabetes, or rheumatoid arthritis.

For clarity, the discussion of occupational performance components and areas focuses on myocardial infarction. The case studies, however, illustrate the effect of a secondary diagnosis, which is a common occurrence.

Sensory Motor: Neuromuscular and Motor Performance

From the onset of an MI, a person's neuromuscular and motor function can be affected. Muscle tone, strength, endurance, and activity tolerance are commonly evaluated and monitored during initial and later stages of cardiac rehabilitation. Fortunately, early mobilization following an MI lessens the negative effects of prolonged bed rest, which in previous years led to a debilitative neuromuscular status. In the last 20 years, cardiac rehabilitation programs have demonstrated that progressive activity programs under supervised conditions can prevent loss of neuromuscular function (3).

However, some individuals develop a "cardiac cripple" mentality as a result of an MI. This term refers to the inaccurate notion that since the heart has been damaged, resumption of normal activity is not possible or safe. The person takes on the "sick role" and lacks the motivation needed to improve health and function.

Regardless of the efforts of cardiac rehabilitation, anxiety from the event leads to fear of resuming previous activity. The impact of inactivity that results from this phenomenon can clearly lead to deficits in neuromuscular function.

Cognitive

Coronary artery disease may affect cognitive function if cerebral arteries are occluded, resulting in interruption of cerebrovascular circulation. (This is dealt with in depth in Chapter 2, "Cerebrovascular Accident.") Cardiac dysfunction without cerebral artery involvement does not usually result in cognitive dysfunction.

Psychosocial Skills and Psychologic Components

White stated 40 years ago that "after MI, the heart may recover more rapidly than the mental state which is so often a complication" (27).

Anxiety and depression are the most common psychologic responses on return home after a MI. A study of individuals 6 months to 1 year following discharge found that 88% reported significant anxiety or depression or both. Most reported frustration from forced inactivity (20). Even though the emotional distress decreases over time following an MI, early maladaptive behaviors are a strong predictor of overall adjustment problems during the course of the illness. Those persons who cannot manage anxiety and depression initially are more likely to have problems later (28).

While the incidence of coronary disease is increasing in the female population, few studies exist regarding psychosocial adjustment in women (29). Where data are available, women demonstrate more difficulty adjusting to an MI than their male counterparts. Stern reported that 80% of women studied experienced anxiety or depression following an MI, fewer than half returned to work, and only 40% resumed sexual activity. These results could not be explained by age, severity of infarct, or presence of risk factors (30). Clearly, further examination of women's response to heart disease is necessary. In addition, there must be further studies on the psychosocial responses of the subgroups of the cardiac population. Differences in adjustment among social class, ethnic, and racial groups have not been a topic of study in the research literature.

Increasing attention to the quality of survival has resulted in an appreciation of the profound effect of psychologic factors on the patient's life. Heart disease often requires both the patient and family to make difficult changes in personality and lifestyle. The rehabilitation team must address these issues in the overall educational program and discharge planning.

IMPACT OF CAD ON OCCUPATIONAL PERFORMANCE AREAS

The impact of coronary artery disease on occupational performance areas is crosscategorical. The level of dysfunction, as in other conditions, is specific to the diagnosis, prognosis, occupational performance components involved and the severity of involvement. For purposes of clarity, the impact of a myocardial infarction on occupational performance areas is described.

Activities of Daily Living

The impact of a myocardial infarction on activities of daily living is an immediate and critical concern of the occupational therapist. In cardiac rehabilitation protocols, activities such as grooming, oral hygiene, dressing, and eating are used as initial guides to determine the functional capacity of the post-MI patient.

Depending on the extent of the MI, there may be great difficulty in initiating and sustaining the physical endurance necessary to perform selected tasks.

Functional mobility is not affected by an MI because of musculoskeletal impairment, rather it is from a lack of physical endurance. Much of the emphasis in cardiac rehabilitation is on progressive attainment of physical capacity. Carefully planned prescriptions of activities and exercises are developed to match the physical capacity and endurance levels.

Resumption of sexual activity is a common concern following an MI. Anxiety and fear about the safety of sex must be addressed. As a guideline, physicians recommended return to sexual activity if the person can walk up and down two flights of stairs without symptoms.

In addition to concerns about the physical safety of resuming sexual activity, the individual may feel less attractive as a result of the MI. Perceived health status has been reported to have an impact on resumption of sexual activity. Gutmann reported that patients who perceived themselves as ill or "damaged" were less likely to resume sexual relations than those who perceived more positive changes in their health. This same correlation was found for socialization (30).

Work Activities

Much of the literature on adjustment to an MI includes return to work in the context of vocation. Return to work in terms of home management, care of others, and educational activities has not been explored.

The degree to which a MI affects return to work depends mostly on physiologic and psychologic factors. In examining psychologic barriers, Garrity explored factors that influence return to work. Patients who initially rated their health as poor at both the acute phase and 6 months postinfarct were least likely to return to work. Gulledge also reported that early maladjustment makes vocational adaptation difficult (32). Patients who attribute their disease to work-related stress are less likely to return to work than those who do not (33).

Physiologic variables have major implications as well in examining the ability to return to work. Analysis of work by MET levels alone cannot determine complete physical capacity. Treadmill tests measure only lower extremity endurance and do not provide a valid assessment of work capacity. The most complete method of determining work capacity uses job analysis to determine which tasks demand the highest energy demand from the heart. Ogden has developed a task analysis that looks at six variables: rate, resistance, muscle groups used, involvement of trunk muscles, arm position, and isometric work. Other aspects that must be examined include temperature, time, and emotional stress related to the task (34). Occupational therapists are becoming more involved in work-capacity assessment with post-MI individuals. Information gathered from job analysis not only determines the person's cardiac capacity to resume work but also determines environmental adaptations that would allow safe, efficient return to work (35).

Leisure Activities

Leisure pursuits will be affected to the degree that the person continues to experience the cycle of anxiety and depression. The health perception concept noted earlier also affects socialization and leisure activities. Persons who continue to perceive that they are ill will essentially "play the role" of a sick individual. In this case, much of the leisure activity the person performs is very passive.

CASE STUDIES

The following cases illustrate the impact of coronary artery disease on occupational performance components and areas.

CASE 1

J.L. is a 54-year-old car salesman admitted to the emergency room 4 days ago following a 5-hour history of chest pain and discomfort in the shoulder, neck, and jaw. He complained of nausea and was diaphoretic and short of breath. He reported that he has felt fatigued for the last 2 weeks and experienced "heartburn" that was relieved with an antacid. J.L. was sitting at home and had finished his evening meal when the pain and shortness of breath occurred. He noted that the shortness of breath persisted even when he tried to lie down and rest.

Upon admission to the ER, he was observed for signs and symptoms of cardiac distress. Auscultation indicated an ectopic or irregular heart rate with blood pressure rate of 140/110. Laboratory tests indicated elevation of CPK and LDH enzymes. ECG studies revealed cardiac arrhythmias and confirmed evidence of an anterolateral myocardial infarction with subsequent complications of left heart failure and arrhythmias.

J.L. is married and has two teenage children. He was recently laid off from a long-held position at an automotive plant and had started a new job in auto sales 2 weeks prior to his hospitalization. The loss of his original job was quite stressful, and he was finding that he was not well-suited for sales. His wife had begun a part-time job as a bookkeeper and managing her new job plus caring for teenage children kept her quite busy. She had never worked outside the home before because J.L. had refused to accept her desire to do so, and this was creating additional problems in the marriage.

Occupational performance components affected by J.L.'s condition include sensorimotor and psychosocial (Table 12.3).

Neuromuscular

The implications of left heart failure include dyspnea, weakness, fatigue, and poor exercise tolerance (21). All these factors create the potential for a reduction in neuromuscular integrity, particularly the complications arising from congestive heart failure. J.L.'s current functional capacity is at the 1.5 MET level (see Table 12.2). He has normal range of motion and muscle strength.

Psychosocial

The immediate inactivity forced on J.L. by hospitalization has caused a loss of role functions. He feels anxious and is angry about the potential of not being able to return to work and provide for his family needs. Because of his current neuromuscular status, he feels that it will limit him in all his activities. He is reluctant to tell the cardiac rehabilitation team about his concerns over resumption of sexual activity. However, he angrily told his wife that "I guess you'll need to find someone else since I won't be able to please you." He stated that "I might as well go to a nursing home and lessen the burden on everyone." While many of his friends and family have called him and sent him cards, he refuses to talk to them, asking to be left alone.

Occupational Performance Areas

ACTIVITIES OF DAILY LIVING

Most areas of ADL are affected by J.L.'s condition. An MET level of 1.5 indicates that he needs frequent rest periods to sustain activity. He can perform grooming, oral hygiene, and eating without discomfort, as these activities do not require sustained effort. Tasks such as dressing, toileting (bowel movements in particular) require more sustained, isometric work and may be more stressful. Issues around sexual activity are of concern because he perceives himself unable to perform sexually.

WORK ACTIVITIES

Because of J.L.'s difficulty with his new job and the apparent stress he perceives from it, his return-to-work potential is affected. He is anxious about his ability to return to his new job and is distressed about his wife having to work to bring in needed income. A thorough analysis of the physical components of work demand cannot be completed until J.L. reaches the 5 MET level. At that time, a job analysis can be completed.

Table 12.3.
Occupational Performance Profile

		Performance Areas			
			Work Activities		
		Vocation	Education	Home Management	Care of Others
OCCUPATIONAL PERFORMANCE COMPONENTS	SENSORIMOTOR — **SENSORY INTEGRATION** Intact				
	NEURO-MUSCULAR Dyspnea, weakness, fatigue, poor exercise tolerance	Job demands need assessment			
	COGNITIVE — **MOTOR** Intact **COGNITIVE**				
	PSYCHOSOCIAL — **PSYCHOLOGIC** Loss of role function, anxious and angry, feels limited, perceives cardiac cripple status	Feels job stressful			Loss of breadwinner role
	SOCIAL Withdrawn, strained family relationships; disinterested in social activity	Withdrawn from co-workers			
	SELF-MANAGEMENT Difficulty coping				

EXTERNAL FACTORS WHICH INFLUENCE PERFORMANCE; CULTURE, ECONOMY, ENVIRONMENT

Grid adapted from Uniform Terminology (2nd ed.) Developed by the occupational therapy faculty at Eastern Michigan University.

LEISURE

J.L. does not have a history of leisure interests and is not willing to explore new ones at this time. He refused to complete a leisure inventory assessment requested by the occupational therapist. He indicated that he was "too worried about his job and family to think about play."

CASE 2

M.M. is a widowed 92-year-old woman with congestive heart failure (CHF) (status post 5 weeks) complicated by pulmonary congestion and a history of rheumatoid arthritis. She is also experiencing a recent and progressive visual loss due to acute glaucoma. Prior to her initial

Client initials: J.L.
Diagnosis:
Age:

Play or Leisure Activities		Activities of Daily Living				
Exploration	Performance	Self-Care	Socialization	Functional Communication	Functional Mobility	Sexual Expression
MET 1.5 = limits	MET 1.5 = limits	MET 1.5 = need for rest periods; dressing, toileting require sustained effort				
Disinterested/feels not important	Disinterested/feels not important		Perceived "illness"/ feels he is a burden			Perceives sexual dysfunction secondary
			Limited social engagement			

hospitalization and subsequent return home, M.M. was an active woman who enjoyed going for short walks, reading, visiting with friends, and a weekly bridge club. She had been independent in most of her activities of daily living, requiring assistance only for some household management requiring heavier maintenance, cleaning, and repairs. Her current condition affects all components of occupational performance (Table 12.4).

Occupational Performance Components

SENSORY MOTOR COMPONENT

M.M. cannot read, watch television, or engage in activities requiring visual acuity because of her advanc-

Table 12.4.
Occupational Performance Profile

OCCUPATIONAL PERFORMANCE COMPONENTS		Performance Areas: Work Activities			
		Vocation	Education	Home Management	Care of Others
SENSORIMOTOR	**SENSORY INTEGRATION** Visual loss; other senses intact			Unable to perform any home management activity	
SENSORIMOTOR	**NEUROMUSCULAR** Severely deconditioned/weak				
SENSORIMOTOR	**MOTOR** Limited ROM UE and LE/pain, crepitation, fatigue				
COGNITIVE	**COGNITIVE** Intermittently intact/diffuse/needs consistent cues, mild confusion/intact for memory events				
PSYCHOSOCIAL	**PSYCHOLOGIC** Anxious about inactivity/feels a burden to daughter, is fearful/reluctant to request assistance				
PSYCHOSOCIAL	**SOCIAL** Limited opportunity for social interaction				
PSYCHOSOCIAL	**SELF-MANAGEMENT** Coping with decreasing function				
	EXTERNAL FACTORS WHICH INFLUENCE PERFORMANCE; CULTURE, ECONOMY, ENVIRONMENT				

Grid adapted from Uniform Terminology (2nd ed.) Developed by the occupational therapy faculty at Eastern Michigan University.

ing visual loss. Her hearing and other senses are intact. As a result of CHF and arthritis, Mrs. M. is severely deconditioned and very weak. She complains of arthritic pain in her shoulders, elbows, hips, and knees. Overall passive and active range of motion is limited, predominantly in the proximal joints. Shoulder motion is limited to 100° of flexion, 65° of internal and external rotation, and 70° of abduction. Hip range of motion is limited to 60° of flexion. Knee flexion is limited to 30° of active motion. Great care had to be taken in pas-

Client initials: M.M.
Diagnosis:
Age:

Play or Leisure Activities		Activities of Daily Living				
Exploration	Performance	Self-Care	Socialization	Functional Communication	Functional Mobility	Sexual Expression
		Deficits in all areas of self-care				
	Weakness/ fatigue				Severely limited/needs assist for all activity	
	Severe ROM limitation				Severely limited/needs assist for all activity	
	Feels cannot perform secondary to physical limits					
				Limited opportunities		

sive joint measurement because of her pain. Pronounced crepitation indicates diminished joint soft tissue integrity. Because of fatigue, she could not tolerate any additional activity following attempts to measure active range of motion.

COGNITIVE INTEGRATION

M.M.'s cognitive status is intermittently intact and diffuse. She is easily aroused and will orient to others, yet a consistent pattern of verbal and tactile cues are required to maintain her attention. She recognizes family and staff without difficulty and can engage in meaningful conversation. Most of what appear to be attention deficits may be caused by physical fatigue making her want to close her eyes and sleep.

Although she demonstrates mild confusion when following instructions, she is generally aware of her errors, often seeking clarification of accuracy in performing a task or exercise. M.M. is able to recall short- and long-term events.

PSYCHOSOCIAL SKILLS AND PSYCHOLOGIC COMPONENTS

M.M. is a friendly, engaging woman who clearly enjoys the social contact from various visiting health-team members. She asks about their families or jobs and shares information about her own family. Visits from other family members (e.g., grandchildren) are infrequent, since they all live out of state. When they have visited her, she reports it as very pleasant for her.

M.M. lives with her daughter, who finds it difficult to meet all of her mother's physical needs. At times, her daughter expresses frustration and anger at the level of care her mother requires. M.M. senses this and is subsequently fearful and reluctant to request things from her daughter.

She expresses concern that she may never resume her previous activity level and notes that her days seem to get longer and longer as her level of inactivity continues. M.M. consistently expresses a concern that she is a major burden on her daughter and clearly hopes she can learn to be more self-sufficient to regain independence.

Occupational Performance Areas

ACTIVITIES OF DAILY LIVING

M.M. is dependent for all activities of daily living. A primary deficit is the lack of functional mobility. M.M. cannot independently change positions in bed and must be repositioned to prevent skin breakdown. She is currently confined to bed, except for being up in a chair for about 30 minutes each day. She cannot transfer from the bed without total assistance of two people. A neighbor helps her daughter put M.M. in the chair and back to bed.

Because she is incontinent, she must wear diapers. She cannot bathe and depends on a daily bed bath, which is done three days a week by the home-health aide and the other days by her daughter.

M.M. can feed herself but often drops her utensil because of lack of endurance for grasping objects.

WORK

M.M. cannot complete any activities related to home management other than money management. She must depend on a cleaning person who works three afternoons a week. Her daughter completes meal preparation and cleanup, shopping, and clothing care.

LEISURE

Due to lack of visual function, immobility, and generalized weakness, it is difficult for M.M. to pursue leisure interests. She cannot visit anyone outside the home at this time, and visits from others are limited. Thus, her opportunity for social interaction is almost nonexistent.

She has enjoyed various handicraft activities in the past but feels she cannot perform these anymore due to her current condition.

REFERENCES

1. Brannon FJ, Geyer MJ, Foley MW. Cardiac rehabilitation. Philadelphia: FA Davis, 1988.
2. Anthony CP, Thibodeau GA. Textbook of anatomy and physiology, St. Louis: CV Mosby, 1983:14–22.
3. Andreoli KG, Fowkes VK, Zipes DR, Wallace AG, eds. Comprehensive cardiac care: a text for nurses, physicians, and other health care practitioners. St. Louis: CV Mosby, 1983.
4. Grollman S. The human body, 4th ed. Macmillan, New York, 1978:85–262.
5. Dubin D. Rapid interpretation of EKG's. Tampa, Florida, 1974, C.O.V.E.R., Inc.
6. Foderaro D. Cardiac dysfunction. In: Pedretti L, ed. Occupational therapy: practice skills for physical dysfunction, St. Louis: CV Mosby, 1985.
7. American Heart Association: Cardiopulmonary resuscitation: advanced life support, JAMA suppl Aug. 1980.
8. Dawber TR. An approach to longitudinal studies in a community: the Framingham Study. Ann NY Acad Sci 1963;107:539.
9. Gordon T, Kannel WWB Predisposition to atherosclerosis in the head, heart, and legs: the Framingham Study. JAMA 1972;221:661.
10. American Heart Association: Fact sheet on heart attack: stroke and risk factors, 1988. Dallas.
11. Vincent MO, Spence MI. Commonsense approach to coronary care. St. Louis: CV Mosby, 1985:160–243.
12. Underhill SL. Diagnosis and treatment of the patient with coronary artery disease and myocardial ischemia. In: Underhill SL, Woods SL, Snarjan ES, Halpenny CJ, eds. Cardiac nursing. Philadelphia: JB Lippincott, 1982.
13. O'Sullivan SB. Coronary artery disease. In: O'Sullivan SB, Schmitz TJ. Physical rehabilitation: assessment and treatment. Philadelphia: FA Davis, 1988.
14. Woods SL, Underhill SL. Coronary heart disease: myocardial ischemia and infarction. In: Patrick ML, et al., eds. Medical surgical nurs-

ing: pathophysiological nursing. Philadelphia: JB Lippincott, 1986.

15. Rothstein JM, Roy SH, Wolf SL. The rehabilitation specialists handbook. Philadelphia: FA Davis, 1991.

16. Heart facts. Dallas: American Heart Association, 1984.

17. Guyton AC. Textbook of medical physiology, 6th ed. Philadelphia: WB Saunders.

18. Long C, ed. Prevention and rehabilitation in ischemic heart disease. Baltimore: Williams and Wilkins, 1980.

19. Wulf KS. Management of the cardiovascular surgery patient. In: Brunner LS, Suddarth SD. Textbook of medical surgical nursing, 5th ed. Philadelphia: JB Lippincott, 1984.

20. Nurse Review: A clinical update system, vol. 1. Cardiac problems. Springhouse, PA: 1986,55–56.

21. Cassem NH and Hackett TP. Psychological rehabilitation of myocardial infarction patients in the acute phase. Heart Lung 1973;2:382.

22. Cornett SJ and Watson JE. Cardiac rehabilitation: an interdisciplinary team approach. New York: John Wiley, 1984.

23. Wilson PW, Anderson KM, Castelli WP. Twelve year incidence of coronary heart disease in middle aged adults during the era of hypertensive therapy: the Framingham offspring study. Am J Med 1991;90(1):11–16.

24. Myers RH, Keily DK, Cupples LA, Kannel WB. Parental history is an independent risk factor for coronary artery disease: the Framingham study. Am Heart J 1990;120(4):963.

25. Kannel WB. CHD risk factors: a Framingham study update. Hosp Pract 1990;25(7):119–127, 130.

26. Miles WM, Zipes DP. Cardiovascular diseases. In: Andreoli TE, Carpenter CJ, Plum F, Smith LH, eds. Cecil essentials of medicine. Philadelphia: WB Saunders, 1986.

27. White PD. Heart disease. New York: Macmillan, 1951.

28. Gundle MJ, Reeves BR, Tate S, Raft D, McLavrin LP. Psychosocial outcome after coronary artery surgery. Am J Psychiatry. 1980;137:(1)591–594.

29. Stallones R. The rise and fall of ischemic heart disease. Psychosom Med 1987;49:109–117.

30. Stern MJ, Pascale L, Ackerman A. Life adjustment, postmyocardial infarction: determining predictive variables. Arch Intern Med 1977;137:1680–1685.

31. Gutmann MC, Knapp DN, Pollock ML, Schmidt D, Simon K, Walcott G. Coronary artery bypass patients and work status. Circulation 1982;66:33–41.

32. Gulledge AD. Psychological aftermaths of myocardial infarction. In: Gentry WD, Williams RB, eds. Psychological aspects of myocardial infarction and coronary care. 2nd ed. St. Louis: CV Mosby, 1979.

33. Kushnir B, Fox KM, Tomlinson IW, Portal RW, Aber CP. The effect of a pre-discharge consultation on the resumption of work, sexual activity and driving following acute myocardial infarction. Scand J Rehabil Med 1975;7:158–162.

34. Ogden LD. Guidelines for analysis and testing of activities of daily living with cardiac patients. Downey, CA: Cardiac Rehabilitation Resources, 1981.

35. Beauchamp N, Creighton C, Summers L. Cardiac work tolerance screening: a case study. Occup Ther Health Care 1984;1(2):99.

Glossary

Anastomosis: Surgical, traumatic, or pathologic formation of a connection between two normally distinct structures.

Aneurysm: A sac formed by the localized dilation of the wall of an artery, vein, or the heart. The chief signs of an arterial aneurysm are the formation of a pulsating tumor and often a bruit heard over the swelling. A true aneurysm results from formation of a sac by the arterial wall with at least one unbroken layer; most often associated with atherosclerosis. A false aneurysm usually is caused by trauma when the wall of the blood vessel is ruptured and blood escapes into surrounding tissues and forms a clot. Aneurysms tend to increase in size, presenting a problem of increasing pressure against adjacent tissues and organs and a danger of rupture.

Angina pectoris: Acute pain in the chest resulting from decreased blood supply to the heart muscle (myocardial ischemia). The disorder is sometimes called cardiac pain of effort and emotion because the pain is brought on by physical activity or emotional stress that places an added burden on the heart and increases the need for additional blood supply to the myocardium.

Arrhythmia: Variation from the normal rhythm, especially of the heartbeat.

Arteriosclerosis: A group of diseases characterized by thickening and loss of elasticity of the arterial walls; popularly called "hardening of the arteries."

Atherosclerosis: An extremely common form of arteriosclerosis in which deposits of yellowing plaques (atheromas) containing cholesterol, other lipoid material, and lipophages are formed within the inner layer (intima) of large and medium-sized arteries.

Auscultation: Listening for sounds produced within the body, chiefly to ascertain the condition of thoracic or abdominal visceral.

Bronchospasm: Bronchial spasm; spasmodic contraction of the muscular coat of the smaller divisions of the bronchi, such as occurs in asthma.

CABG: Coronary artery bypass grafting.

Crepitation: A dry, crackling sound or sensation, such as that produced by the grating of the ends of a fractured bone.

Depolarization: The process that takes place when neurotransmitter molecules diffuse across a synaptic cleft of a nerve cell and bind with specific receptors on the postsynaptic membrane, thereby transmitting nerve impulses.

Diastole: The phase of the cardiac cycle in which the heart relaxes between contractions; specifically, the period when the two ventricles are dilated by the blood flowing into them.

Dyspnea: Labored or difficult breathing. A symptom of a variety of disorders and primarily an indication of inadequate ventilation or of insufficient amounts of oxygen in the circulating blood.

Ectopic: Arising or produced at an abnormal site or in a tissue where it is not normally found.

Edema: An abnormal accumulation of fluid in the intercellular spaces of the body.

Pedal edema: Swelling of the feet and ankles.

Endocardium: The endothelial lining membrane of the cavities of the heart and the connective tissue bed on which it lies.

Epicardium: The inner layer of the serous pericardium, which is in contact with the heart.

Fibrillation: A small, local, involuntary, muscular contraction, due to spontaneous activation of single muscle cells or muscle fibers. Atrial: A cardiac arrhythmia marked by rapid randomized contractions of the atrial myocardium, causing a totally irregular, often rapid, ventricular rate. Ventricular: A cardiac arrhythmia marked by fibrillary contractions of the ventricular muscle due to rapid repetitive excitation of myocardial fibers without coordinated ventricular contraction.

Fistula: Any abnormal, tubelike passage within body tissue, usually between two internal organs, or leading from an internal organ to the body surface.

Friedreich's ataxia: A hereditary sclerosis of the dorsal and lateral columns of the spinal cord, usually beginning in childhood or youth, with resultant progressive ataxia, speech impairments, scoliosis, and peculiar swaying and irregular movements, with paralysis of the muscles, especially of the lower extremities.

Hypertrophy: Increase in volume of a tissue or organ produced entirely by enlargement of existing cells.

Immunosuppression: Inhibition of the formation of antibodies; used in transplant procedures to prevent rejection of the transplanted organ or tissue.

Infarct: A localized area of ischemic necrosis produced by occlusion of the arterial supply or the venous drainage of the part.

Intima: The innermost coat of a blood vessel; also called the tunic intima.

Ischemia: Deficiency of blood in a part, due to a functional constriction or actual obstruction of a blood vessel.

Isoenzymes: Any of the several forms of an enzyme, all of which catalyze the same reaction, but which may differ in reaction rate, inhibition by various substances, electrophoretic mobility, or immunologic properties. Several enzymes, particularly alkaline phosphatase, lactate dehydrogenase, and creatine kinase, have clinically important isoenzymes. Isoenzymes are separated by electrophoresis, and the pattern indicates which damaged organ has released the enzymes.

Muscular dystrophy: A group of genetically determined, painless, degenerative myopathies that are progressively crippling as muscles gradually weaken and atrophy.

Myocardium: The middle and thickest layer of the heart wall, composed of cardiac muscle.

Necrosis: The morphologic changes indicative of cell death caused by enzymatic degradation.

PTCA (percutaneous transluminal coronary angioplasty): A procedure to enlarge the lumen of a sclerotic coronary artery by using a balloon-tipped catheter that is guided under fluoroscopy to the site of an atheromatous lesion. It provides an alternative to by-pass cardiac surgery for selected patients with ischemic heart disease.

Plaque: Any patch of flat area. Atheromatous plaque: A deposit of predominantly fatty material in the lining of blood vessels occurring in atherosclerosis.

Purkinje fibers: Modified cardiac muscle fibers in the subendothelial tissue, concerned with conducting impulses to the heart.

Systole: The contraction, or period of contraction, of the heart, especially of the ventricles, during which blood is forced into the aorta and pulmonary artery.

Tachycardia: Abnormally rapid heart rate, usually taken to be over 100 beats per minute.

Thrombocytopenia: Decrease in number of platelets in circulating blood, which can cause excessive bleeding during trauma.

Thrombus: An aggregation of blood factors, primarily platelets and fibrin with entrapment of cellular elements, frequently causing vascular obstruction at the point of its formation. Mural thrombus: One attached to the wall of the endocardium in a diseased area. Venous thrombus: One attached to the wall of a vein.

Tremor: An involuntary trembling of the body or limbs, occurring either at rest or during activity, depending on the origin of the lesion.

Vertigo: A sensation of rotation or movement of one's self (subjective) or of one's surroundings (objective) in any plane. The term is sometimes used erroneously as a synonym for dizziness. Vertigo may result from diseases of the inner ear or may be due to disturbances of the vestibular centers or pathways in the central nervous system.

Medications

I. NITRATES

	Nitroglycerin	Isosorbide dinitrate	Nitroglycerin (topical)	Nitroglycerin (transdermal patches)
Generic name	Nitroglycerin	Isosorbide dinitrate	Nitroglycerin (topical)	Nitroglycerin (transdermal patches)
Brand name	Nitrostat	Isordil	Nitro-Bid, Nitrol	Nitro-Dur, Transderm-Nitro
Indication	Vasodilator—reduces myocardial O_2 demand		Vasodilator—reduces myocardial O_2 demand	Vasodilator—reduces myocardial O_2 demand
Potential side effects	Tachycardia, hypotension, flushing, headache		Tachycardia, hypotension, flushing, headache	Tachycardia, hypotension, flushing, headache
Usual adult dosage-mode	Sublingual 1/100–1/400 gr p.r.n. IV dosage titrated	Sublingual chewable: 2.5–5.0 mg	Topical: 1/1–4 inch ribbon of ointment	Topical patch: (q.d.) 26–154 mg

II. β-BLOCKING AGENTS

	Propranolol	Metoprolol	Nadolol	Timolol
Generic name	Propranolol	Metoprolol	Nadolol	Timolol
Brand name	Inderal	Lopressor	Corgard	Biocadren
Indication	Hypertension; angina, some arrhythmias postinfarct to prevent reinfarction; migraines	Hypertension; angina, some arrhythmias	Hypertension; angina, some arrhythmias	Hypertension; angina. Post infarct to prevent reinfarction. To decrease intraocular pressure
Potential side effects	Bronchospasm, hypotension, drug fever, GI disturbances transient thrombocytopenia, fatigue, and sleep disorders	SAME	Bronchospasm, hypotension, drug fever, GI disturbances transient thrombocytopenia, fatigue, and sleep disorders	SAME

	Limit smoking as it may result in elevated blood pressure. Sudden d/c of drugs may cause increased angina		Limit smoking as it may result in elevated blood pressure. Sudden d/c of drugs may cause increased angina	
Usual adult dosage-mode	10–12 mg b.i.d. to q.i.d. Extremely variable dosage and variable uses	100–450 mg/day single dose or t.i.d.	40–320 mg/day single dose or t.i.d.	10 mg b.i.d. ophthalmic 0.25% solution

III. CALCIUM-CHANNEL BLOCKERS

Generic name	Diltiazem	Nifedipine	Verapamil
Brand name	Cardizem	Procardia	Calan, Isoptin
Indication	Angina; hypertension	Angina; hypertension	Angina; tachycardia
Potential side effects	Hypotension, reflex tachycardia, peripheral edema, and headache; CNS signs—tremors, mood changes, and fatigue	SAME plus pedal edema	SAME
Usual adult dosage	30 mg t.i.d. to q.i.d.	SAME	320–480 divided doses

IV. COMMON ANTIARRHYTHMICS: CLASS II/III

Generic name	Lidocaine (class II)	Propranolol (class III)	Bretylium (class IV)	Verapamil (class V)
Brand name	Xylocaine	Inderal	Bretylol	Calan, Isoptin
Indication	Treatment and control of ventricular arrhythmias. Decreases/eliminates ventricular ectopy	β-Blockers—block sympathetic stimulation at SA node—slows ventricular response	Acute mgmt of refractory ventricular tachycardia	Antiarrhythmic, controls atrial fibrillation
Potential side effects	Disorientation, seizures, hypotension	Exacerbation of CHF side effects of other β-blockers	Hypotension, vertigo light-headedness	Hypotension, vertigo constipation

Usual adult dosage	50–100 mg rapidly. Repeat if necessary followed by IV drip titrated to control PVCs	10–30 mg t.i.d. or q.i.d.	5–10 mg/kg IV over 30 min (acute care only)	IV 0.1 to 0.15 mg/kg to treat SVT maintenance oral dose 40–160 mg q. 8 hr

V. COMMON ANTIARRHYTHMICS: CLASS I

Generic name	Quinidine sulfate	Quinidine gluconate	Procainamide hydrochloride	Disopyramide
Brand name	Quinidex	Quinaglute	Pronestyl	Norpace
Indication	Alter conductivity of myocardium to correct abnormal electrical activity Restores normal heart rhythm	SAME	SAME	Alter conductivity of myocardium to correct abnormal electrical activity Restores normal heart rhythm
Potential side effects	Severe nausea, diarrhea	SAME	GI disturbances; fatigue severe hypotension; systemic lupus syndrome may develop	Specific for ventricular arrhythmias Cardiac decompensation
Usual adult dosage	200–400 mg q. 4–6 hr	324 mg q. 6 hr	250–500 mg q 3–4 hr	400–800 mg/day divided doses

13

Rheumatoid Arthritis

CYNTHIA D. BATTS

Lauren, a 32-year-old certified public accountant, mother of two small children, woke again with severe pain and stiffness as she had every morning for the past few weeks. Her hands were swollen and warm to the touch. She thought, I was hoping the last time I felt like this was the last time. Her husband convinced her to see a doctor for an evaluation. She did, and was diagnosed with rheumatoid arthritis (RA).

A.J. Landnia-Beauvais is given credit for the earliest description of RA in his Paris thesis of 1800. However, it was not until 1858 that A.B. Garrod coined the actual phrase *rheumatoid arthritis,* and not until 1941 that the American Rheumatism Association adopted the terminology (1).

RA is only one of 109 different forms of arthritis. Of the eight major categories into which arthritis is divided, RA is included under the synovitis category (2). Even though less common than other forms of the disease, such as osteoarthritis, it is potentially more serious. According to an American National Health Interview conducted by the Arthritis Foundation, RA is America's number one ranked crippling disease, costing the economy $14 billion in lost wages and medical bills (3).

ANATOMY

It is important to have an accurate concept of the joint anatomy and its related structures (Fig. 13.1) before discussing the etiology, signs and symptoms, and course of RA. The word *arthritis* comes from the Greek words "anthron" (which means joint) and "itis" (which means inflammation or infection). Therefore, the word is defined as "inflammation or infection of the joint" (4). In addition, the base word "rheum" in rheumatoid refers to the stiffness, general aching, weakness, and fatigue that is experienced throughout the body.

The anatomy of a healthy joint (Fig. 13.1) should be kept in mind later in the chapter when the disease process and its effect on the joint are discussed. Refer to the glossary for specific anatomical definitions.

ETIOLOGY

The cause of RA is unknown. RA is currently thought to be associated with a malfunctioning immune system. It is also speculated that RA may be caused by a virus or bacterium (5, 6). A high proportion of individuals with RA demonstrate circulating antibodies to an antigen present in the Epstein-Barr (EB) virus (7). The inflammatory problem involves a "triggering" of a chronic inflammation that begins in the synovial membrane of the joints and progresses to erosion of the joint capsule, tendons, ligaments, and eventually cartilage and bone. The inflammation usually spreads to other joints, resulting in further joint damage (8) (Fig. 13.2). Further, since this disease is systemic, chronic involvement includes manifestations that affect the lungs, the cardiovascular system, and the eyes.

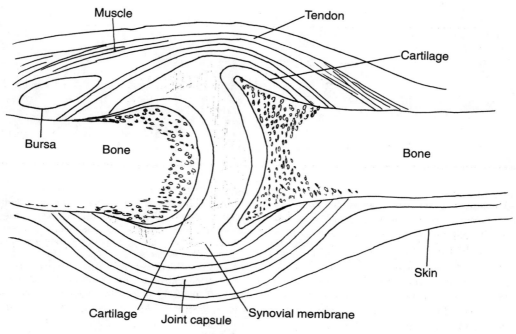

Figure 13.1. Anatomy of a joint.

Research indicates that genetic factors may influence the disease. Leukocytes (white blood cells) have been studied for hereditary factors that predispose a person to RA.

One type of leukocyte, the T cell, matures under the influence of the thymus and mediates cellular immunity. This cell-mediated immunity provides the body's main defense against intracellular organisms and involves the identification and removal of foreign substances (antigens) from the body. The entire process depends upon the interaction of the antigen with receptors on the surface of the T cell; therefore, T cells are further categorized into genetic classes containing human leukocyte antigen (HLA) receptors. A large accumulation of data links specific HLA antigens with particular disease states in the human (7).

The T cell has a binding cleft (receptor site) with specific sensitivity to certain antigens and complimentary to the structures found in antibodies. One particular class, the HLA-DR4 type, does not distinguish between antigens and healthy tissue and is associated with a susceptibility to rheumatoid arthritis. As a result, substances that facilitate inflammation of the synovial lining are released.

The following description helps to provide an understanding of the molecular process. Initially, an antigen such as the EB virus comes in contact with the T cell receptor; the T cell membrane becomes activated, and the T cell is transformed into a large blast cell which then proliferates. The sensitized T cells indirectly stimulate macrophage-like cells of the synovial lining of the joints. During this inflammatory phase, the affected joint demonstrates increased heat, swelling, pain, redness, and decreased range of motion (9).

Later, there is a proliferation of connective tissue and a heavy infiltration by more lymphocytes as well as plasma cells. The activated synovial cells grow out as a malignant pannus (cover) (Fig. 13.3) over the cartilage, leading to cartilage breakdown. This granulation tissue continues

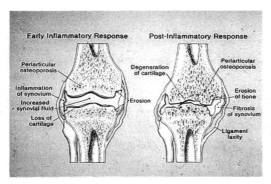

Figure 13.2. The postinflammatory response to joint inflammation is fibrosis, not unlike the scarring (fibrosis) that results from a surgical incision. The function of the postinflammatory joint depends on the degree of fibrosis and the destruction that occurred during the inflammatory stage. The damage influences the alignment, angle of tendon pull (joint integrity), range of motion, and stability. (From the AHPA Arthritis Teaching Slide Collection, 2nd ed., copyright 1988. Used with permission of the Arthritis Foundation.)

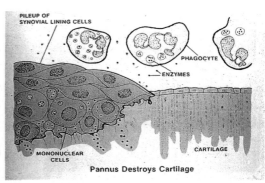

Figure 13.3. Synovial lining cells multiply, creating a mass called pannus. Substances in this mass further damage the underlying cartilage, which softens, weakens, and ultimately is destroyed. The waste products of cartilage cell destruction further stimulate the inflammatory process. New phagocytes rush to the area to clean up the debris. Some lymphocytes and other mononuclear cells are mistakenly rendered capable of attacking cartilage. Lysosomal enzymes and collagenase are released, thus perpetuating the abnormal process. (From the AHPA Arthritis Teaching Slide Collection, 2nd ed., copyright 1988. Used by permission of the Arthritis Foundation.)

to spread, the joint space is slowly effaced by fibrous adhesions, and eventually fibrous ankylosis appears. The by-product of the synovial lining destruction further stimulates the inflammation process, leading to more tissue damage than tissue repair (10) (Fig. 13.4).

JUVENILE RHEUMATOID ARTHRITIS

Etiology

Juvenile Rheumatoid Arthritis (JRA), of which there are three known types, begins in a variety of ways:

Systemic JRA affects 20% of children with JRA. It is characterized by fluctuating high fevers followed by chills and shaking. Children with systemic JRA often experience a rash with the high fever; the rash may be present only when temperature is elevated. Systemic JRA usually affects many joints and may facilitate other problems, such as pericarditis, pleuritis, stomach pain, anemia, and an increase in white blood cells (11, 12). General feelings of fatigue, weakness, and weight loss may be experienced as well.

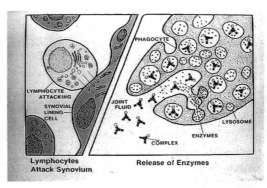

Figure 13.4. In the development of inflammatory rheumatic diseases, the normal protective process of inflammation goes awry. Lymphocytes can no longer distinguish between antigens and healthy tissue and secrete substances that cause the synovial lining to become inflamed. Phagocytes become overloaded with immune complexes and release lysosomal enzymes into the joint fluid. The enzymes then attack and destroy cells of the joint lining. (From the AHPA Arthritis Teaching Slide Collection, 2nd ed., copyright 1988. Used with permission of the Arthritis Foundation.)

Polyarticular JRA affects approximately 40–50% of children with JRA and is initiated in several joints at once (5 or more). The course usually involves the small joints of the hands and fingers, but it can also affect the weight-bearing joints. The joints are typically affected symmetrically and fevers may be present. Many children with polyarticular arthritis have a positive blood test for the rheumatoid factor and are likely to develop nodules on the parts of their bodies that experience a significant amount of pressure (e.g., elbows) (11, 13).

Pauciarticular arthritis or oligoarthritis accounts for 30–40% of those with JRA. This type of JRA characteristically affects the large joints such as the knees, ankles, or elbows and engages only a few joints (4 or fewer) at a time. Boys with pauciarticular arthritis also have hip and low back stiffness. Some children (more often girls) may be afflicted with an eye condition called iridocyclitis which displays red eyes, eye pain, and failing vision as symptoms (11, 13).

INCIDENCE AND PREVALENCE

Arthritis is widely prevalent, affecting approximately 14.6% (34.7 million persons) of the United States population, based on the National Health Interview Survey of 1987 (14). Approximately 12.1% of those affected with an arthritic condition consulted a physician. Specifically, rheumatoid arthritis affects 2.1 million people in the United States, based on statistics reported from the National Institute of Arthritis, Musculoskeletal, and Skin Disease National Advisory Board in conjunction with the Arthritis Foundation (15).

This study also reported that 71,000 children have juvenile rheumatoid arthritis (JRA), with girls being affected seven times more often than boys. Women are three times more commonly affected than men. Onset may be at any age, but it most often occurs between the ages of 30 and 50 (5). Racial factors also appear relevant

in RA. American blacks have a lower occurrence of RA than whites (16). North American Indians have a higher prevalence of RA, while native Japanese and Chinese may have a lower prevalence than whites (17). Reasons for these variations are currently unknown and may be attributed to both genetic and environmental factors.

SIGNS, SYMPTOMS, AND GENERAL MANIFESTATIONS

Onset of symptoms may be sudden and vary in degree. RA is frequently characterized by exacerbations (flare-ups) and remissions, in which the disease appears to be quiet and nonexistent.

Most often, RA affects more than one joint at the same time. In two-thirds of patients, an exacerbation is initiated by feelings of fatigue, generalized weakness, weight loss, malaise, and vague musculoskeletal symptoms until synovitis becomes more obvious. Although joint involvement is generally symmetrical, some patients may experience an asymmetrical pattern.

Discussion of joint involvement can be divided into two sections: stages of inflammatory joint disease as experienced overall, and specific manifestations to particular joints.

Articular and Periarticular Involvement

STAGES

Table 13.1 describes the stages of the inflammatory process as: (*a*) acute, (*b*) subacute, (*c*) chronic-active, and (*d*) chronic-inactive.

As mentioned earlier, onset may be sudden, with inflammation occurring in many joints at once. In the acute and subacute phases, various degrees of general fatigue, soreness, stiffness, and aching are followed by progressive localized symptoms of pain, inflammation, warmth, and tenderness in a joint or multiple joints.

Pain originates primarily from the joint capsule, which is abundantly supplied with

Table 13.1.
Stages of Inflammatory Joint Disease

Stages	Objective Signs	Subjective Symptoms
Acute	Limited range of motion	Pain at rest and movement most severe
	Fever	
	Decreased muscle strength	Tenderness most severe
	Possible cold, sweaty hands	Inflammation most severe
	Overall stiffness	Hot, red joints
	Gel phenomenon most prominent	Decreased function
	Weight loss	Tingling and numbness in hands and feel
	Decreased appetite	
Subacute	Decreased range of motion	Pain and tenderness at rest and movement decreases
	Endurance poor	
	Mild fever	Joints warm and pink
	Decreased muscle strength	Inflammation sudsiding
	Morning stiffness	Decreased function
	Gel phenomenon	Tingling and numbness in hands and feet
	Weight loss	
	Decreased appetite	
Chronic-active	Decreased range of motion	Pain and tenderness at rest minimal
	Fever has subsided	
	Muscle strength decreased	Pain on motion decreases
	Endurance low	Inflammation, low-grade
		Increased activity noted, due to adjustment to pain
		Tingling and numbness decreases
Chronic-inactive	Limited range of motion	Pain at motion due to stiffness from disuse during previous stages and instability of joint
	Muscle atrophy	
	Decreased endurance from limited activity in previous stages	No inflammation
		Residuals seen from above stages
	Residuals seen from above stages	
	Potential contracture	Functioning may be decreased due to fear of pain

pain fibers and is highly sensitive to stretching and distention.

Joint swelling results from the accumulation of synovial fluid, hypertrophy of the synovium, and thickening of the joint capsule.

In addition, there is usually decreased joint motion, decreased muscle strength and endurance, and a loss of appetite and weight. Patients frequently experience chills in their hands and feet, as well as numbness and tingling. As motion is limited by pain, the inflamed joint is usually held in flexion to maximize joint volume and minimize distention of the capsule (18).

Various degrees of generalized stiffness occurs, including the "gel phenomenon," which is the inability to move joints after prolonged rest (13). Morning stiffness of greater than 1 hour duration is an almost uniform feature of inflammatory arthritis, which distinguishes it from noninflammatory disorders. The length and intensity of the stiffness can be used as a gross assessment of disease activity.

Fatigue may be extensive enough to cause disability from disuse of joint motion and strength before joint changes actually occur.

Once the acute and subacute stages have subsided, the limited joint range of motion facilitates the formation of contractures. Contractures are due to adhesions that are formed when the patient avoids movement during the acute, painful phase. Limitations in range of motion result from ankylosis, subluxation, or dislocation. Also, muscle atrophy in chronic

stages results from disuse in the earlier, more acute stages.

SPECIFIC JOINT MANIFESTATIONS

Hand

The hands are by far the most severely affected sites of RA. Table 13.2 shows data from two studies, supporting this (19). Joints with the highest synovium to cartilage ratio are those most frequently affected by the disease.

Fusiform or spindle-shaped fingers, a typical sign of RA, result from swelling in the proximal interphalangeal (PIP) joints (Fig. 13.5). This is usually related to bilateral and symmetrical swelling of the metacarpophalangeal (MCP) joints. Pressure on these joints elicits tenderness. Distal interphalangeal (DIP) joints are rarely involved, which discriminates between RA and osteoarthritis (20).

Boutonnière and swan-neck deformities are two other common hand disfigurements seen resulting from RA. A boutonnière deformity is a combination of PIP joint flexion and DIP joint hyperextension (Fig. 13.6). More descriptively, it is flexion of the PIP joint through the detached central slip of the extensor tendon, which serves as a "button-hole" through which the joint can pop. The DIP joint is then forced into hyperextension (5).

Swan-neck deformities result from contractures of the interosseus and flexor muscles and tendons, which in turn produce a flexure contracture of the MCP joint, compensatory hyperextension of the

Table 13.2.
Characteristics of Onset of Rheumatoid Arthritis[a]

Method of Onset (%)		Area of Onset (%)		Pattern of Onset (%)	
Rapid (days or weeks)	46	Small joints	32	Monarticular	21
Insidious	54	Medium sized joints	16	Oligoarticular	44
		Large joints	29	Polyarticular	35
		Combined	26		

[a]Adapted from information in Fallahi S, Halla JT, Hardin JG, A reassessment of the nature of onset of rheumatoid arthritis (abstract). Clin Res 1983; 31:650A.

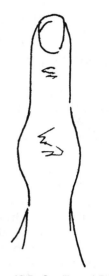

Figure 13.5. Swelling of PIP.

PIP joint, and flexion of the DIP joint (Fig. 13.7).

Thumb deformities associated with RA have been classified into three categories by E.A. Nalebuff. In type I, MCP inflammation leads to stretching of the joint capsule and boutonnière-like deformity. In type II, edema of the carpometacarpal (CMC) joint leads to volar subluxation during ankylosis of the adductor pollicis. In type III, after sustained disease of both MCP joints, exaggerated adduction of the first metacarpus, flexion of the MCP joint, and hyperextension of the DIP joint result from the patient's need to establish a compensatory method to pinch (Fig. 13.8) (5, 21).

De Quervain's tenosynovitis, which involves extensors at the thumb, causes se-

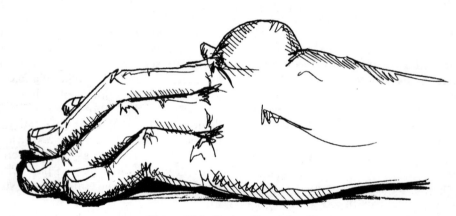

Figure 13.6. Boutonnière deformity.

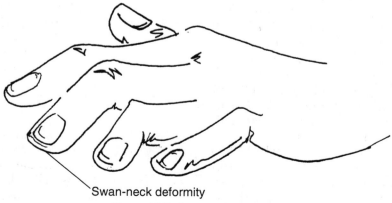

Swan-neck deformity
Figure 13.7. Swan-neck deformity.

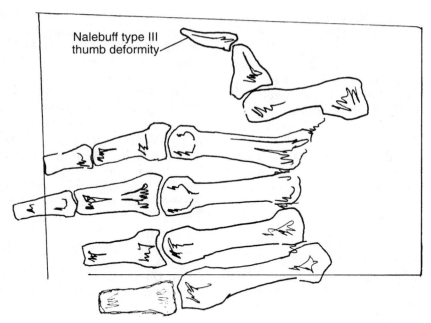

Nalebuff type III
thumb deformity

Figure 13.8. Thumb deformity-type III.

vere pain and discomfort resulting in a decrease in hand function and ability to grip (Fig. 13.9).

Wrists

Ulnar deviations and volar subluxation at the MCP joints or radiocarpal deviation are characteristic signs of RA at the wrist. These problems result from severe tenosynovitis and inflammation where the ligaments surround the joint, and eventually lead to edema, joint laxity, erosion of the tendons and ligaments, and muscle imbalance. When ulnar deviation of the MCP is present with radial deviation at the radiocarpal joint, a "zig-zag" presentation of the hand is seen (Fig. 13.10). Dorsiflexion of the wrist is often one of the first movements to be limited (22). Carpal tunnel syndrome is commonly diagnosed, resulting from synovial proliferations on the volar aspect of the wrist, which then impinges upon the median nerve (23). This causes paresthesia of the palmar aspect of the thumb, the second and third digits, and the radial aspect of the fourth digit.

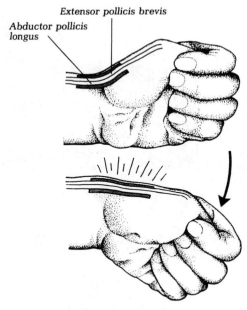

Extensor pollicis brevis

Abductor pollicis longus

Figure 13.9. Finklestein's test for de Quervain's disease.

Elbows

Loss of motion due to flexion contractures in addition to inflammation are the most prevalent problems of elbow involvement. Synovial swelling and thickening may be observed in the lateral area between the radial head and the olecranon. A bulge will be seen. Thickening of the fluid in the olecranon bursa and rheumatoid nodules that are painful if irritated by pressure are customary as well (24). Lateral epicondylitis, more often referred to as tennis elbow, is reported as sharply painful when firm pressure is placed on this specific area.

Synovitis in the radiohumeral joint can result in decreased motion during pronation and supination of the forearm (22).

Shoulders

Shoulder involvement is common and can be complicated as the RA disease process progresses. The glenohumeral, acromioclavicular, and thoracoscapular joints are the most susceptible. Since the shoulder relies on extensive coordinated movement, when any one of these joints becomes affected, dysfunction in activities of daily living will be seen.

Localized pain and tenderness, resulting from tendonitis in the glenohumeral area where the supraspinatus muscle or the long head of the biceps tendon inserts, are frequently seen. Rotator cuff tears are likely where the rotator cuff tendon inserts into the greater tuberosity. Erosion is triggered by the proliferative synovitis that develops there (Fig. 13.11) (25). Tendonitis, capsulitis, and bursitis (grouped under the "local conditions" of arthritis categories) are more frequently diagnosed causes of shoulder pain than synovitis (20).

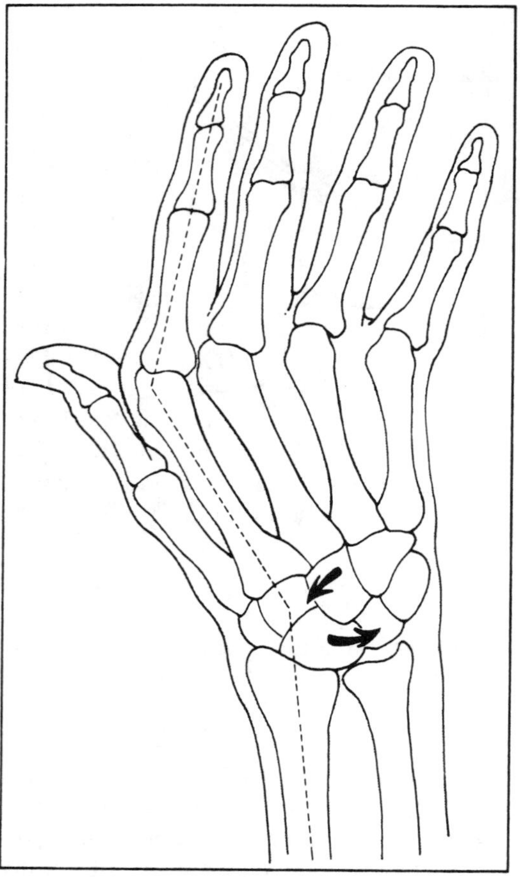

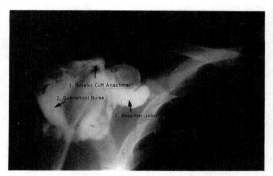

Figure 13.11. The supraspinatus, infraspinatus, and teres minor tendons make up a tendinous envelope commonly called the rotator cuff. This structure aids in the rotation of the humeral head and approximates the head to the glenoid fossa permitting the deltoid to abduct and forward flex the arm. The rotator cuff can undergo degenerative changes. Under conditions of trauma or repetitive stress, it may rupture. In incomplete tears, the patient may have only mild pain, atrophy of muscles in the shoulder region, and slight weakness on abduction. When the rupture is complete, the patient is unable to abduct the arm from 0° to 90° but can hold the arm above that level by deltoid muscle action.

This contrast arthrogram shows abnormal communication between the shoulder joint space (1) and the subdeltoid bursae (2). The rotator cuff (3) usually prevents the contrast media, injected into the shoulder joint itself, from entering the bursal space. Presence of contrast in the bursa confirms partial or complete tear. (From the AHPA Arthritis Teaching Slide Collection, 2nd ed., copyright 1988. Used by permission of the Arthritis Foundation.)

Figure 13.10. Radial deviation of wrist.

Synovitis of the glenohumeral area is seen occasionally in those with RA and is observed as a bulge in the anterior or lateral superior area of the shoulder.

Loss of motion results as a complication of shoulder synovitis, which is seen in progressed cases and is known as a "frozen shoulder."

Head, Neck, and Cervical Spine

During radiologic examination of this area (Fig. 13.12) in advanced cases of RA, the lower cervical and odontoid processes often appear eroded, as do the cervical apophyseal and intervertebral joints. The first to the fourth cervical joints are those most commonly affected by inflammation and pain. Involvement of the upper cervical spine in advanced cases leads to subluxation, whereas lower cervical spine involvement produces symptoms of cord-root compression (5, 20). For example, with a C5 root compression, problems are (a) sensation on the radial aspect of the forearm, (b) muscle weakness with abduction of the shoulder and flexion of the

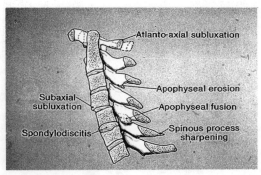

Figure 13.12. Neck abnormalities in rheumatoid arthritis. The neck is commonly involved in adult and juvenile rheumatoid arthritis. The most common disorder is subluxation of the atlantoaxial joint, which occurs particularly on flexion of the neck. C1 moves forward on C2, and the odontoid process can actually cause pressure to the spinal cord posteriorly.
Other findings include erosions at the apophyseal joints, fusion of the apophyseal joint, which occurs particularly in juvenile rheumatoid arthritis, and subluxation at other levels. Disc involvement may also occur, and erosive changes and resorption can cause sharpening of the spinous process. (From the AHPA Arthritis Teaching Slide Collection, 2nd ed., copyright 1988. Used by permission of the Arthritis Foundation.)

elbow, and (c) decreased biceps jerk reflex. Subluxation can also cause twisting and compression of the vertebral arteries, which leads to vertebrobasilar insufficiency. This may be facilitated by syncope on a downward gaze. Flexion and extension of the cervical spine are usually less affected.

Temporomandibular joints (TMJ) have varied involvement in RA, ranging from 1 to 60%. Women are affected three times more often than men. Both TM joints are usually involved. Pain, swelling, and stiffness are the most common symptoms (23).

Hoarseness occurs in up to 30% of rheumatoid patients. This stems from inflamed cricoarytenoid joints, which rotate with the vocal cords as they abduct and adduct to vary pitch and tone of the voice.

Hips

Approximately one-half of the patients diagnosed with RA have radiographic evidence of hip disease. People with hip involvement often have an abnormal gait pattern, possibly a limp (24). This can result from a variety of factors including: pain, flexion contractures, muscle weakness, or hip instability. Fibrous contractures in flexion or external rotation are standard if restriction of motion is prolonged. Since the hip joint capsule is limited in its ability to stretch, severe RA involvement followed by swelling and massive effusion of synovium into the joint capsule may be extremely painful. Also, hip involvement will result in discomfort and pain in the groin and the medial side of the knee.

As involvement increases (e.g., increased flexion contractures), further functional problems will be experienced in activities such as donning pants, sitting in a chair comfortably, walking upstairs, and positioning during sexual relations.

Knees

Hypertrophy and effusion of large amounts of synovium into the joint capsule are common in the knee joint and are more readily demonstrated in the knee than in the hip. Synovial fluid in the knee in excess of 5 ml may be observed as a "bulge" sign; bulges occur behind the patella when fluid is pushed into the suprapatellar pouch and then back into the joint. Swelling, quadriceps muscle atrophy, ligamentous laxity, and joint instability may be more obvious when the patient stands or walks. Pain and swelling on the posterior knee may be caused by marked increases in the intra-articular pressure during flexion, which produces an out-pouching or Baker's cyst. Popliteal cysts, such as these, may impede superior venous flow in the thigh, producing a dilation of veins and edema. When the joint capsule is stretched, a reflex spasm triggers in the hamstring muscles. To relieve joint pain and tension, patients will hold their hips and knees in a flexion pattern that facilitates contractures in those positions. These contractures will cause difficulty in all weight-bearing activities (24, 26).

Ankles and Feet

True rheumatic disease is less common in the ankle than in other areas of the body; however, tibiotalar swelling and loss of subtalar motion can develop. Ankle synovitis can be palpitated in front of, behind, and below the malleoli. It is often very tender and sensitive.

Symptomatic involvement of the feet is reported by 30 to 90% of those 2.1 million who have RA (27). Rheumatoid arthritis of the toes involving the metatarsophalangeal (MTP) joints results in changes similar to those in the hands. When the MTP joints are affected, normal gait is disrupted. Problems will be observed during the push-off phase of ambulation, causing compensatory action with other weight-bearing joints.

Characteristic manifestations of the feet include claw toes, hammer toes, cock-up toes, and hallux valgus (Fig. 13.13) (13). Claw toes result from the hyperextension of the MTP joints and the flexion of the PIP and DIP joints. Hammer toes differ from claw toes in that the DIP joint is hyperextended (Fig. 13.14). Cocking-up of the toes may be associated with subluxation of the metatarsal heads and finally a claw-like appearance with an elevation of the tip of the toe above the surface on which the foot is resting. Hal-

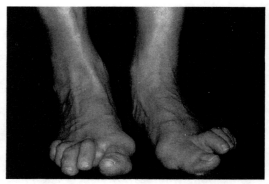

Figure 13.13. Hallux valgus and hammer toes are among the common foot deformities in patients with rheumatoid arthritis. The cockup toe deformities in this patient are associated with subluxation of the metatarsophalangeal joints. Painful corns and bunions are made worse from irritation due to improper shoes. (From the AHPA Arthritis Teaching Slide Collection, 2nd ed., copyright 1988. Used by permission of the Arthritis Foundation.)

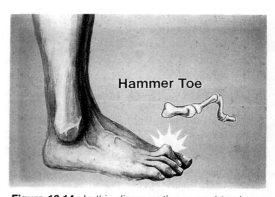

Figure 13.14. In this diagram, the second toe has a cockup deformity, which is similar to the boutonnière abnormality of the hand. Often, this deformity is associated with subluxation of the corresponding metatarsophalangeal joints. This deformity may be hastened in a patient who wears shoes that are too small. Rubbing of the proximal interphalangeal joints on the shoe causes pain, callus formation, and possibly ulceration. This abnormality is not restricted to patients with rheumatoid arthritis. (From the AHPA Arthritis Teaching Slide Collection, 2nd ed., copyright 1988. Used by permission of the Arthritis Foundation.)

lux valgus is a common event in which fibular deviation of the first through the fourth toes occurs. This is similar to ulnar deviation of the hands (Fig. 13.15).

Rheumatoid nodules develop over bony prominences that bear more than normal pressure. For those affected by painful forefoot weight bearing, rheumatoid nodules can occur on the heels due to increased weight bearing on this area.

Tarsal joint involvement does not occur as often as that of the forefoot; however, it can be quite detrimental to a person's ability to ambulate. As the longitudinal arch in the foot flattens and hindfoot valgus occurs, weight-bearing pressure tends to shift medially. This, in turn, facilitates the possible development of callositas and more rheumatoid nodule formations (28).

Muscle Involvement

Most patients with RA have muscle involvement, including muscle weakness. Recent studies suggest at least five stages of muscle disease in the RA process: (19, 29)

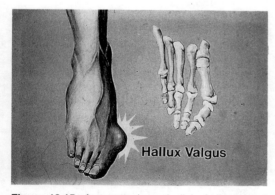

Figure 13.15. An anatomic and clinical diagram of hallux valgus. Pes planus and ligamentous laxity lead to lateral deviation of the great toe with a resultant hallux valgus. This deformity can be hastened by the wearing of narrow-toed shoes. Rubbing of the bunion on the shoe surface produces pain, and the lateral deviation of the great toe may impinge on other digits of the foot. This abnormality is not restricted to patients with rheumatoid arthritis. (From the AHPA Arthritis Teaching Slide Collection, 2nd ed., copyright 1988. Used by permission of the Arthritis Foundation.)

1. Reduction of muscle bulk associated with muscle atrophy that accompanies the inflammatory process due to disuse, bed rest, vascular events, and drug effects (30). A muscle can lose 30% of its bulk in 1 week (31). Loss of muscle bulk is associated with functional decrease (32).
2. Peripheral neuromyopathy, usually due to mononeuritis multiplex, which is frequently associated with rheumatoid vasculitis involving localized sensory loss (a complication of RA).
3. Steroid myopathy.
4. Active myositis and muscle necrosis (or muscle fiber inflammation resulting in destruction of the muscle fibers).
5. Chronic myopathy resembling a dystrophic process.

EXTRA-ARTICULAR SYSTEMIC MANIFESTATIONS

As previously described, RA not only affects the joint but also is systemic. The number and the severity of extra-articular features vary with the duration and extent of the disease, and tend to occur in individuals with higher levels of rheumatoid factor (RA factor) in their blood. The following are additional manifestations that may exist in those with RA.

Rheumatoid or Subcutaneous Nodules

These develop in approximately 20 to 30% of those with RA, usually in those whose disease is more destructive and progressed (5). Periarticular structures, extensor surfaces, and areas subject to pressure such as the olecranon, the proximal ulna, the Achilles' tendon, the occiput, and the sacrum are primary sites for those growths (33). Most can develop insidiously and regress at any time.

Pulmonary Manifestations

Pleuritis, interstitial fibrosis, pulmonary nodules, pneumonitis, and other forms of pulmonary obstructive disease occur more frequently in those with RA than in the normal population (34, 35). Evidence of pleuritis is most often found upon autopsy, because the disease is usually asymptomatic during life (9). In few cases, upper airway obstruction from cricoarytenoid arthritis or laryngeal nodules may develop (27). Others believe that small airway dysfunction is related to factors other than RA.

Felty's Syndrome

The condition of leukopenia associated with collagen-vascular disorders is termed Felty's syndrome. This syndrome is usually found in those who have progressed and chronic RA, as well as those who have high levels of the RA factor (5). Splenomegaly, leukopenia, anemia, neutropenia, thrombocytopenia, and granulocytopenia are also features of this syndrome (27). Although hypersplenism is proposed as one of the causes of the leukopenia, splenectomies do not correct the abnormality in many patients.

Cardiac Manifestations

Asymptomatic pericarditis is found in nearly 50% of autopsied cases (24). Most pericardial disease develops with synovitis several years into the course of RA. Manifestations may vary from mild to being the cause of death.

Other forms of cardiac disease in RA include rheumatoid carditis, endocardial (valve) inflammation, conduction defects, coronary arteritis, and granulomatous aortitis (29, 36).

Nervous System Manifestations

Neurologic manifestations may occur from cervical spine subluxation. As briefly described in the neck/cervical spine and wrist sections, nerve entrapment secondary to proliferative synovitis or joint deformities may facilitate neuropathies of the median, ulnar, radial, or anterior tibial nerves. In aggressive forms of vasculitis (Fig. 13.16), polyneuropathy and mono-

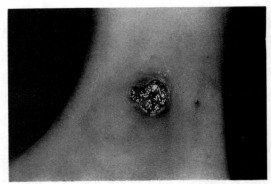

Figure 13.16. Vasculitis, defined as inflammation of the small vessels, is common in rheumatoid arthritis. The most common vascular abnormality in rheumatoid arthritis patients is leg ulceration, which may be indolent and very difficult to heal. Ulcers are not usually associated with either arterial or venous insufficiency. Other vasculitis problems in rheumatoid arthritis patients include benign digital (fingertip) ulceration and severe systemic vasculitis similar to polyarteritis nodosa. (From the AHPA Arthritis Teaching Slide Collection, 2nd ed., copyright 1988. Used by permission of the Arthritis Foundation.)

neuritis multiplex may result (5). Central nervous system involvement does not appear to occur directly, but vasculitis (as discussed above) and rheumatoid nodule-like granulomas can irregularly occur in the meninges (1).

Ophthalmologic Manifestations

The rheumatoid process involves the eye in less than 1% of patients. Sjögren's syndrome (Fig. 13.17) is a chronic disease of unknown etiology causing corneal and conjunctual lesions and characterized by dry eyes and mouth (37). Eye discomfort includes inability to cry and a sandy feeling in the eye when blinking. Scleritis, which involves the deeper coats of the eye, may cause pain and visual impairment. Episcleritis is a less serious inflammatory condition, and is usually temporary.

CLINICAL COURSE AND PROGNOSIS

The effects of RA differ significantly from person to person. Onset of the disease is usually gradual or insidious, although it

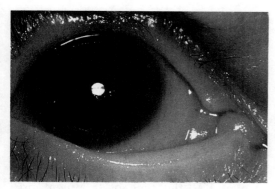

Figure 13.17. Rheumatoid arthritis patients may also have Sjögren's syndrome. Sjögren's syndrome is a chronic inflammatory disorder characterized by diminished lacrimal and salivary gland secretions (sicca complex), resulting in keratoconjunctivitis sicca and xerostomia. Patients may complain that the eyes feel "as if there were sand in them." The syndrome may also include decreased vaginal lubrication. Keratoconjunctivitis sicca is demonstrated here by flecks of reddish-purple discoloration in the lower portion of the cornea and conjunctiva, which were stained with rose bengal dye.
One-half of all Sjögren's syndrome patient have rheumatoid arthritis or some other connective tissue disease, particularly systemic lupus erythematosus or systemic sclerosis. More than 90% of these patients are women, with a mean age of 50 years at the time of diagnosis. Keratoconjunctivitis sicca develops in 10 to 15% of all rheumatoid arthritis patients. (From the AHPA Arthritis Teaching Slide Collection, 2nd ed., copyright 1988. Used by permission of the Arthritis Foundation.)

may be abrupt. Due to the cyclical nature of the RA process, an individual's ability to function can fluctuate according to the stage and severity of the disease. Researchers have found that approximately two-thirds of those with RA do not seek medical treatment and are able to care for themselves through conservative measures (e.g., rest, aspirin, rehabilitation therapy, etc.). Five years after the initial onset of RA, data suggest that the disease may be present in only one-third of all individuals.

Features that appear to have prognostic importance are: (*a*) number and length of remissions (Table 13.3), (*b*) levels of rheumatoid factor, (*c*) presence of subcutaneous nodules, (*d*) extent of bone erosion seen radiographically at initial evaluation, and (*e*) sustained disease activity for more than one year.

Classification and prognosis of RA can also be assessed by functional analysis (Table 13.4). The functional capacity of an individual declines as the disease becomes more prevalent.

Even though there is no cure for RA, treatment methods continue to improve. Data suggest that individuals currently admitted to the hospital for RA are likely

Table 13.3.
Proposed Criteria for Clinical Remission in Rheumatoid Arthritis[a]

Five or more of the following requirements must be fulfilled for at least 2 consecutive months:

1. Duration of morning stiffness not exceeding 15 minutes
2. No fatigue
3. No joint pain (by history)
4. No joint tenderness or pain on motion
5. No soft tissue swelling in joints of tendon sheaths
6. Erythrocyte sedimentation rate (Westergren method) less than 30 mm/hr for a female or 20 mm/hr for a male

[a]These criteria are intended to describe either spontaneous remission or drug-induced disease suppression, which simulates spontaneous remission. To be considered for this designation a patient must have met the ARA criteria for definite or classic rheumatoid arthritis at some time in the past. No alternative explanation may be invoked to account for the failure to meet a particular requirement. For instance, in the presence of knee pain, which might be related to degenerative arthritis, a point for "no joint pain" may not be awarded.

Exclusions: Clinical manifestations of active vasculitis, pericarditis pleuritis, or myositis, and unexplained recent weight loss or fever attributed to RA will prohibit a designation of complete clinical remission.

to have a decreased number of contractures and less fusion of peripheral joints at admission than patients 20 years ago (19). The median life expectancy of individuals with RA is shortened by 3 to 7 years (5). Upon completion of a thorough evaluation by a physician, early diagnosis can assist with developing a treatment approach to diminish joint pain, impede the disease process, and decrease joint deformity. Early classification of the disease facilitates earlier intervention and possibly

a "retarding of the disease process" (Table 13.5).

Emotional and financial support for treatment both contribute to the prognostic outcome for an individual. Studies have demonstrated a high incidence of depression, decreased self-esteem, and social withdrawal. Also, more than one-half of the individuals with RA report a major change in income, marital, or work status (38, 39). In those with a progressed case of RA, the type of treatment pre-

Table 13.4.
Classification of Functional Capacity in Rheumatoid Arthritis

Class I:	Complete functional capacity with the ability to carry on all usual duties without handicaps
Class II:	Functional capacity adequate to conduct normal activities despite handicap of discomfort or limited mobility of one or more joints
Class III:	Functional capacity adequate to perform only few or none of the duties of usual occupation or self-care
Class IV:	Largely or wholly incapacitated, with patient bedridden or confined to wheelchair, permitting little or no self-care

Table 13.5.
Classification of Progression of Rheumatoid Arthritis[a]

Stage I, Early
*1. No destructive changes on roentgenographic examination
 2. Roentgenologic evidence of osteoporosis may be present

Stage II, Moderate
*1. Roentgenologic evidence of osteoporosis with or without slight subchondral bone destruction; slight cartilage destruction may be present
*2. No joint deformities, although limitation of joint mobility may be present
 3. Extensive muscle atrophy
 4. Extra-articular soft tissue lesions such as nodules and tenosynovitis may be present

Stage III, Severe
*1. Roentgenologic evidence of cartilage and bone destruction in addition to osteoporosis
*2. Joint deformity such as subluxation, ulnar deviation, or hyperextension, without fibrous or bony ankylosis
 3. Extensive muscle atrophy
 4. Extraarticular soft tissue lesions, such as nodules and tenosynovitis may be present

Stage IV, Terminal
*1. Fibrous or bone ankylosis
 2. Criteria of stage III

[a]An asterisk marks criteria required for classification in the particular stage.

scribed plays a key part in life expectancy. For example, drug therapy, especially the more aggressive, systematic corticosteroid drugs may play a role in the increase of mortality rates.

DIAGNOSTICS

Individuals with joint disease delay seeking medical care on an average of 2 to 4 years (5). It is much more difficult to establish a diagnosis of RA in the early development of the disease than in the more progressed, later stages. Several visits to a physician for evaluation and testing may be needed prior to a confirmed diagnosis. The American Rheumatism Association first developed diagnostic criteria for the classification of RA in 1958 with revisions in 1987 (Table 13.6). Originally, these criteria were guidelines for classification of

disease syndromes to facilitate a correct diagnosis in individuals taking part in clinical research investigations. However, the criteria have also been used as guidelines for the specific diagnosis of general individuals (1). See Appendix 13.2 for a detailed description of diagnostic tests.

DRUG THERAPY

Many different drugs are used in the medical management of rheumatoid arthritis. Treatment is focused on antiinflammatory and immunosuppressive effects to prevent destruction of the joint as well as pain control (39). Treatment of rheumatoid arthritis should not be limited to drug therapy. As frequently seen in the pyramid approach (Fig. 13.18), medical management should begin with the most conservative method and as-

Table 13.6.
1987 ARA Revised Criteria for the Classification of Rheumatoid Arthritis[a]

Criterion	Definition
1. Morning stiffness	Morning stiffness in and around the joints lasting at least 1 hour before maximal improvement
2. Arthritis of 3 or more joint areas	At least 3 joint areas at the same time have had soft tissue swelling or fluid observed by a physician. The 14 possible areas are right or left PIP, MCP, wrist, elbow, knee, ankle, and MTP joints
3. Arthritis of hand joints	At least 1 area swollen in a wrist, MCP, or PIP joint
4. Symmetric arthritis	Simultaneous involvement of the same joint areas on both sides of the body (bilateral involvement of PIPs, MCPs, or MTPS is acceptable without absolute symmetry)
5. Rheumatoid nodules	Subcutaneous nodules over bony prominences or extensor surfaces or in juxtaarticular regions, observed by a physician
6. Serum rheumatoid factor	Demonstration of abnormal amounts of serum rheumatoid factor by any method for which the result has been positive in 5% of normal subjects
7. Radiographic changes	Radiographic changes typical of RA on posteranterior hand and wrist x-rays, which must include erosions or unequivocal bony decalcification localized in (or most marked adjacent to) the involved joints.

[a]A person is to be diagnosed with RA if he or she has met at least 4 out of 7 of the established criteria. The criteria of morning stiffness, arthritis of 3 or more joint areas, at least 1 area swollen in the hand joints, and presence of symmetrical involvement must be present for at least 6 weeks to establish a diagnosis of RA as well. Note that failure to meet these criteria, especially in the early stages does not exclude the diagnosis. Patients with 2 clinical diagnoses are not excluded. Designation as classic, definite, or probable RA is not to be made.

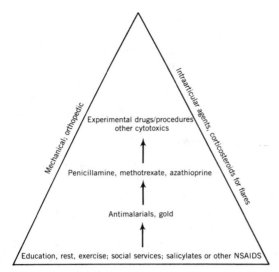

Figure 13.18. Treatment pyramid for rheumatoid arthritis. (From the primer on the rheumatic diseases, 9th ed., copyright 1988. Used by permission of the Arthritis Foundation.)

sume a more aggressive approach as the disease progresses (40, 41).

Salicylates (e.g., aspirin) or the newer nonsteroidal antiinflammatory drugs (NSAIDs) are the primary and less toxic drugs available for rheumatoid arthritis treatment. They provide relief from pain, reduce inflammation, and are fairly inexpensive.

Remission-inducing drugs (disease-modifying antirheumatic drugs (DMARDS)) are the best line of management. If the salicylates and NSAIDS have not yielded good disease control, one must consider the use of the slow-acting drugs that affect the immune response, which appear to induce remission in some patients. These drugs include the antimalarials, gold, penicillamine, and cytotoxic agents. These drugs display more serious side effects such as possible blindness, rashes, diarrhea, and bone marrow suppression.

Corticosteroids are related to cortisone (a natural hormone produced by the body's adrenal glands) and are often not used because of powerful and serious side effects. These drugs give short-term relief at the expense of long-term toxicity and

are used with individuals with serious extra-articular manifestations. If used for a long time, the side effects accumulate and cause such problems as bone erosion, diabetes, cataracts, weight gain, emotional problems, and high blood pressure.

OCCUPATIONAL PERFORMANCE COMPONENTS

Effects on occupational performance for those with RA are usually disruptive but not life-threatening. A person with RA will experience varying degrees of improvement, depending on the progression of the disease, the anatomical structures involved, the systemic problems the person is experiencing, the financial support available, and psychologic outlook (Table 13.7).

Sensory Integration

Sensory processing may be affected, specifically tactile, proprioceptive, visual, and auditory. Nerve impingement from the loss of soft tissue integrity can affect tactile and proprioceptive processing throughout both proximal and peripheral joints. Visual changes occur in 1% of the population, resulting from iridocyclitis (described above). Auditory changes can result from inflammation of the inner ear bone joints.

Neuromuscular

The most prominent deficit in the neuromuscular component is decreased range of motion in the major joints, with subsequent muscle weakness. Joint deformities are common, especially in the direction of flexion. The inflammation of rheumatoid arthritis causes joint swelling. Joint stiffness, especially in the morning, is a common complaint. The cumulative effects of immobility, stiffness, and pain result in generalized fatigue that exacerbates the mobility impairment.

Motor

The most likely motor impairment will be depressed activity tolerance due to the

Table 13.7.
Occupational Performance Components Affected by Rheumatoid Arthritis[a]

Sensory Motor Component		Cognitive Integration & Cognitive Components	Psychosocial Skills & Psychologic Components
1. **Sensory integration**		1. Level of arousal	1. **Psychologic**
a. Sensory awareness		2. Orientation	*a. **Roles**
*b. **Sensory processing**		3. Recognition	b. Values
*1. **Tactile**	(*D)	4. **Attention span**	*c. **Interests**
*2. **Proprioceptive**		5. Memory	*d. **Initiation of activity**
3. Vestibular	(*D)	a. **Short-term**	*e. **Termination of activity**
*4. **Visual (only 1%)**		b. Long-term	*f. **Self-concept**
*5. **Auditory**		c. Remote	2. **Social**
6. Gustatory	(*D)	6. **Sequencing**	*a. **Social conduct**
7. Olfactory		7. Categorization	*b. **Conversation**
c. Perceptual skills		8. Concept formation	*c. **Self-management**
*1. **Sterognosis**		9. Intellectual operations in space	3. **Self-management**
*2. **Kinesthesia**		10. **Problem solving**	*a. **Coping skills**
3. Body scheme		11. Generalization of learning	*b. **Time-management**
4. Right-left discrimination	(*D)	12. Integration of learning	*c. **Self-concept**
5. Form constancy		13. Synthesis of learning	
6. Position in space			
7. Visual closure			
8. Figure ground			
9. Depth perception			
10. Topographic orientation	(*D)	due to depression rather than to progression of RA	

2. **Neuromuscular**
  *a. **Reflex**
  *b. **Range of motion**
  *c. **Muscle tone**
  *d. **Strength**
  *e. **Endurance**
  *f. **Postural control**
  *g. **Soft tissue integration**
3. **Motor**
  *a. **Activity tolerance**
  *b. **Gross motor coordination**
  *c. **Crossing the midline**
  *d. **Laterality**
  *e. **Bilateral integration**
  f. Praxia
  *g. **Fine motor coordination**
  h. Visual motor integration

From AOTA Uniform Terminology (2nd ed.). *Note:* All these may or may not be involved at one time, depending on the progression and/or acuteness of the disease process decreased neuromuscular status. Gross and fine coordination deficits occur as well.

Cognitive

RA has no direct cognitive effects. However, difficulty with attention span, short-term memory, sequencing, and problem solving may be caused by depression.

Psychosocial Skills and Psychologic Components

It is not unusual for an individual with RA to have an exacerbation of the disease as a result of major psychologic stressors. The breakdown in coping mechanisms may lead to feelings of hopelessness and helplessness, which creates a reduction in self-management and self-concept. Depres-

sion and anxiety are other potential problems (42).

CASE STUDIES

The following case studies show how individuals with RA can be affected in work tasks, activities of daily living, and leisure activities.

Case 1

M.C. is a 37-year-old housewife and mother of an energetic 10-year-old son and a 8-year-old daughter. She was diagnosed with RA 5 years ago and has, until her most recent flare-ups, been able to take care of her home and her own self-care responsibilities.

Prior to this exacerbation, M.C. had always been very involved with her children and their activities. In addition, she did volunteer secretarial work at the local Arthritis Foundation and taught Sunday School. M.C. enjoyed doing needlework and went golfing with

Table 13.8.
Occupational Performance Profile

			Performance Areas			
				Work Activities		
			Vocation	Education	Home Management	Care of Others
OCCUPATIONAL PERFORMANCE COMPONENTS / SENSORIMOTOR	**SENSORY INTEGRATION**	Intact				
	NEURO-MUSCULAR	*Active ROM:* Full flexion 3/4 active extension in B hands, wrists, and elbows *Muscle strength:* G- in flexion, F in extension of shoulder, elbows, hands *Grip:* Decreased from normal *Endurance:* Fatigue experienced after 1 1/2 hours of minimal-to-moderate exertion	Unable to complete volunteer secretarial responsibilities Able to teach Sunday School		Unable to perform heavy cleaning, vacuuming, laundry, lawn work Able to complete bill paying	Unable to be as involved in physical activities with the children; unable to braid daughter's hair
	MOTOR	*Activity tolerance:* Fair for 1 1/2 hr light activity, poor for moderate exertion *Fine coordination:* Decreased & slowed due to joint stiffness	Unable to type, file, etc. due to hand pain and decreased coordination		Able to perform simple meal prep; fine coordination tasks are difficult, (peeling, opening boxes and jars, etc.)	Able to perform small grocery shopping trips Able to drive family to activities for short distances

a friend. M.C. did most of the household maintenance because her husband is a salesman who travels and works long hours.

Since her last flare-up, M.C.'s lifestyle has been dramatically affected in all occupational performance areas. (See Table 13.8 for a chart of her occupational performance deficit profile.)

M.C. displays moderate involvement in the neuromuscular and motor areas. Range of motion and muscle strength are affected in all movement of extension in her elbows, wrists, and hands. A slight ulnar drift is noted at the MP joints. Prehension skills are within normal limits, but grip strength is below normal. Endurance has declined to 1.5 hours of light activities before fatigue is experienced. Due to pain and stiffness in the small joints of the hands, fine coordination has become significantly slowed. M.C. has left most of the housekeeping chores (e.g., laundry, vacuuming, and lawn cutting) to her husband, children, and supportive sister, because of her declined activity tolerance and pain. She has been able to continue her

own self-care, simple meal preparations (using many convenience items), light housework with several rest breaks, and teaching Sunday School. She has completely discontinued her volunteer activities, her needlework, and her golfing.

Due to the effects of the neuromuscular and motor problems, M.C. is having difficulty adjusting psychologically and socially. Previously, M.C. exhibited a high level of self-esteem for her flexibility, planning skills, and ability to cope with the unexpected events that occur in raising a family. Now she has difficulty concentrating for long periods of time and has a poor appetite. She feels guilty and angry about no longer being the "supermom" she once thought herself to be. She feels that she is a burden to others, especially to her husband who must now add most of the household chores to his already busy and tiring schedule. She also is very frustrated by the fact that she was once a great source of support and motivation for others with arthritis and is now "letting them down."

Client initials: M.C.
Diagnosis:
Age:

Play or Leisure Activities		Activities of Daily Living				
Exploration	Performance	Self-care	Socialization	Functional Communication	Functional Mobility	Sexual Expression
	Unable to engage in needlework or golfing due to pain, fatigue, and stiffness	Is able to perform grooming and dressing activities independently, however is slowed Buttoning, zipping, hair washing, makeup application are the most difficult Overhead dressing is painful			Able to walk and drive Decreased endurance and tolerance	

Table 13.8.   (Continued)
Occupational Performance Profile

			Performance Areas			
				Work Activities		
			Vocation	Education	Home Management	Care of Others
COGNITIVE	**COGNITIVE**	Decreased attention span and problem-solving abilities due to depression	Difficulty concentrating on work activity, increased errors made			
	PSYCHOLOGIC	Decreased self-esteem due to others helping her with her role and responsibilities	Depression felt due to her inability to volunteer since others were counting on her & this was a positive stroke to her self-esteem		Experiencing depression since family members must help with household tasks	Fears children will love her less if she can't be "supermom" Fears decreased relationship with husband since he has to take on more responsibility
PSYCHOSOCIAL	**SOCIAL**	Engages less frequently in conversations with others due to depression				
	SELF-MANAGEMENT	Difficulty in managing stress and managing time due to fluctuating endurance				

EXTERNAL FACTORS WHICH INFLUENCE PERFORMANCE; CULTURE, ECONOMY, ENVIRONMENT

Grid adapted from Uniform Terminology (2nd ed.) Developed by the occupational therapy faculty at Eastern Michigan University.

Case 2

M.S. was a fairly normal 9-year-old fourth grader who enjoyed swimming, soccer, collecting baseball cards, and science class. He is the third of 4 children (2 boys and 2 girls). M.S.'s mother is a part-time teacher and his father is a banker.

Three months ago, M.S. was diagnosed with juvenile rheumatoid arthritis (JRA) of the pauciarticular type (4 or fewer joints are involved). The diagnosis was made after a series of laboratory tests, x-rays, and physical examinations by his pediatrician. Prior to the diagnosis, M.S. had been complaining of intermittent mild pain and stiffness in his lower back and hips for approximately 2 months.

Play, activities of daily living, and education are the areas primarily affected. The intensity of his symptoms fluctuate significantly. (See Table 13.9 for a chart of his occupational performance deficit profile.)

Involved neuromuscular components include hip and trunk range of motion, lower extremity muscle strength, endurance, and occasionally postural control. Hip range-of-motion is limited, and muscles appear "stiff" in the last quarter of the range early in the morning, after sitting for more than 45 minutes, and before going to bed. Muscle strength is measured as fair/fair+ on hip flexion and extension, and fair+ for trunk extension. At the highest degree of hip and trunk stiffness, his postural control is compromised and he cannot react quickly during play. His musculoskeletal endurance decreases in the afternoon, especially after a morning of school activities.

M.S.'s gross motor coordination (and activity tolerance) declines on "bad days," which significantly

Client initials: M.C.
Diagnosis:
Age:

Play or Leisure Activities		Activities of Daily Living				
Exploration	Performance	Self-care	Socialization	Functional Communication	Functional Mobility	Sexual Expression
Has no interest in pursuing new leisure endeavors due to decreasing self esteem	Relationship with golfing friend has become difficult since friend does not understand the effects of arthritis					

affects his ability to play on the school soccer team. M.S.'s parents have met with his teachers to explain his special needs, so he can function at his optimal level. The teachers must allow M.S. to walk around the classroom from time to time to prevent stiffness and rest more frequently if he is doing a great deal of walking on a field trip.

On a functional level, M.S. can dress and bathe independently; however, some days it takes him much longer, due to stiffness. Feeding and grooming present no problems at this point. Functional mobility is affected after M.S. has been sitting for a time. He experiences increased stiffness and even walks with a limp when his back pain increases.

For the most part, M.S. has been able to maintain most of his leisure interests except soccer. His regular swim session at the local Y.M.C.A. helps to de-

crease pain and stiffness in his hips and back. The whole family has become involved at the open swim night, which has helped promote good family fun and relations.

Psychosocially, M.S. has had some difficulty adjusting to limitations, even though his parents have been very supportive. To maintain his role within the family, M.S.'s parents have attempted to treat him as they do their other children so he is not perceived as the "special" or "sick" child. M.S.'s self-esteem fluctuates, depending on his ability to participate in activities with his friends. M.S. has not told his friends that he has JRA. He fears that they will not want to play with him, will avoid him because he has a contagious disease, or will make fun of him. The time that he was devoting to soccer he now spends with the science club at school at his mother's insistence. M.S.

Table 13.9.
Occupational Performance Profile

		Performance Areas			
			Work Activities		
		Vocation	Education	Home Management	Care of Others
SENSORY INTEGRATION	Intact				
NEURO-MUSCULAR	*Active ROM:* LE pain upon movement in the morning & after sitting in hips & on trunk flexion & extension *Muscle strength:* Hip flexion/extension & trunk flexion and fair to fair+ & rest is good *Postural control:* declined with increased stiffness		Able to sit through class if allowed to walk when necessary to ease hip and trunk pain & stiffness	Able to help clean own room and do simple chores around the house like his sisters & brothers	Able to assist sister with baby sitting of young children in the neighborhood
MOTOR	*Activity tolerance:* Fluctuated greatly; tolerance declined from normal for prolonged standing & sitting LE gross coordination fair		De-creased activity tolerance displayed in after-noon at school Difficulty partici-pating in all gym activities		
COGNITIVE	Attention span de-creased with pain or stiffness experi-enced from pro-longed sitting		Displays difficulty concen-trating in class & on home-work when hip stiffness is at its peak		

Vertical row labels: OCCUPATIONAL PERFORMANCE COMPONENTS — SENSORIMOTOR — COGNITIVE

Client initials: M.S.
Diagnosis:
Age:

| Play or Leisure Activities | | Activities of Daily Living | | | | |
Exploration	Performance	Self-care	Socialization	Functional Communication	Functional Mobility	Sexual Expression
	Is able to perform many premorbid play activities (except soccer) with appropriate pacing	Performs bathing & dressing activities independently but is slower than normal with LE activities			Walks with a limp with increased hip or back pain	
	Unable to participate in soccer due to decreased LE gross motor coordination & decreased tolerance	Independent with feeding and grooming			Transfers independently	
	Able to participate fully in swim program					
					Occasionally displays difficulty with long distance walking on class field trips	
Has been able to explore new activities, e.g., science club						

Table 13.9.   (Continued)
Occupational Performance Profile

		Performance Areas			
			Work Activities		
		Vocation	Education	Home Management	Care of Others
PSYCHOLOGIC	*Role:* Unsure of role in family, school due to self-doubt *Self-concept:* Fluctuates on activity and good vs. bad day				
SOCIAL	Able to socialize in some groups but fears not "being one of the guys" due to his "sickness"		Fears telling other kids of his "sickness" Tries to always "keep up"		
SELF-MANAGEMENT	At times displays poor coping strategies Parents display good coping mechanisms				

(PSYCHOSOCIAL — vertical label at left)

EXTERNAL FACTORS WHICH INFLUENCE
PERFORMANCE; CULTURE, ECONOMY, ENVIRONMENT

[a]Grid adapted from Uniform Terminology (2nd ed.) Developed by the occupational therapy faculty at Eastern Michigan University.

has periodic temper tantrums and displays anger about JRA and sometimes refuses to take his medications. M.S. and his parents attend a family support group for children with JRA, where the whole family has met new friends and has been able to share their feelings in a nonthreatening environment.

CONCLUSION

Researchers continue to seek the cause of, and a cure for, RA. In the meantime, the challenge is for physicians and allied health professionals, including occupational and physical therapists, to assist those with RA to "take charge" of their lives and to learn to live with it as comfortably and independently as possible. Rehabilitation professionals can help with specific interventions including: (*a*) exercises; (*b*) joint protection and energy conservation; (*c*) techniques for self-care and daily living using adaptive devices; (*d*) pain control; and (*e*) development of coping strategies and skill in solving problems. All interventions require a great deal of patience and support from a therapist; however, the rewards from assisting those with arthritis to regain self-confidence and to manage their lives with a positive outlook are truly gratifying.

ACKNOWLEDGMENTS

I would like to express my thanks to my family, colleagues, and the Arthritis

Client initials: M.S.
Diagnosis:
Age:

| Play or Leisure Activities | | Activities of Daily Living | | | | |
Exploration	Performance	Self-care	Socialization	Functional Communication	Functional Mobility	Sexual Expression
	His inability to compete with his friends in soccer has decreased his self-concept Swim program has helped family relations and his ability to be an important part of the family unit		Will not share his feelings about JRA with his friends in fear he will lose them Breaks out in temper tantrums & outbursts over anger at having JRA			
Family & RA support group has helped to develop better coping strategies and improve self-concept		When feeling depressed, becomes angry about taking his medication	Socializes in support group, school, science club, family			

Foundation–National Office and Michigan Chapter for their assistance and support during the work on this chapter. A special thanks is also given to Gary Nederveld and Associates and Mercy Hospital, Port Huron for allowing me to continue to focus energy toward developing resources, programs, and community activities to help individuals and their families to attempt to effectively cope with rheumatoid arthritis.

REFERENCES

1. Schumacher HR Jr, Klippel JH, Robinson DR. Primer on the rheumatic diseases, 9th ed. Atlanta: Arthritis Foundation, 1988.
2. Fries JF. Arthritis: a comprehensive guide, 5th ed. Reading, MA: Addison-Wesley, 1983.
3. National Center for Health Statistics. National Health Interview Survey, Rheumatoid arthritis in adults, 1960–62. Series 11:17, 1966.
4. Lorig L, Fries JF. The arthritis helpbook, 3rd ed. Reading, MA: Addison-Wesley, 1990.
5. Lipsky P. Rheumatoid arthritis. In: Harrison TR, Braunwald E. Principles of internal medicine, 11th ed. New York: McGraw-Hill, 1987.
6. Winchester R. Studying genetic susceptibility to rheumatoid arthritis. Joint Movement 1989;1:4.
7. Roitt I. Essential immunology, 4th ed. Boston: Blackwell Scientific Publications, 1980:85, 287,321.
8. Anonymous. The immune system [Abstract]. Joint Movement 1989;1:4.
9. Anonymous. Inflammation [Abstract]. Joint Movement 1989;1:2.

10. Silverman EH. Rheumatic diseases: evaluation and treatment. In: Logigian MK, ed. Adult rehabilitation: a team approach for therapists. Boston: Little, Brown & Co., 1981:111–115.

11. Singsen BH. Pediatric hematic diseases: nonarticular rheumatism, juvenile rheumatoid arthritis, juvenile spondylarthropies. In: Schumacher EH, Klippel JH, Robinson DR. Primer on the rheumatic diseases, 9th ed. Atlanta: Arthritis Foundation, 1983.

12. Rosenberg A. Living with your arthritis. New York: Arco, 1979:23.

13. Cassidy JT, Levinson JE Jr, Brewer EJ. The development of classification criteria for children with juvenile rheumatoid arthritis. Bull Rheum Dis 1989;38:6.

14. LaPlante MP. Data on disability from the National Health Interview Survey, 1983–85. Washington D.C.: National Institute on Disability and Rehabilitation Research, 1988.

15. Lawrence RC, Hunchberg MC, Kelsey JL, McDuffie FC, Medsger TA Jr, Felts WR, Shulman LE. Estimates of the prevalence of selected arthritis and musculoskeletal diseases in the United States. J Rheumatology 1989;16:427–441.

16. Cunningham LS, Keesley JL. Epidemiology of musculoskeletal impairments and associated disability. Am J Public Health 1984;74:574–579.

17. Beasley RP, Bennett PH, Len CC. Low prevalence of rheumatoid arthritis in Chinese: prevalence survey in a rural community. J Rheumatoid 1983;10:11–15.

18. Talbott JH. Clinical rheumatology, 2nd ed. New York: Eiserview, 1981.

19. Fallahi S, Halla JT, Hardin JG. Clinical Research 31:650,1983.

20. Melvin JL. Rheumatic disease: occupational therapy and rehabilitation, 2nd ed. Philadelphia: FA Davis, 1982.

21. Nalebuff EA. Diagnosis, classification, and management of rheumatoid thumb deformities. Bull Hosp Joint Dis 1968;24:119.

22. Pedretti LW. Occupational therapy: practice skills for physical dysfunction, 2nd ed. St. Louis: CV Mosby, 1985:291–306.

23. Ryan D. Painful temporomandibular joint. In: McCarty DJ, ed. Arthritis and allied conditions. 11th ed. Philadelphia: Lea & Febiger, 1989.

24. Berkow R, Talbott JH. Merck manual, 13th ed. Rahway, NJ: Merck, 1977:1312,1331,1656–1675.

25. Post M. The shoulder: surgical and non-surgical management. Philadelphia: Lea & Febiger, 1978.

26. Bennett JC. Rheumatoid arthritis: clinical features. In: Schumacher HR, Klipper JH, Robinson DR, eds. Primer on rheumatic diseases, 9th ed. Atlanta: Arthritis Foundation, 1988.

27. Valniok K. The rheumatoid foot, a clinical study with pathological roentgenological comments. Am Clin Gynecol 1956;45:1–5 (supp.).

28. Frieberg RA, Moncur C. Arthritis of the foot. Bull Rheum Dis 1991;40:1.

29. Pearson CM. Polymyositis and dermatomyositis. In: McCarthy DJ, ed. Arthritis and allied conditions, 9th ed. Philadelphia: Lea & Febiger, 1978.

30. Mullen EA. Influence of training and activity on muscle strength. Arch Phys Med Rehabil 1990;51:449–469.

31. Kottle F. The effects of limitation of activity on the human body. JAMA 196:825–830,1966.

32. Harris E. Rheumatic arthritis: the clinical spectrum. In: Kelly WH, ed. Textbook of rheumatology. Philadelphia: WB Saunders, 1981.

33. Jurik AG, Davison D, Graudal H. Prevalence of pulmonary involvement in rheumatoid arthritis and its relationship to some characteristics of the patients. Scand J Rheumatol 1982;11:217–224.

34. Hunninghald GW, Fauci HS. Pulmonary involvement in the collagen vascular diseases. Am Rev Resp Dis 1979;119:471–503.

35. Robert WC, Kehoe JA, Carpenter DF. Cardiac valvular lesion in rheumatoid arthritis. Arch Intern Med 1968;122:141–146.

36. Talal N. Sjögren's syndrome. In: Rose N, Mackey I, eds. The autoimmune diseases. New York: Academic Press, 1985:145–159.

37. Yelin E, Mechan R, Nevitt M. Work disability in rheumatoid arthritis: effects of disease, social and work factors. Ann Intern Med 1980;93:551–556.

38. Yelin E, Henkle C, Epstein W. The work dynamics of the person with rheumatoid arthritis. Arthritis Rheum 1987;30:507–512.

39. Fries JF. Arthritis: a comprehensive guide to understanding your arthritis, 3rd ed. Reading, MA: Addison-Wesley, 1990.

40. Gall EP. Drug treatment of arthritis. In: Postgraduate advances in arthritis for health professionals. Berryville, VA: Forum Medicum, 1988.

41. Hess EV. Rheumatoid arthritis: treatment. In: Schumacher HR, Kuppel JH, Robinson DR, eds. Primer on the rheumatic diseases, 9th ed. Atlanta: Arthritis Foundation, 1988.

42. Rudolph M. The psychosocial affects of rheumatoid arthritis. O.T. Forum 1987;2:24.

Suggested Readings

Brattström M. Joint protection and rehabilitation in chronic rheumatic disorders. Rockville, MD: Aspen, 1987.

Canthum CJ, Clawson DL, Decker JL. Functional assessment of the rheumatoid hand. Am J Occup Ther 1969;23:122.

Chronic disease report: deaths from nine chronic diseases—United States. MMWR 1990;39(2):17–20.

Ehrlich GE, ed. Rehabilitation management of rheumatic conditions. 2nd ed. Baltimore: Williams & Wilkins, 1986.

Flatt AE. Care of the rheumatoid hand. St. Louis: CV Mosby, 1974.

Fries JF. Aging well. Reading, MA: Addison-Wesley, 1989.

Gerber LH. Rehabilitative therapies for patients with rheumatic disease. In: Schumacher HR, Wippel JH, Robertson DR, eds. Primer on the rheumatic diseases. 9th ed. Atlanta: Arthritis Foundation, 1988.

Hoppenfeld S. Physical examination of the spine and extremities. New York: Appleton-Century-Crofts, 1976.

Kate WA. Diagnosis and management of rheumatic diseases. 2nd ed. Philadelphia: JB Lippincott, 1988.

Lawrence RC. Estimates of the prevalence of selected arthritic and musculoskeletal disease in the United States. J Rheumatol 1989;16(4):427–440.

McCarty DJ, ed. Arthritis and allied conditions. 11th ed. Philadelphia: Lea & Febiger, 1989.

Melvin JL. Rheumatic disease in the adult and child: Occupational therapy and rehabilitation. 3rd ed. Philadelphia: FA Davis, 1989.

National Commission on Arthritis and Musculoskeletal Diseases. Report to congress. Arthritis: out of the maze. Volume I. The arthritis plan. Washington, D.C.: U.S. Dept. of Health, Education and Welfare, April, 1976.

Peck JR, Smith TW, Ward JR, Milano R. Disability and depression in rheumatoid arthritis. Arthritis Rheum 1989;32(9):1100–1106.

Phillips RH. Coping with rheumatoid arthritis. Garden City Park, NY: Avery, 1988.

Polatin PB. The functional restoration approach to chronic low back pain. J Musculoskeletal Med 1990;1:.

Riggs GK, Gall EP, eds. Rheumatic disease: rehabilitation and management. Boston, MA: Butterworth, 1984.

Sartoris DJ, Nesnick D. Magnetic resonance imaging of the foot. J Musculoskeletal Med 1990;1.

Sine RO, Holcomb JD, Rousch RE, Less SE, Wilson GB. Basic rehabilitation techniques: a self instructional guide. Rockville, MD: Aspen, 1981.

Smith CJ, Freyberg RH, McEwen C. History of rheumatology in the United States. Atlanta: Arthritis Foundation, 1985.

Wright V, Woen S. Effect of rheumatoid arthritis on the social situation of housewifes. Rheumatol Rehabil 1976;15:156.

RESOURCES

Informational Booklets Available through the Arthritis Foundation

Arthritis and employment
Arthritis and farmers
Arthritis and vocational rehabilitation
Aspirin and related medications
Arthritis in children
Back pain
Basic facts about arthritis
Carpal tunnel syndrome
Coping with pain
Coping with stress
Diet and arthritis
Guide to insurance for people with arthritis
Guide to medications
Help yourself to a better relationship
Juvenile rheumatoid arthritis
Rheumatoid arthritis
Sjögren's syndrome
Taking charge (learning to live with arthritis)
When your student has arthritis

Adaptive Aids

Aids for Arthritis, Inc.
3 Little Knoll Court
Medford, NJ 08055

Be O.K. Sales Co./Fred Sammons
Box 32
Brookfield, IL

Guide to Independent Living for People with Arthritis.

Atlanta: Arthritis Foundation, 1314 Spring Street, NW, Atlanta, GA 30309

Support Groups

Contact the Arthritis Foundation for local groups across the United States

Informational Association & Memberships/Support Resources

American Juvenile Arthritis Organization (AJAO)
1314 Spring Street, NW
Atlanta, GA 30309 (404) 872-7100

AJAO is a membership organization of AF which represents the special needs of children with arthritis and their families

American Rheumatism Association (ARA)
17 Executive Drive, NE, Suite 480
Atlanta, GA 30309 (404) 633-3777

A professional society of physicians specializing in rheumatic diseases

Arthritis Foundation
1314 Spring Street, NW
Atlanta, GA 30309 (404) 872-7100

Arthritis Health Professionals Association (AHPA)
1314 Spring Street, NW
Atlanta, GA 30309 (404) 872-7100

AHPA is the professional section of the Arthritis Foundation

HEALTH (Higher Education and Adult Training for People with Handicaps)
1 Dupont Circle, Suite 800
Washington, D.C. 20036-1193 1-800-544-3284

National Chronic Pain Outreach
4922 Hampden Lane
Bethesda, MD 20814 (301) 652-4948

National Institute of Arthritis and Musculoskeletal
Diseases (NIAMS)
Building 31
Bethesda, MD 20892

NIAMS, a member institute of the National Institutes of Health (NIH), conducts research in all
aspects of the rheumatic diseases and provides information through the Arthritis Information Clearing House

NIAMS Clearing House
Box AMS
Bethesda, MD 20892

Journals/Newsletters

Arthritis Care and Research
Elsevier Science Publishing Co., Inc.
Journal Information Center
P.O. Box 882
Madison Square Station
New York, NY 10159

Arthritis Today Magazine
Arthritis Foundation
1314 Spring Street, NW
Atlanta, GA 30309

Arthritis Today Newsletter (Free)
University of Alabama at Birmingham
108 Basic Health Science Building
VAB Station
Birmingham, AL 35294

Bulletin on the Rheumatic Diseases (Free)
Arthritis Foundation
1314 Spring Street, NW
Atlanta, GA 30309

Disabled USA (Free)
The President's Committee on Employment of the
Handicapped
Washington, D.C. 20210

Joint Movement Newsletter (Free)
Arthritis Foundation
1314 Spring Street, NW
Atlanta, GA 30309 1-800-283-7800

Perspectives
Arthritis Health Professionals Association
Arthritis Foundation
1314 Spring Street, NW
Atlanta, GA 30309

Glossary

Anemia: A reduction below normal in the number of erythrocytes or in the quantity of hemoglobin in the blood. Anemia is not a disease but a symptom of any of a number of different disorders that upset the balance between blood loss through bleeding or destruction of blood cells and blood production in the bone marrow.

Ankylosis: Immobility and consolidation of a joint because of disease, injury, or surgical procedure. In arthritis, there is destruction of articular cartilage, allowing bony surfaces to fuse. Bony ankylosis: Union of the bones of a joint by proliferation of bone cells, resulting in complete immobility. Fibrous ankylosis: Reduced joint mobility due to proliferation of fibrous tissue. Also called false ankylosis.

Antibodies: Special proteins produced by the body (plasma cells) in response to infectious agents or other foreign matter (antigens). Antibodies are immunoglobulin molecules having a specific amino acid sequence that gives each antibody the ability to adhere to and interact only with the antigen that induced its synthesis, thereby neutralizing or facilitating the destruction of the antigen.

Antigen: A foreign protein or protein polysaccharide complex that stimulates a specific immune response.

Antinuclear antibodies (ANA): A group of abnormal antibodies found in most people with systemic lupus erythematosus, Sjögren's syndrome, and scleroderma. Also found in juvenile and rheumatoid arthritis cases. ANAs are autoantibodies directed against components of the cell nucleus, e.g., DNA, RNA, and histones.

Apophyseal: Pertaining to any outgrowth or swelling, especially a bony outgrowth that has never been entirely separated from the bone of which it forms a part, such as a process, tubercle, or tuberosity.

Artheritis: Inflammation of an artery.

Arthritis: Inflammation of a joint. Arthritis and rheumatic diseases in general constitute the major cause of chronic disability in the U.S., with osteoarthritis and rheumatoid arthritis the most common forms.

Autoimmune disease: A disease in which the immune system malfunctions and attacks tissues of the body, causing tissue injury and inflammation.

B cells: Lymphocytes capable of becoming antibody-secreting plasma cells.

Binding cleft: A biochemical term describing the cleft area of the human leukocyte antigen molecule that appears to determine whether or not an antibody will react (bind) with an antigen.

Boutonnière deformity: A finger deformity in which flexion of the proximal interphalangeal joint and hyperextension of the distal interphalangeal joint occurs.

Bursa: A small sac (like a water balloon) that is not part of the joint but is located around the joints where tendons, ligaments, and bone rub against each other. Bursae contain a fluid that lubricates the movement of muscles and are similar to synovial sacs. There are over 140 bursae located throughout the body.

Callositas (callosity): Circumscribed thickening and hypertrophy of the horny layer of the skin. Usually appear on flexor surfaces of hands and feet, caused by friction, pressure, or other irritation.

Capsule: A band of cartilaginous, fatty, fibrous, membranous tissue enveloping a joint. Articular capsule: A sac-like envelope enclosing the cavity of a synovial joint.

Carpal tunnel syndrome: Compression of the median nerve in the carpal tunnel of the wrist, causing atrophy in the thenar area and paralysis, as well as trophic changes of the fingertips and sensory deficits of the first three fingers.

Cartilage: A specialized, fibrous connective tissue that covers the ends of bones to help them glide smoothly and also absorbs shock to a joint by acting as a "sponge" to release and reabsorb.

Chronic pulmonary obstructive disease: Generalized airway obstruction, particularly of small airways, associated with varying combinations of chronic bronchitis, asthma, and emphysema. The term COPD was introduced because these conditions often coexist, and it may be difficult to decide which is the major one producing the obstruction.

Cock-up toe: Deformity with dorsiflexion of the metatarsophalangeal joint and flexion of the interphalangeal/distal interphalangeal joint.

Complete blood count (CBC): Diagnostic test showing the number of different cellular components of the blood, such as white blood cells, red blood cells, and platelets.

Conduction: Conveyance of energy, as of heat, sound, or electricity.

Contracture: A permanent muscular contraction resulting from a tonic spasm or loss of muscular equilibrium, the antagonists being paralyzed.

Cricoarytenoid: Pertaining to the cricoid and arytenoid cartilages. Cricoid cartilage: A ring-like cartilage forming the lower and back part of the larynx. Arytenoid cartilage: Shaped like a jug or pitcher, as in the cartilage of the larynx.

De Quervain's disease: Stenosing (constricting) tenosynovitis of the dorsal compartment of the wrist involving the abductor pollicis longus and extensor pollicis brevis.

Endomysium: The sheath of delicate reticular (resembling a net) fibrils that surround each muscle fiber.

Episcleritis: Inflammation of the loose connective tissue forming the sclera and the conjunctiva of the eye.

Epstein-Barr virus (EBV): A herpesvirus that is the etiologic agent of infectious mononucleosis. It has been isolated from cells cultured from Burkitt's lymphoma (an undifferentiated malignant form usually found in central Africa) and has been found in certain cases of nasopharyngeal cancer. EBV has been implicated in cases of chronic fatigue and a high proportion of individuals with RA have circulating antibodies in response to the antigen present in the EBV.

Erythrocyte sedimentation rate (ESR): A diagnostic test that measures how fast red blood cells fall to the bottom of a tube; it indicates the presence and degree of inflammation.

Exacerbation: A flare-up, a period during which disease symptoms reappear or become worse systematically or local to a finger joint.

Felty's syndrome: A disease consisting of rheumatoid arthritis, splenomegaly, anemia, and leukopenia.

Fibrosis: Formation of fibrous tissue; fibroid degeneration.

Fusiform: Tapering at both ends; spindle-shaped.

Granulocytopenia: An acute or chronic reduction in peripheral blood granulocytes resulting in increased susceptibility to bacterial infection and mucous membrane ulcerations.

Granulomatous: Composed of granulomas or nodules representing a chronic inflammatory response associated with infectious (disease) or noninfectious (foreign body) agents. Granulomatous aortitis: Inflammatory nodule in the aorta.

Hallux valgus: Lateral deviation at the first metatarsophalangeal joint.

Hemoglobin: A substance in red blood cells that transports oxygen through the body.

HLA-DR4: A genetic marker associated with increased risk of development of rheumatoid arthritis.

Human leukocyte antigens (HLA): Specific genetic markers on the white blood cells (leukocytes), several of which are related to an increased tendency to develop certain rheumatic diseases.

Immune system: The body's natural defense system against injury or infection.

Inflammation: A local response to injury, characterized by swelling, pain, increased temperature, and redness in the region of injury due to increased local blood flow.

Joint: A meeting of two bones for the purpose of allowing movement.

Juvenile rheumatoid arthritis (JRA): Polyarticular (more than four joints) is the most common form. Pauciarticular (four or fewer joints) the second most common. Systemic JRA affects many parts of the body including organs and joints and is the least common form.

Juxta-articular: Situated near (adjoining) or in the region of a joint.

Keratoconjunctivitis: Inflammation of the cornea and conjunctiva (the delicate membrane lining the eyelids and covering the eyeball).

Leukocyte: White blood cell; a colorless blood corpuscle whose chief function is to protect the body against microorganisms causing disease.

Leukopenia: Reduction of the number of leukocytes in the blood.

Ligament: A band of short, fibrous, elastic-like tissue that helps hold tendons in proper alignment and stabilizes joints by attaching one bone to another. The joint capsule is considered a ligament. Capsular ligament: Fibrous layer of a joint capsule.

Lymphocyte: A type of leukocyte responsible for specific defenses of the body against foreign matter divided into two classes, B (humoral) and T (cellular) lymphocytes. Lymph nodes: Small organs containing lymphocytes.

Mononeuritis multiplex: Simultaneous inflammation of several nerves remote from one another with sensory, motor, reflex, or vasomotor symptoms, and/or a combination of these.

Muscle: Elastic tissue that moves the joints by helping them flex, extend, or rotate, depending on how the joints are designed.

Myositis: Inflammation of a voluntary muscle.

Neuromyopathy: A disease of the nervous system and muscle.

Neutropenia: Diminished number of neutrophils in the blood.

Osteoarthritis: A noninflammatory joint disease marked by degeneration of the articular cartilage, hypertrophy of bone at the margins, and changes in the synovial membrane; also called degenerative joint disease (DJD).

Pannus: An inflammatory exudate overlying synovial cells on the inside of a joint capsule, which can damage the cartilage, usually occurring in rheumatoid arthritis or related articular rheumatism.

Paresthesia: Morbid or perverted sensation; an abnormal sensation as burning, prickling, formication, due to a disorder of the central nervous system.

Pleuritis: Inflammation of the pleura which may be caused by infection, injury, or tumor.

Polymyositis: A chronic, progressive inflammatory disease of skeletal muscle, occurring in both children and adults, and characterized by symmetric weakness of the limb girdles, neck, and pharynx, usually associated with pain and tenderness, and sometimes preceded or followed by manifestations typical of scleroderma, arthritis, systemic lupus erythematous, or Sjögren's syndrome.

Pneumonitis: Inflammation of lung tissue.

Rheumatoid arthritis (RA): A chronic, inflammatory systemic disease that causes pain, inflammation, mobility limitations, and joint deformity, with problems also seen with the tendons, sheaths, nerves, and muscles.

Rheumatoid carditis: Inflammation of the heart due to a rheumatic disorder.

Rheumatoid factor (RH) factor: An abnormal antibody often present in people with RA.

Roentgenology: That branch of radiology dealing with the diagnostic and therapeutic use of roentgen rays (x-rays).

Scleritis: Inflammation of the sclera, the tough, white outer coat of the eyeball.

Scleroderma: Chronic hardening and shrinking of the connective tissues of any organs of the body, including the skin, heart, esophagus, kidney, and lung. It may be generalized (systemic) or localized. Milder forms are most often seen in persons in the 30- to 50-year-old age group, and affect twice as many women as men; however, the severest forms usually affect men, blacks, and older persons. It is difficult to diagnose as it mimics symptoms of other diseases such as osteoarthritis and rheumatoid arthritis and other collagen disorders.

Sjögren's syndrome: A chronic disease of unknown etiology, usually occurring in middle-aged or older women, marked by the triad of keratoconjunctivitis with or without lacrimal gland enlargement, xerostomia with or without salivary gland enlargement, and the presence of a connective tissue disease, usually rheumatoid arthritis but sometimes systemic lupus erythematosus, scleroderma, or polymyositis. An abnormal immune response has been implicated and symptoms include dry eyes and mouth.

Splenomegaly: Enlargement of the spleen.

Steroid myopathy: A disease of the muscle due to the ingestion of steroids, complex molecules important in body chemistry.

Subluxation: Incomplete or partial dislocation.

Subchondral: Below the cartilage.

Swan-neck deformity: A finger deformity involving hyperextension of the proximal interphalangeal joint and flexion of the distal interphalangeal joint.

Synovial membrane: The inner of the two layers of the articular capsule of a synovial joint, composed of loose connective tissue with a free smooth surface that lines the joint cavity. Each joint capsule is lined with synovium for protection of the joint. Synovial tissue is also found on muscle, tendons, bursae, and some organs of the body. The synovial lining produces "fluid" to fill the joint space and aids the cartilage in absorbing shock. It also provides nourishment and aids in removing excess fluids from the joint.

T cells: Specialized lymphocytes that help remove antigens from the body or interact with B cells.

Tendon: A cord or band of strong, white, fibrous tissue that attaches muscles to bone. When the muscle contracts or shortens, it pulls on the tendon, which moves the bone.

Tendonitis: Inflammation of a tendon.

Tenosynovitis: Inflammation of a tendon and its sheath, the lubricated layer of tissue in which the tendon is housed and through which it moves. It occurs most frequently in the hands and wrists or feet and ankles, and is often the result of intense and continued use. Rheumatoid and other types of arthritis frequently involve tendon sheaths. Treatment is by immobilization of the limb or, in severe cases, by surgery for the purpose of draining an infected sheath or releasing a tendon from a constricting sheath.

Thrombocytopenia: A decrease in number of platelets in circulating blood, which can be caused by infections.

Ulnar drift: Abnormal ulnar deviation of the fingers at the metacarpophalangeal joints.

Valgus: Bent outward; twisted; denoting a deformity in which the angulation is away from the midline of the body, as in talipes valgus.

Xerostomia: Dryness of the mouth from salivary gland infection such as found in Sjögren's syndrome.

APPENDIX **13.2**

Diagnostic Tests

RHEUMATOID ARTHRITIS PATIENT HISTORY

Evaluation requires an extensive history and physical examination. Even though some symptoms appear localized, an evaluation of the entire body and assessment of various systems must be completed. Coexistent conditions or therapy must be documented, since they may influence manifestations. Other symptoms of systemic disease could suggest a rheumatic disease process.

Musculoskeletal pain must be assessed to determine whether the pain is specific to the joints or surrounding tissues and whether a single joint or area of the body is involved or symptoms are more generalized. An individual should report details about the pattern of onset and the course of the pain.

Edema and stiffness must be evaluated carefully to determine patterns and specific areas that may be involved. Addi-

tional complaints and symptoms of fatigue, fever, weakness, and functional problems should be addressed as well.

A detailed history of psychologic effects of the disease process, previous attempts at treatment and rehabilitation, previous drug reactions and allergies, as well as a family history should be taken.

LABORATORY TESTS

Several blood tests (40, 41) can assist in making diagnosis of RA. The most common include the following:

Rheumatoid Factor (RF)

The immune system does not ordinarily attack the body's own cells. However, 80% of the people with RA have a "renegade" antibody to their own immunoglobulin, which normally helps the body fight infection. This antibody is referred to as the rheumatoid factor (RF). RF can also occur in other diseases such as lupus erythematous and mononucleosis. A blood test is performed on a venous blood sample, and if the RF factor is present, the individual is described as sero-positive.

Erythrocyte Sedimentation Rate (SED Rate or ESR)

This test is used to screen for inflammation and infection, not to diagnose a specific disease. This procedure measures how fast red blood cells fall to the bottom of a glass tube. People with chronic inflammation have cells that fall faster than normal. Inflammation and infections increase the blood's protein content, making the red blood cells stick together, so they settle to the bottom of the tube faster. Generally, as inflammation responds to medication, the SED rate declines.

Hematocrit (HCT) and Hemoglobin (Hgb) Counts

These tests measure the number and quality of red blood cells. Low hematocrit or hemoglobin counts usually indicate anemia.

White Blood Count (WBC)

This test measures the total number of white blood cells in a specific amount of blood, as well as the percentage of each type. There is normally one white blood cell for every 500 red blood cells, but if a bacterial infection is present, the number of white blood cells may increase dramatically. In the case of RA, if a WBC below 2000/mm is found, a diagnosis of RA would be unlikely.

Antinuclear Antibodies (ANA)

This test is performed on a venous sample in the same way as that for RF and is used to determine whether the immune system is producing additional antibodies (ANAs) against the body's own tissues. Polymositis (anti-JO-1 or anti-PM/Dcl) and Sjögren's syndrome (anti-RO/

SSA and anti-La/SSB) are two conditions that can be evaluated by tests.

Human Leukocyte Antigen (HLA) Tissue Typing

These tests detect whether certain genetic markers or traits are present in the blood. B-13 a genetic marker that tends to be present in people with arthritis.

Urinalysis

A urine test shows whether the urine contains red blood cells, protein, or other substances not normally present. Detection of these substances may indicate kidney damage from a rheumatic disease.

Synovial Fluid Analysis

A sample of synovial fluid can assist a physician in diagnosing RA, infection, arthritis as a result of an injury, or other types of joint problems. One portion of the joint fluid sample is used for a series of immediate tests for bacteria, blood cells, or crystals. Another portion is examined in a laboratory to determine possibilities for various joint conditions, including RA. Perhaps the most frequent use of synovial fluid analysis is to differentiate between inflammatory and noninflammatory arthritis. As previously stated, with a white blood count below 2000/mm, a diagnosis of RA is unlikely.

Radiographic Testing

In the later stages, RA may irreversibly alter a joint and interfere with its expected mechanical functioning. When this happens, compensatory degenerative changes may occur and can be observed through x-rays. Cartilage thinning or bone erosion generally takes at least 3 months to appear.

Bone erosion will be seen on x-rays near the attachments of the joint capsule where the articular cartilage ends and the synovial reflection begins (41). In the areas where bones are not covered by articular cartilage, bone erosion will be seen most readily (e.g., at the IP joints). Other examples include:

Area	Specific Site
Thumb	Ulnar side of the distal phalanx
Ulna	Ulna styloid
Radius	Distal radioulnar joint
Feet	Medial aspect of 1–4 metatarsal heads
	Lateral aspect of the 5th metatarsal
Cervical spine	Lower cervical and odontoid processes
	Cervical apophyseal

Ankylosis of bones may be observed in the tarsal and carpal bones.

Biopsies

To help confirm a diagnosis, the physician may order a skin or muscle biopsy to assess for signs of damage.

Magnetic Resonance Imaging (MRI)

MRI is based on the interaction of radio waves with hydrogen nuclei in the presence of a strong magnetic field (1). MRI scanners have been shown to be superior to other imaging modalities in the diagnosis of ischemic necrosis of bone.

As a newer diagnostic tool with rheumatoid arthritis, early evidence suggests that a diminished overall radio wave signal intensity of the hyaline cartilage occurs in an affected joint. Abnormalities in soft tissues secondary to the rheumatoid process, such as synovial thickening, can be viewed.

Cervical spine involvement and vertebral subluxation that results in compression of the underlying brainstem and cervical spinal cord can be easily seen on MRI.

Generic Name	Brand Name	Action	Indication	Potential Side Effects	Usual Adult Dose & Availability	Comments
ASPIRIN (Acetylsalicylic acid)	Anacin Bayer Bufferin Ecotrin	Analgesic Antipyretic Antiinflammatory Antiplatelet	Pain relief	Increased night sweating; tinnitus; dizziness; gastrointestinal distress; decreased hearing; constipation; liver abnormalities	*For pain:* two 5-grain tablets (10 grains) every 4 hours; *for antiinflammatory action,* 3–4 tablets, 4–6 times daily; continue only with medical supervision Over the counter	Overdose can cause very rapid and heavy breathing leading to unconsciousness & coma
CHOLINE MAGNESIUM TRISALICYLATE	Trilisate	Analgesic Antiinflammatory	Relief of mild pain due to cartilage degeneration, local conditions. Antiinflammatory due to synovitis	Nausea; vomiting; tinnitus; decreased hearing	*For pain:* 1 to 2 tablets (500 mg/ea) every 12 hours; *for antiinflammatory activity,* 2 to 3 tablets every 12 hours; maximum effect is reached in 2 hours for pain and in to 6 weeks for antiinflammatory action	Overdose can cause very rapid and heavy breathing
PHENYL-BUTAZONE, OXYPHEN-BUTAZONE	Butazolidine Tandearil	Antiinflammatory	To reduce inflammation when it is causing harm	May destroy red or white blood cells; irritation of stomach with nausea, heartburn, indigestion and occasional vomiting; possible fluid retention	Prescription 3 or 4 100-mg capsules spread throughout the day Prescription	On rare occasions, this drug can be hazardous, destroying all red or white blood cells

SULINDAC	Clinoril	Analgesic Antinflammatory	To reduce inflammation and for mild pain relief	Gastrointestinal side effects with irritation of the stomach lining are most common: e.g., nausea, indigestion, heartburn, stomach pain, stomach ulcer; diarrhea; tinnitus; fluid retention; nervousness; rash	One 150-mg tablet twice a day; dosage may be increased to a 200-mg tablet if needed; maximum recommended dosage is 400 mg per day Prescription
PIROXICAM	Feldene	Analgesic Antinflammatory	As above	Gastrointestinal symptoms, e.g., nausea, stomach lining irritation, heartburn, peptic ulceration; headache; dizziness	One 20-mg tablet once daily; it is recommended not to exceed this doage since it is long-acting Prescription
INDOMETH-ACIN	Indocin	Analgesic Antinflammatory	As above	Irritation of stomach lining, e.g., nausea, indigestion, heartburn, headache; dizziness	One 25-mg capsule 3 to 4 times daily; for men or larger women, doses totaling as high as 150 to 200 mg may be required and tolerated each day Prescription
MECLOFEN-AMATE	Meclomen	Analgesic Antinflammatory	As above	Gastrointestinal effects, e.g., nausea, diarrhea	The total daily dosage is 200 mg to 400 mg, usually taken in 3 or 4 equal doses; maximum effect is achieved about 6 weeks after initiation Prescription
IBUPROFEN	Motrin Rufen	Analgesic Antinflammatory	As above	Gastrointestinal effects, e.g., irritation of	One or two 400-mg tablets 3 times daily;

Generic Name	Brand Name	Action	Indication	Potential Side Effects	Usual Adult Dose & Availability	Comments
				stomach lining, nausea, heartburn, indigestion, aseptic meningitis syndrome possible; fluid retention; rash	maximum daily recommended dosage is 2400 mg (6 tablets); maximum effect is achieved after 6 weeks of treatment / Over the counter	
FENOPROFEN	Nalfon	Analgesic Antiinflammatory	To reduce inflammation and for mild-to-moderate pain relief	Irritation of stomach lining, nausea, heartburn, vomiting; fluid retention	One or two 300-mg capsules, 3 to 4 times daily; maximum recommended dosage is 10 tables daily; maximum effect may take 6 weeks / Prescription	
NAPROXEN	Naprosyn	Analgesic Antiinflammatory	As above	Gastrointestinal side effects, e.g., nausea indigestion, irritation of stomach lining, heartburn; fluid retention	One 250-mg tablet 2 to 3 times a day; maximum recommended dosage is 1000 mg / Prescription	
TOLMETIN SODIUM	Tolectin	Analgesic Antiinflammatory	To reduce inflammation and for mild pain relief	Gastrointestinal effects, e.g., nausea, heartburn, upset stomach, indigestion, fluid retention	Two 200-mg tablets 3 to 4 times each day; maximum recommended dosage is 2000 mg (10 tablets) / Prescription	
PREDNISONE	Prednisone (corticosteroid)	Antiinflammatory, suppress immunologic responses	To reduce inflammation	Related to dose and duration, effects worsen with time; ulcers, mental changes,	Low dose = 5–10 mg/day; moderate dose = 15–130 mg/day; high dose = 40–60>	Possible psychologic dependency

Drug	Brand Names	Type	Purpose	Side Effects	Dosage
				infection with bacterial, acne, weight gain, increased facial and skin hair, bruises easily, stretch marks, calcium loss, cataracts, thinning of the skin, hardening of the arteries	mg/day; more effective when given in several doses throughout the day Prescription
METHYPREDNI- SOLONE ACETATE	Depo-Medrol	Antiinflammatory	To reduce noninfectious inflammation and pain in a specific body area	If a specific area is injected many times, the injection appears to cause damage in that area	Varies depending upon preparation and purpose desired; the frequency of injection is important, and should not be repeated more than every six weeks with a limit of three injections in one area Physician injected
GOLD SALTS	Myochrysine, Solganal	Antiinflammatory	R.A. that is not responsive to less hazardous medications or is severe & rapidly progressive	Rash, itchy skin, kidney damage, mouth ulcers, nausea, liver damage, mouth ulcers, nausea, & liver damage usually occur after a long period of time	50 mg per week by intramuscular injection for 20 weeks, then 1 to 2 injections per month thereafter; a maintenance dosage may be from 10 to 20 mg
AURANOFIN	Ridaura	Antiinflammatory	To reduce inflammation	Diarrhea, rash, kidney problems, blood platelet level problems	6 mg daily; takes weeks to months to achieve full therapeutic effectiveness Prescription
PENCILLAMINE	Cuprimine	Antiinflammatory	R.A. that is not responsive to less hazardous	Rash, protein leakage in the urine, decrease in	Usually 250 mg per day for one month (one 250-

Physician injected

Generic Name	Brand Name	Action	Indication	Potential Side Effects	Usual Adult Dose & Availability	Comments
			medications or is severe and rapidly progressive	production of blood cells, nausea, metallic taste in mouth, decreased sense of taste, weakened connective tissue, slowed blood clotting process	mg or two 125-mg tablets), then two tablets (500 mg) a day for one month, then three tablets (250 mg) a day for one month and, finally, four tablets (1000 mg) a day Prescription	
ACETAMINO-PHEN	Tylenol	Analgesic	For mild, temporary pain	Minimal to none	Two tablets (10 grains) every 4 hours as needed Over the counter	
PROPOXYPHENE	Darvon Compound or Darvocet	Analgesic	For short-term, mild pain relief	Mentally dull feeling; dizziness; headache; sedation; somnolence; paradoxical excitement; rash; gastrointestinal disturbances	One-half grain (32 mg) or one grain (65 mg) every 4 hours as needed Prescription	Possible dependence after long-term use
CODEINE	Empirin Aspirin with codeine	Analgesic	For short-term moderate pain relief	Proportional to the dosage; constipation; diverticulitis; depression; sedation	#3 tablet (32 mg codeine) every 4 hours as needed Prescription	Possible addiction
OXYCODONE PERCOGESIC Phenyltoloxamine Citrate	Percobarb, Percodan	Analgesic	For short-term moderate-to-severe pain	Depression; sedation	One tablet every 6 hours Prescription	Possible addiction

14

Multiple Sclerosis

TRISHA MOZDZIERZ

Multiple sclerosis (MS) is by far the most common demyelinating CNS disease in the United States (1, 2). Because of its prevalence and the pervasive dysfunction that results, occupational therapists frequently work with individuals who have this disease.

> A staff occupational therapist (OT) working in a rehabilitation center found out that a high school classmate had been admitted to the main hospital for "tests." When the OT went to visit her 23-year-old friend and asked her what was happening, the friend said, "Gosh, I don't know. I've been having some trouble with my eyes and some funny tingling in my arms. And they just keep running all these tests on me. This morning they told me that they think I may have something called multiple sclerosis. What is that, anyway?" The OT's mind raced as she tried to sort out how best to answer her friend. The information in this chapter contains some of the facts the OT reviewed in formulating an answer.

INCIDENCE AND PREVALENCE

Approximately 500,000 American men and women have been diagnosed as having multiple sclerosis. It is usually first diagnosed between the ages of 20 and 40, occurring slightly more often among women (60% of cases) (3). About 8000 new diagnoses of this disease are made each year (4).

ETIOLOGY

Although there are many speculations, the etiology of MS is still unknown. Epidemiologic studies over the last 50 years have revealed a clear geographic distribution, with higher prevalence in the northern United States and northern Europe. Analysis of data indicates that the risk of developing MS is (a function of) where the individual lived up to age 15. This phenomenon has lead to several speculations about its etiology including factors related to geomagnetic latitudes, climate, and dietary patterns. Because the patterns of prevalence of MS parallel that of poliomyelitis prior to the Salk vaccine, there is also a possibility that MS is caused by a virus that remains latent in the CNS for many years (5).

If the etiology of multiple sclerosis is viral, the destruction of the myelin may be caused by an autoimmune response. Genetic susceptibility and familial links are also suspected because of the tendency for the disease to be more prevalent among certain families and among persons with specific tissue types (5, 6). For example, MS occurs more frequently among people of European ancestry than other white racial groups, is twice as common among white individuals, and is rare among Japanese and Chinese people. Also, immediate relatives of a person who has MS are 12 to 20 times more likely to develop the disease than an unrelated person living in the same climate and of the same ethnicity.

Recent studies implicate a retrovirus as the cause of MS (4, 7). A retrovirus enzymatically changes RNA, its genetic material, to DNA. The DNA of the virus then integrates into the person's DNA. It can then remain silent in the host for years, without causing any symptoms at all. This retrovirus is called human T-lymphotropicovirus 1 (HTLV 1) and is being studied for its possible connection to MS.

In 1990 researchers at the University of Vermont in Burlington discovered that T lymphocyte immune cells in blood of persons with MS react to myelin basic protein (6). Myelin protein is found in the protective sheaths that cover the nerve fibers in the spinal cord and brain. The T lymphocytes respond to this protein by proliferating and releasing substances that damage or destroy the myelin. In the normal CNS, impulses are transmitted along the nerve fibers at speeds exceeding 200 mph. This speed is achieved primarily because of the insulating properties of myelin (5). When the myelin is destroyed, neurotransmissions along these nerves are disrupted.

Although the etiology of MS is not definite, the pathology is known. The myelin sheath that surrounds the axons of the nerve fibers in the CNS is destroyed. Initially, the myelin sheath swells and then reduces in thickness. With continued exacerbations, the myelin sheath is destroyed and the damaged myelin is removed by scavenger cells called astrocytes. These astrocytes also form a sclerotic scar called a plaque, causing slowing or cessation of nerve impulse transmission. This demyelination is irreversible and occurs predominantly in the white matter of the CNS.

SIGNS AND SYMPTOMS

Some of the more common symptoms of MS include visual deficits, sensory disturbances such as dysesthesia or paresthesia, urinary incontinence or retention,

muscle weakness and/or spasticity, gross and fine motor incoordination, fatigue, ataxia, dysphagia, dysarthria, and cognitive or mental disturbances. Each person with MS has specific symptoms that result from lesions in specific areas of the CNS. The types of symptoms, their intensity, and the effects on the person's functional status are highly individualized. For example, if the basal ganglia or cerebellum are affected, the individual experiences intention tremors and ataxia, whereas involvement of the corticospinal tract results in weakness and/or spasticity (3). See Table 14.1 for a summary of common signs and symptoms.

Visual disturbances are often some of the earliest signs of MS. These are usually manifested by a partial loss of vision (scotoma), double or blurred vision, or ocular pain. Sudden loss of vision with pain in or behind the eye is caused by optic neuritis. These early symptoms may sub-

Table 14.1.
Common Signs and Symptoms of Multiple Sclerosis[a]

Tactile awareness
  Numbness
  Disturbances in pain sensation
  Hypersensitivity

Motor
  Spasticity
  Limitations in tolerance/low energy
  Weakness
  Ataxic-like symptoms
    Intention tremor
    Nystagmus

Visual
  Double vision
  Pain behind the eyes
  Blurred vision
  Partial blindness—scotoma

Cognitive
  Memory loss or disturbance
  Difficulty with complex ideas
  Decreased attention span

Psychologic
  Depression or euphoria
  Impulsivity
  Lability

[a]Taken in part from Umphred DA, ed. Neurological rehabilitation. 1st ed. St. Louis: CV Mosby, 1985:401.

side after 3 to 6 weeks without any residual deficit. For others, visual loss may be insidious and painless. Nonetheless, nearly 80% of all persons who have MS have some loss of visual acuity.

Oculomotor control can also be affected, due to lesions of the supranuclear connection to the oculomotor nuclei in the brainstem. As a result, the person loses horizontal eye movement either unilaterally or bilaterally.

With MS the individual can experience a variety of other sensory disturbances such as numbness, impairment of vibratory, proprioceptive, pain, touch, and/or temperature sensation; and distortion of superficial sensation. Because of these sensory losses, the person also may lose various perceptual skills such as stereognosis, kinesthesia, and body scheme (5).

Fatigue is the most common complaint and is often identified as the most debilitating symptom (1, 3). Increased energy is required for nerves to conduct their impulses in a demyelinated nervous system, making it difficult for the individual to initiate movement and perform sustained activities. Closely associated is the muscle weakness that the individual may experience. As the disease progresses, the person requires more frequent rest periods between activities, and decreased levels of activity lead to further debilitation.

Persons with MS often have urinary dysfunction that can range from urgency, frequency, hesitancy, and retention to incontinence or a combination of these symptoms. Involvement of the sensory and/or motor pathways to the bladder causes these disturbances, which over 80% of persons with MS experience at some time. In addition, the person with a neurogenic bladder is more prone to urinary tract infections (UTI) (8), and because there is often sensory loss as well, the UTI can go undetected until it becomes a major complication.

Bowel dysfunction can also become a problem, leading to constipation and impaction if left untreated.

Because of sensory and motor changes in the genital area, the individual may also experience a disturbance in, or total loss of, sexual function. Of course, these problems may also be the result of medications.

Some persons with MS experience dysarthria and/or dysphagia from the loss of sensory and motor control of the oral cavity, pharynx, and larynx.

Approximately 50% of individuals with MS experience some change in cognitive ability. For some it is difficulty with verbal or spatial-motor memory (3). Others have disorders of judgment, decreased attention and concentration, various types of agnosia, or diminished ability to think conceptually (2).

An emotional component to this disease results in some individuals having bouts of depression, euphoria, or lability (2), thought to be caused by lesions in the frontal lobe of the brain.

Factors that increase or exacerbate symptoms are excessive fatigue, emotional or physical trauma, heat, and pregnancy. Increase in either internal temperature because of fever or external temperature because of hot weather or a hot bath can cause the person's symptoms to worsen, but there are no reliable predictors of this increased symptomatology.

PROGRESSION AND PROGNOSIS

The clinical course of this disease can be roughly organized into four types or patterns. The first is benign, in which the person experiences one or two episodes of neurologic deficits with no residual impairments. This person's chance of remaining symptom-free increases with each nonsymptomatic year. The next pattern of progression is relapsing-remitting-nonprogressive. In this pattern the person returns to the previous level of function after each exacerbation. With the third type, relapsing-remitting-progressive, however, the person has some residual impairments with each remission. Finally, there is the progressive pattern, which involves a steady decline in function without remissions and exacerbations. Individuals with MS may shift from one pattern to another with no reliable predictors of these shifts (1, 8, 10).

In 1976, a London physician described two patients he had treated at opposite ends of this spectrum. He "met a patient who started with diplopia at the age of 22, who had 10 incapacitating episodes . . . in rapid succession over the course of the next six weeks." This person had no remissions and never recovered. He also had "a patient who had her first episode of diplopia at the age of 23 on the first night of her honeymoon after eating for the first time in her life a lobster supper." This person recovered completely from this episode and did not have a second episode until age 65, from which she also recovered completely. A third episode at age 71, following an operation, resulted in a slight paraplegia. However, she left the hospital with no neurologic disability and died at the age of 73 from other causes (11).

Overall, about 60% of individuals with MS remain fully functional up to 10 years

after their first exacerbation, and about 30% remain functional 30 years after their first attack (12). In a longitudinal study conducted in 1971, over two-thirds of the subjects were ambulatory 25 years after onset (13). In spite of the seriousness of this disease, it does not decrease the person's life expectancy greatly. However, a few people do become severely disabled and die prematurely because of recurring infections or complications resulting from inactivity (5, 12).

Inactivity and bed rest cause further physiologic changes that complicate the total medical picture. These complications are not unique to MS; they occur as a result of any extended period of inactivity. A list of the possible changes that can occur is contained in Table 14.2.

DIAGNOSIS AND MEDICATIONS

Since there are no definitive laboratory tests to diagnose MS, the diagnosis depends upon a composite of clinical findings. It is based upon three types of evidence: multiple CNS lesions, distinct episodes of neurologic dysfunction, and compatibility of the various signs and

Table 14.2.
Complications of Inactivity[a]

Cardiovascular	Respiratory
Decreased cardiac output	Relative hypoxemia
Thrombophlebitis	Upper respiratory infection
Pulmonary infarction	Bronchitis
	Bronchopneumonia
Musculoskeletal	**Gastrointestinal**
Muscle atrophy and loss of strength	Constipation
Decreased muscle oxidation capacity	Impaction
Bone loss (osteoporosis)	
Joint contractures	
Osteoarthritis	
Psychologic	**Genitourinary**
Sensory deprivation (e.g., unable to enjoy human touch, hold your children)	Renal calculi
	Urinary tract infection
Sensory systems	
Sensory deprivation (e.g., paresthesia, dysethesia)	**Skin**
	Decubitus ulcers
	Chronic sepsis
	Amyloidosis

[a] Taken in part from Umphred DA, ed. Neurological rehabilitation. St. Louis: CV Mosby, 1985:401,404.

symptoms with MS. It is also used when there is no better neurologic explanation for the signs and symptoms the individual has (5).

Many of the diagnostic procedures are used to rule out other neurologic diseases. Such procedures include: evoked potentials (visual, auditory, and somatosensory), oligoclonal banding, myelogram, high-dose delayed computed tomography (CT) scan, and magnetic resonance imaging (MRI). (See Appendix 14.2 for explanations of each of these tests.)

A definite diagnosis of MS is made when the person has episodes of exacerbation and remission, slow or step-by-step progression over 6 months, neurologic signs that are evidence of lesions in more than one site in the white matter, an onset of symptoms between the ages of 10 and 50, and no better neurologic explanation for the clinical picture (5).

Medications (Appendix 14.3) commonly used to alleviate the symptoms of MS include Baclofen, propantheline bromide, oxybutynin chloride, Tegretol, laxatives, and stool softeners. Antidepressants are prescribed when indicated. (See Chapter 6, "Mood Disorders" for more details about this group of medications.)

OCCUPATIONAL PERFORMANCE AREAS AND COMPONENTS

Since MS can be progressive, it can affect all the performance components and occupational performance areas. As was noted previously, the types and severity of dysfunction that the individual has depend upon the location and extent of lesions in the CNS. In this section the most common deficits are described.

Table 14.3 lists all the performance components and highlights those that might be affected. An individual with this condition can have any combination of the deficits listed.

Activities of Daily Living

Self-care skills are mainly affected by changes in the person's sensorimotor skills.

Changes are most commonly noted in sensation, gross and fine motor coordination, bilateral integration, postural control, muscle tone, and endurance.

Toileting can become problematic due to the loss of bladder and bowel control. The individual may experience any combination of the complications noted earlier in this chapter. Eating may become difficult either because the person loses the strength and/or coordination to self-feed or because of chewing and/or swallowing difficulties. Dysphagia, swallowing difficulty, is caused by weakness or incoordination of the pharyngeal musculature, and can also make it difficult for an individual to ingest oral medications.

Difficulty with short-term memory can limit independence in this area because of the inability to recall what has transpired in the recent past. "Did I take my pills, or not?"

Dysarthria or imperfect articulation is caused by a lack of control of the tongue and other oral muscles essential to speech. This problem can affect the person's ability to communicate thoughts, needs, and desires and also limit social interaction. The individual may lose upper extremity function, making it difficult to compensate for speaking problems by substituting some sort of written communication.

Functional mobility is another critical concern. Neuromuscular and motor problems make ambulation difficult or impossible, either independently or with assistive devices, even in an electrically propelled wheelchair. Acquiring alternate methods of mobility requires the ability to adapt. The person must be able to change motor patterns, requiring concurrent new and varied perceptual and cognitive strategies. At the same time the person is challenged psychologically to make the necessary adjustments to new and different types of mobility. As the person's function decreases, issues of home and work accessibility must be considered and the necessary adaptations made to maintain critical occupational performance.

Due to depression and diminished self-concept, the person may no longer feel attractive, causing problems in sexual expression. In addition, demyelination of specific sensory and motor pathways can also affect physical performance.

Bladder dysfunction, sexual inadequacy, and eating, communication, or mobility problems all impinge upon the person's normal socialization with individuals or groups. This leads to secondary psychosocial problems because of lifestyle

Table 14.3.
Occupational Performance Components

Sensory Motor Component	Cognitive Integration & Cognitive Components	Psychosocial Skills & Psychologic Components

1. Sensory integration
 a. Sensory awareness
 b. **Sensory processing**
  1. **Tactile**
  2. Proprioceptive
  3. Vestibular
  4. **Visual**
  5. Auditory
  6. Gustatory
  7. Olfactory
 c. Perceptual skills
  1. Stereognosis
  2. Kinesthesia
  3. Body scheme
  4. Right-left discrimination
  5. Form constancy
  6. Position in space
  7. Visual-closure
  8. Figure ground
  9. Depth perception
  10. Topographic orientation
 	
2. **Neuromuscular**
 a. **Reflex**
 b. **Range of motion**
 c. **Muscle tone**
 d. **Strength**
 e. **Endurance**
 f. **Postural control**
 g. **Soft tissue integrity**
 	
3. **Motor**
 a. **Activity tolerance**
 b. **Gross motor coordination**
 c. **Crossing the midline**
 d. **Laterality**
 e. **Bilateral integration**
 f. Praxis
 g. **Fine motor coordination**
 h. **Visual-motor integration**
 i. **Oral-motor control**
	1. Level of arousal
	2. Orientation
	3. Recognition
	4. Attention span
	5. **Memory**
	 a. Short-term
	 b. Long-term
	 c. Remote
	 d. **Recent**
	6. Sequencing
	7. Categorization
	8. Concept formation
	9. Intellectual operations in space
	10. **Problem solving**
	11. Generalization of learning
	12. Integration of learning
	13. Synthesis of learning
		1. **Psychologic**
		 a. **Roles**
		 a. **Values**
		 c. **Interests**
		 d. Initiation of activity
		 f. **Self-concept**
		2. **Social**
		 a. **Social conduct**
		 b. **Conversation**
		 c. **Self-expression**
		3. **Self-management**
		 a. **Coping skills**
		 b. **Time management**
		 c. Self-control

Table 14.3. (Continued)
Occupational Therapy Performance Areas
(Effects depend on degree of disability)

Activities of Daily Living	Work Activities	Play/Leisure Activities
1. Grooming	1. Home management	1. Play or leisure exploration
2. Oral hygiene	a. Clothing care	2. Play or leisure performance
3. Bathing	b. Cleaning	
4. Toilet hygiene	c. Meal preparation and cleanup	
5. Dressing	d. Shopping	
6. Feeding and eating	e. Money management	
7. Medication routine	f. Household maintenance	
8. Socialization	g. Safety procedures	
9. Functional communication	2. Care of others	
10. Functional mobility	3. Educational activities	
11. Sexual expression	4. Vocational activities	
	a. Vocational exploration	
	b. Job acquisition	
	c. Work or job performance	
	d. Retirement planning	

changes. MS not only requires an initial social-psychologic adjustment, but it may also require continual readjustment, due to erratic appearance and disappearance of symptoms. A person who was active and outgoing will probably have a diminished self-concept because of an inability to engage in activities that were once of interest and value. The result is a variety of role changes in the family or society.

Role expectations exist in every social situation and are ways of behaving or reacting that fit with one's self-image and the expectations of others. This includes attitudes, activities, patterns of decision-making, expressing feelings, and meeting the needs of significant others (14). Some individuals with loss of bladder control may avoid going out in public. Mothers may not be able to care for their children. Some may come to see themselves as no longer useful or attractive to others. Marriages can break up under the strain of living with MS. Occasionally, individuals with MS threaten suicide. An individual with MS must think seriously about current role expectations and how they might be threatened by MS (14).

In some ways, the effects of MS are no different than those of other severe disabilities. Based on self-concept as a key indicator, Matson and Brooks (15) conducted an exploratory survey using patient reports which proposed a model of adjustment to MS. Stages include denial (It's not true; it can't be happening), resistance (It won't get me down), affirmation (I guess I have to face it), and integration (I know it's there, but I don't think much about it). The researchers suggest that this model can be used for any chronic illness that appears in adulthood. However, the long-term experience of living with MS and its exacerbation/remission cycle not only requires an initial acceptance stage, but "also demands a flexibility (in adjustment) made necessary by a lack of closure" (15). Individuals may not follow the stages in order nor progress through all the stages; they may regress when exacerbation occurs, or they may remain forever in one stage. Approaches used to cope with MS seem to match the personalities of different patients. However, the findings of the study indicate that an adjustment is achieved in full by many individuals, which led the authors to suggest that, over time, the self-concept gets better and in many cases, markedly better.

Work

All performance components have the potential to affect work activities. Since MS is a disease of adults, work is a crucial area of occupational performance. For many adults it is an important part of their self-identity.

As sensorimotor skills decline, the ability to perform specific work tasks also declines. "Invisible symptoms" such as fatigue, weak or blurred vision, and difficulties with bladder control often confound the issue. Co-workers may not un-

Table 14.4.
Occupational Performance Profile

			Performance Areas			
			Work Activities			
		Vocation	Education	Home Management	Care of Others
PERFORMANCE COMPONENTS — SENSORY MOTOR	**SENSORY INTEGRATION**			Difficulty reading recipes, directions	
	NEURO-MUSCULAR			Fatigues doing light housework; falls from chair while trying to perform	Unable to meet the needs of her family
	MOTOR				
PERFORMANCE COMPONENTS — COGNITIVE	**COGNITIVE** Intact				
PERFORMANCE COMPONENTS — PSYCHOSOCIAL	**PSYCHOLOGIC**			Frustrated and depressed over her changing role and decreased functioning	
	SOCIAL				
	SELF-MANAGEMENT			Doesn't understand the disease and how to cope with it	
	EXTERNAL FACTORS WHICH INFLUENCE PERFORMANCE; CULTURE, ECONOMY, ENVIRONMENT				

Grid adapted from Uniform Terminology (2nd ed.) Developed by the occupational therapy faculty at Eastern Michigan University.

derstand why someone can't work who doesn't look ill. Again, this affects the person psychologically, with changes in societal roles and self-concept. This is particularly true for an individual whose job requires a high degree of physical stamina and skill. For example, assembly workers or truck drivers may lose their jobs fairly early in the course of the disease. An individual who has been the breadwinner of the family and whose identity is closely tied to physical strength and endurance will have serious adjustment problems. Cognitive deficits will also

Client initials: **M.A.**
Diagnosis: **MS**
Age: 28

Play or Leisure Activities		Activities of Daily Living				
Exploration	Performance	Self-care	Socialization	Functional Communication	Functional Mobility	Sexual Expression
	Unable to knit	Difficulty with small closures				Decreased enjoyment (secondary to loss of light touch)
		Fatigues with performance; difficulty maintaining balance while dressing; poor coordination of a task		Dysarthric	Able to self-propel wheelchair short distances only	Fatigue, poor postural control, decreased gross motor coordination all impact on performance

make it difficult for the person to function and continue to find satisfaction in work.

A normal work activity for most persons with MS is the care of others—including a spouse or significant other, children, or older dependent adults. The individual with MS will have increasing difficulty fulfilling this role and may have to rely on these care receivers to provide support and care, creating a major role reversal. These changes in responsibilities are very stressful for all concerned and challenge everyone's ability to maintain the integrity of relationships.

Play and Leisure

Alternative leisure activities must be explored as more and more performance

Table 14.5.
Occupational Performance Profile

		Performance Areas		
		Work Activities		
	Vocation	Education	Home Management	Care of Others
SENSORY INTEGRATION	Difficulty seeing the computer screen			
NEURO-MUSCULAR	Ataxia & intention tremors impair computer programming ability		Ataxia, tremors, fatigue impact ability to make small household repairs	
MOTOR				
COGNITIVE Intact				
PSYCHOLOGIC	Depression over being unable to keep up at work			Feeling inadequate to provide for family
SOCIAL				
SELF-MANAGEMENT				Feelings of inadequacy

(left margin labels, top to bottom: PERFORMANCE COMPONENTS; SENSORIMOTOR; COGNITIVE; PSYCHOSOCIAL)

EXTERNAL FACTORS WHICH INFLUENCE PERFORMANCE; CULTURE, ECONOMY, ENVIRONMENT

Grid adapted from Uniform Terminology (2nd ed.) Developed by the occupational therapy faculty at Eastern Michigan University.

deficits occur. A balance between work and play should be maintained as long as possible. However, if the person can no longer engage in usual work and daily living activities, it is even more critical to have meaningful and fulfilling leisure pursuits. These activities will become increasingly important as a means of self-actualization and satisfaction.

MS may cause dysfunction in all performance components and occupational performance areas. Because of the unpredictable nature of the exacerbation/remission pattern of MS, potential depen-

Client initials:	**L.S.**
Diagnosis:	**MS**
Age:	**41**

Play or Leisure Activities		Activities of Daily Living				
Exploration	Performance	Self-care	Socialization	Functional Communication	Functional Mobility	Sexual Expression
	Visual deficits impair hunting ability					Decreased enjoyment (secondary to loss of light touch)
	Deficits impair hunting safety			Decreased ability to type on computer to communicate at work	Ataxia, tremors, fatigue impair ability to ambulate	
		Inability to hook closures secondary to decreased fine motor coordination			Fatigue	
	Depression over being unable to perform leisure tasks				Avoids going places where increased walking is required	

dency issues are ongoing problems. The following cases illustrate how this condition changed two people's lives.

CASE STUDIES

Case 1

M.A. is a 28-year-old woman who was diagnosed with MS 5 years prior to this hospital admission. She was admitted because she has noticed a progressive deterioration of function over the past 6 months. The main problems she identifies are an increase in fatigue, difficulty with bowel and bladder function, and numerous falls from her wheelchair. She also has grade II decubitus ulcers on her buttocks, bilaterally, and on her left calf. She reports that they happened after she was left on a bed pan too long.

She is married and has two children—a girl 11 years old and a boy 5 years old. She is not employed outside the home. Her husband works full time and has been very supportive. At the time of admission he seemed overwhelmed.

M.A. tries to do her morning self-care but is finding it increasingly difficult and frustrating. Getting dressed is particularly fatiguing, and she admits that at times she goes to bed fully dressed to avoid having to get dressed in the morning. She has been using a manual wheelchair for the past 3 years.

Her daughter is currently helping with the laundry, cooking, and simple cleaning. M.A. states that she has problems doing household tasks because she must hold onto something stable before reaching for, or lifting, an object.

She currently has no leisure activities that she enjoys. At one time, she liked to knit, but it has become too frustrating to be pleasurable.

She complains of bladder urgency but often cannot void. She also has a mild dysarthria, spasticity of the lower extremities, weakness of the upper extremities (able to move against gravity against minimal resistance), poor sitting balance, poor fine and gross motor coordination, blurred vision, and loss of stereognosis and light touch.

When the occupational therapist spoke with her, it became apparent that she does not comprehend the nature and course of MS. She is feeling frustrated and depressed about her recent decline of function.

She is currently taking Tylenol, Senokot, Metamucil, Colace, heparin, multivitamins and Dulcolax suppositories.

Table 14.4 is a summary of the effects of MS on M.A.'s occupational performance.

Case 2

L.S. is a 41-year-old male who has been experiencing transient upper and lower extremity weakness and transient ocular pain and blurred vision for the past 3 years. He was diagnosed as having MS 6 months ago. He also has numbness in both hands, bilateral upper extremity weakness (can move against gravity but with only minimal resistance), intention tremors in both upper extremities, and a slightly ataxic gait.

His active range-of-motion is within normal limits. He has good dynamic sitting balance and fair dynamic standing balance. He can ambulate for short distances but fatigues easily. He avoids going places where he would have to walk any distance.

He can do all self-care activities independently except manipulating small closures (buttons, snaps, zippers). Occasionally he drops utensils while eating, because of intention tremors. L.S. is employed as a computer programmer but complains that the intention tremors interfere with his ability to type at the keyboard. His main leisure interests are fishing and hunting.

L.S., his wife, and his 10-year-son live in a trilevel home. He has difficulty ascending and descending the stairs and must use both hands on the railings for stability. He has fallen on the stairs once.

He is currently very worried about his ability to provide for his family and about the kind of role model that he can provide for his son. He is very afraid of becoming disabled and dependent upon others.

Table 14.5 is a summary of L.S.'s deficits in the occupational performance areas.

REFERENCES

1. Maloney PF, Burks JS, Ringel SP, eds. Interdisciplinary rehabilitation of multiple sclerosis and neuromuscular disorders. Philadelphia: JB Lippincott, 1985.
2. Chusid JG. Correlative neuroanatomy and functional neurology, 16th ed. Los Altos, CA: Lange Medical Publications, 1976.
3. Delisa JA, Hammond MD, Mikulic MA, Miller RM. Multiple sclerosis: part 1. Common physical disabilities and rehabilitation. Am Fam Physician 1985;32(4):157–163.
4. Patlak M. M.S. The puzzling picture of multiple sclerosis. FDA Consumer 1989;23(6):17–21.
5. Umphred DA, ed. Neurological rehabilitation, 2nd ed. St Louis: CV Mosby, 1990.
6. Fackelmann KA. MS researcher finds missing immune link. Science News 1990;137:86.
7. Morgante LA, Madonna MG, Pokoluk R. Research and treatment in multiple sclerosis: implications for nursing practice. J Neurosci Nurs 1989;21(5):285–289.
8. Ferguson JM. Helping an MS patient live a better life. RN 1987;50(12):22–27.
9. Samonds RJ, Cammermeyer M. The patient with multiple sclerosis. Nursing '85 1985;15:60–64.
10. Delisa JA, Miller RM, Mikulic MA, Hammond MD. Multiple sclerosis: part 2. Common func-

tional problems and rehabilitation. Am Fam Physician 1985;32(5):127–132.

11. Kelly R. Management of MS. Nurs Mirror 1976;143(6):48–56.

12. Andreoli TE, Carpenter CC, Plum F, Smith LH. Cecil essentials of medicine, Philadelphia: WB Saunders, 1986.

13. Percy AK. Multiple sclerosis in Rochester, Minnesota: a 60 year appraisal. Arch Neurol 1971;25:105.

14. Holland NJ, Kaplan SR. Social adaptations. In: Scheinberg LC, Holland NJ. Multiple sclerosis: a guide for patients and their families. New York: Raven Press, 1987:219.

15. Matson RR, Brooks NA. Adjusting to multiple sclerosis: an exploratory study. Soc Sci Med 1977;11:245–250.

16. Andreoli TE, Carpenter CCJ, Plum F, Smith LH, eds. Cecil essentials of medicine. Philadelphia: WB Saunders, 1986.

Glossary

Agnosia: Inability to recognize the import of sensory impressions despite being able to recognize the elemental sensation of a stimulus. Language deficits must be absent for this diagnosis; the varieties correspond to several senses and are distinguished as auditory (acoustic), gustatory, olfactory, tactile, and visual. Specific sensory agnosias can occur when the connections are interrupted between the primary cortical receptor region for a stimulus and the memory of that abstraction (parietal lobe damage). An example is the incapacity to identify familiar faces despite perceiving them.

Amyloidosis: The deposition in various tissues of amyloid, fibrils of identical polypeptide chains arranged in stacked sheets. This protein is almost insoluble, and after it infiltrates the tissues they become waxy and nonfunctional. Primary amyloidosis is due to a metabolic disturbance and affects cardiac, smooth, and skeletal muscle; it cannot be cured, and heart failure is usually the cause of death. Secondary amyloidosis is related to tuberculosis, lung abcess, osteomyelitis, or bronchiectasis; treatment involves treating the underlying cause. It may also occur with inflammatory disease such as rheumatoid arthritis. The most common sites of deposition are the spleen, kidney, liver, and adrenal cortex.

Ataxia: Incoordination occurring in the absence of apraxia, paresis, rigidity, spasticity, or involuntary movement manifested when voluntary muscular movements are attempted. In posterior column damage of the spinal cord, there is a loss of proprioception and incoordination due to misjudgment of limb position with balance problems. Cerebellar ataxia produces a reeling, wide-based gait.

Atelectasis: A collapsed or airless state of all or part of the lung, which may be acute or chronic. Primary cause is obstruction of the bronchus serving the affected area. In chronic form, symptoms include gradually developing dyspnea and weakness.

Clonus: Alternate involuntary muscular contraction and relaxation in rapid succession.

Demyelination: Destruction, removal, or loss of the myelin sheath of a nerve or nerves.

Dysesthesia: Impairment of any sense, especially of the sense of touch; a painful, persistent sensation induced by a gentle touch of the skin.

Dysarthria: Imperfect articulation of speech due to disturbances of muscular control resulting from central or peripheral nervous system damage.

Dysphagia: Difficulty in swallowing. The condition can range from mild discomfort, such as a feeling that there is a lump in the throat, to a severe inability to control the muscles needed for chewing and swallowing.

Euphoria: A pervasive and sustained emotion of intense elation with feelings of grandeur.

Exacerbation: An increase in severity of a disease or any of its symptoms.

Hypoxemia: Deficient oxygenation of the blood.

Infarction: A localized area of ischemic necrosis produced by occlusion of the arterial supply or the venous drainage of the heart.

Intranuclear ophthalmoplegia: Paralysis of the eye muscles relative to involvement of the brainstem tracts connecting motor cranial nerve nuclei 3, 4, and 6. This condition can be transient with accompanying diplopia (double vision).

Kinesthesia: The ability and sense by which position, weight, and movement are perceived. Kinesiology: Scientific study of movement of body parts.

Lability: The quality of being unstable or fluctuating. In psychiatry, emotional instability; a tendency to show alternating states of gaiety and somberness.

Lymphotropic: Having an affinity for lymphatic tissue.

Myelin: The lipid substance forming a sheath around the axons of certain nerve fibers, occurring predominantly in the cranial and spinal nerves that compose the white matter of the brain and spinal cord. The myelin sheath is formed by a glial cell, either an oligodendrocyte (in the CNS) or Schwann cell (in the PNS).

Myelogram: A graphic representation of the differential count of cells found in a stained representation of bone marrow.

Neurogenic bowel/bladder: Dysfunction resulting from congenital abnormality, injury, or disease process of the brain, spinal cord, or local nerve supply to the urinary bladder or rectum and their respective outlets. The dysfunction may manifest as partial or complete retention, incontinence, or frequency of elimination.

Optic neuritis: Inflammation of the optic nerve, affecting the part of the nerve within the eyeball (neuropapillitis) or the part behind the eyeball (retrobulbar neuritis), usually causing pain and partial blindness in one eye.

Orthostatic intolerance: An inability to tolerate sitting upright or standing, related to a fall in blood pressure causing dizziness, syncope, and blurred vision.

Osteoporosis: A decreased mass per unit volume of normally mineralized bone compared with age- and sex-matched controls. Related to disuse, as much as 30–40% of initial bone mass may be lost after 6 months of total immobilization, as in paraplegia or quadriplegia. There must be movement, weight-bearing activity, and the use of antigravity muscles to maintain healthy bones.

Paresthesia: Morbid or perverted sensation; an abnormal sensation as burning, prickling, formication, due to a disorder of the central nervous system.

Plaque: Any patch of flat area.

Proprioception: From the Latin word for "one's own." Interpretation of stimuli originating in muscles, joints, and other internal tissues that give information about the position of one body part in relation to another. Perception is mediated by sensory nerve endings, chiefly in muscles, tendons, and the labyrinth. Proprioceptive input tells the brain when and how muscles are contracting or stretching, and when and how joints are bending, extending, or being pulled or compressed.

Remission: Diminution or abatement of the symptoms of a disease; the period during which diminution occurs.

Retrovirus: A large group of RNA viruses that includes the leukoviruses and lentiviruses; so called because they carry reverse transcriptase.

Scotoma: An area of lost or depressed vision within the visual field, surrounded by an area of less depressed or of normal vision.

Sepsis: The presence in the blood or other tissues of pathogenic microorganisms or their toxins; the condition associated with such presence.

Stereognosis: The sense by which the form of objects is perceived, such as the ability to judge the shape of an object pressed against the skin.

Tachycardia: Abnormally rapid heart rate, usually taken to be over 100 beats per minute.

Thrombocytopenia: Decrease in number of platelets in circulating blood, which can cause excessive bleeding during trauma.

Thrombophlebitis: Inflammation of a vein, associated with thrombus formation.

Tremor: An involuntary trembling of the body or limbs, occurring either at rest or during activity, depending on the origin of the lesion.

APPENDIX **14.2**

Diagnostic Procedures

1. Evoked potentials: Through repeated stimulation of specific receptors the subsequent response (evoked potential) of a particular area of the brain is measured. For example, the retina is repeatedly stimulated with light flashes and then the evoked electrical response is measured. Computers are used to average the response and to dampen the normal electroencephalographic activity (2).

2. Oligoclonal banding: A specific laboratory test of spinal fluid. Multiple, discrete (oligoclonal) bands are highly supportive of a diagnosis of multiple sclerosis (16).

3. Myelography: A procedure used to examine the spinal cord. A substance that is opaque to x-rays (radiography) is injected into the subarachnoid space. The area(s) are then x-rayed and examined on film for structural abnormalities (2).

4. High-dose delayed computed tomography scan (CT): A method of recording x-ray photon accumulation after an area(s) of the body have had successive layers of narrow-beam x-ray exposure. These data are collected and translated into an internal, three-dimensional image of the exposed structures. This technique identifies hypodense areas that may be indicative of multiple sclerosis.

5. Magnetic resonance imaging (MRI): Although similar to CT, this technique is much more sensitive and can be used to identify discrete patches of demyelination (16).

Medications

Generic Name	Brand Name	Action	Indication	Potential Side Effects	Usual Adult Dose
BACLOFEN	Lioresal	Skeletal muscle relaxant & antispastic	Decreases number and severity of muscle spasms; relieves associated pain, clonus and muscle rigidity	Weakness, fatigue, drowsiness, nausea, dry mouth	Prescription only Optimal dosage requires individual titration; total daily dose should not exceed 80 mg; supplied in tables of 10 and 20 mg
PROPANTHE-LINE BROMIDE	Pro-Banthine	Antimuscarinic, gastrointestinal antispasmodic	Decreases GI motility & inhibits gastric acid secretion	Headache, drowsiness, dry mouth, urinary hesitancy	Prescription only Dosage: one tablet 30 min before each meal and 30 mg h.s.; supplied in 15-mg tablets
OXYBUTYNIN CHLORIDE	Ditropan	Antispasmodic for neurogenic bladder	Decreases urge to void and increases bladder capacity	Drowsiness, dizziness, tachycardia, dry mouth, rash	Prescription only Dosage: one 5-mg tablet 2–3×/day or one teaspoon syrup 2–3×/day

Generic Name	Brand Name	Action	Indication	Potential Side Effects	Usual Adult Dose
CARBAMAZEPINE	Tegretol	Anticonvulsant, analgesic specific to trigeminal neuralgia	Treatment of psychomotor and grand mal seizures & trigeminal neuralgia	Dizziness, aplastic anemia, thrombo-cytopenia, fatigue, ataxia, dry mouth, nausea, urinary frequency	Prescription only Dosage: individual, but should not exceed 1200 mg daily in patients over 15 years of age; supplied in 100- & 200-mg tablets
HEPARIN	Heparin sodium injection	Inhibits reactions that lead to blood clotting & formation of fibrin clots	Prevention and treatment of deep vein thrombosis (DVT)	Hemorrhage	Prescription only Individual dosage and variable supply
LAXATIVES	Senokot & Dulcolax, stimulant laxatives; Colace, stool softener; Metamucil, bulk-forming	Increases bowel movement	Constipation	Diarrhea, abdominal cramps	Prescription Dosage: Senokot, two tablets; Dulcolax suppositories, one tablet, 10 mg daily; Colace, caplets & syrup 50–200 mg daily; Metamucil, follow directions

Index

Page numbers in *italics* denote figures; those followed by "t" denote tables.